Nutritional Oncology

Nutritional Oncology

Editor: Erik Coleman

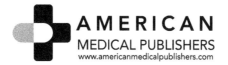

AMERICAN
MEDICAL PUBLISHERS
www.americanmedicalpublishers.com

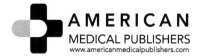

Cataloging-in-Publication Data

Nutritional oncology / edited by Erik Coleman.
    p. cm.
Includes bibliographical references and index.
ISBN 978-1-63927-767-4
1. Cancer--Nutritional aspects. 2. Cancer--Diet therapy.
3. Diet in disease. 4. Nutrition. I. Coleman, Erik.
RC26845 .N88 2023
616.994 065 4--dc23

American Medical Publishers,
41 Flatbush Avenue,
1st Floor, New York,
NY 11217, USA

ISBN 978-1-63927-767-4 (Hardback)

Contents

Preface

This book was inspired by the evolution of our times; to answer the curiosity of inquisitive minds. Many developments have occurred across the globe in the recent past which has transformed the progress in the field.

Nutritional oncology refers to an increasingly active interdisciplinary field in which cancer is studied as a local and systemic disease. Cancer originates due to the changes in the genome and develops as a multi-step process. It might be affected at certain points in its natural history through nutritional factors, which can decrease the risk of cancer in swiftly increasing population of cancer survivors. Nutritional oncology can prevent cancer and is helpful in enhancing the quality of life of cancer patients, by calculating energy requirements, diet planning and counseling. Nutrition problems generally occur in tumors related to the neck, stomach, head, esophagus, intestines, liver or pancreas. Cancer treatments like stem cell transplant, chemotherapy, radiation therapy, immunotherapy and hormone therapy can affect normal eating in patients. Some changes in diet can be done to aid the patient in getting the proper required nutrients. The foods which are high in vitamins, calories, minerals and protein are crucial for health of cancer patients. The various advancements in nutritional oncology are glanced at and their applications as well as ramifications are looked at in detail within this book. It will serve as a reference to a broad spectrum of readers.

This book was developed from a mere concept to drafts to chapters and finally compiled together as a complete text to benefit the readers across all nations. To ensure the quality of the content we instilled two significant steps in our procedure. The first was to appoint an editorial team that would verify the data and statistics provided in the book and also select the most appropriate and valuable contributions from the plentiful contributions we received from authors worldwide. The next step was to appoint an expert of the topic as the Editor-in-Chief, who would head the project and finally make the necessary amendments and modifications to make the text reader-friendly. I was then commissioned to examine all the material to present the topics in the most comprehensible and productive format.

I would like to take this opportunity to thank all the contributing authors who were supportive enough to contribute their time and knowledge to this project. I also wish to convey my regards to my family who have been extremely supportive during the entire project.

Editor

Integrating Nutrition into Outpatient Oncology Care—A Pilot Trial of the NutriCare Program

Laura Keaver [1,2,*]**(iD)**, **Ioanna Yiannakou** [3] **and Fang Fang Zhang** [2]**(iD)**

[1]   Department of Health and Nutritional Science, Institute of Technology Sligo, FP1 YW50 Sligo, Ireland
[2]   Friedman School of Nutrition Science and Policy, Tufts University, Boston, MA 02111, USA; Fang_Fang.Zhang@tufts.edu
[3]   Department of Medicine, Boston University, Boston, MA 02215, USA; ioannay@bu.edu
[*]   Correspondence: Keaver.laura@itsligo.ie

Abstract: Nutrition is an essential part of oncology care; however, nutrition advice and guidance are not always provided. This six-week pilot pretest-posttest intervention was designed to test the feasibility and effectiveness of integrating a nutrition education program (NutriCare) into outpatient oncology care. Twenty breast cancer survivors were recruited through Tufts Medical Centre. Nutrition impact symptoms and demographics were collected at baseline, dietary quality and quality of life measures were collected pre and post-intervention and an evaluation form was completed post-intervention. Forty-four percent of eligible participants were recruited, and 90% of those completed the study. The NutriCare program was well received with participants reporting that goals were feasible (94.4%), the program had a positive impact on their diet (77.8%), and over 80% would recommend the program. There was an interest in continuing with the program (89%) and in receiving additional guidance from the healthcare team (83%). There was a significant improvement ($p = 0.04$) in physical function over the six weeks; however, no additional significant differences in quality of life or dietary quality were seen. In conclusion, cancer survivors were positive about the NutriCare program and its integration into practice.

Keywords: diet quality; cancer survivor; nutrition intervention; oncology care; quality of life

1. Introduction

Nutrition is extremely important in the management of cancer. It is well recognized that some treatments could have detrimental effects on patients' dietary intake [1,2], which can negatively impact the patient's nutritional status and outcomes. It is also known that maintaining muscle mass is of utmost importance as reduced muscle mass as a result of cachexia [3] and/or sarcopenia is associated with fatigue, impaired physical function, reduced tolerance to treatments, impaired quality of life and reduced survival [4]. Therefore, it is important to deliver this information to all rather than waiting until a patient requests it or they have experienced substantial weight loss. However, in some cases, muscle wasting is not evident, for example, in those who have obesity [4]. Recent work has shown that cancer survivors who received nutritional information more often changed their dietary behavior, regardless of whether they had nutritional information needs [5]. Survivors, when compared to the general population, have a diet of poorer quality [6] and they can experience weight gain from early in treatment right into survivorship [7]. As cancer survivors are already at an increased risk of additional cardiovascular disease risk factors such as hypertension and type 2 diabetes [8], it is important that this is addressed early on to ensure the best outcomes in terms of recurrence and development of additional conditions.

Continued active clinical support and education for cancer survivors should be considered an essential element in the cancer journey to address patient well-being [9]. The NutriCare program was developed to address this gap by proving easy to use evidence-based nutrition information and a step-by-step process for clinicians and healthcare professionals to follow in order to ensure that oncology patients and survivors receive nutrition advice and guidance as part of oncology care. The aim of this study was to determine the feasibility of the NutriCare program as well as any changes in quality of life and dietary quality that occurred over the course of the six-week pilot intervention.

2. Materials and Methods

2.1. Study Design and Population

NutriCare is a program designed to integrate nutrition into oncology care. The components of this intervention have been published elsewhere [10] and have been briefly outlined below. This pilot consisted of a six-week oncology clinic study to determine the feasibility of integrating this model into outpatient oncology care. The study design was a pretest-posttest intervention. Study recruitment took place at Tufts Medical Centre through the oncology team at the Breast Health Clinic between July and August 2018, and 20 women were enrolled in the study. The inclusion criteria were (1) 21 years or older, (2) not undergoing active treatment, (3) not palliative (4) not currently enrolled in a weight management program or receiving nutritional counseling and (5) could read and speak English. Any advanced nutrition-related issues or a requirement for supplements or enteral feeding were to be referred to a dietitian, as outlined in the Health Care Professional (HCP) toolkit.

2.2. Intervention

As mentioned previously, the NutriCare model has previously been reported, but in short, it utilizes the 5-A model (Ask, Advise, Assess, Assist, Arrange) to integrate nutrition care into the oncology setting. This model has previously been utilized in smoking cessation [11], obesity counseling [12], and the development of nutrition interventions for adolescent athletes [13]. We refined this model based on feedback from focus groups [10], and an overview of the process used in this pilot can be seen in Figure 1. It was initially designed to be fully delivered by the oncology team, however, based on feedback, it was refined to be introduced by the oncology team and was then delivered by a registered dietitian (LK). A Nutrition Assessment for Cancer Patients (NACP) questionnaire was completed by all individuals at baseline, and this formed the basis of the intervention. The symptoms list was chosen from nutrition impact symptoms commonly reported by cancer patients [14,15]. Questions on food groups were adapted from the validated Rapid Eating Assessments for Patients (REAP) [16]. Each individual then set their own Specific, Measurable, Achievable, Realistic and Timely (SMART) goals with guidance from the dietitian, and these were noted on a Nutrition prescription pad (Figure 2). A patient toolkit was provided to all participants to help them to implement these goals. This toolkit consisted of the following nutritional and educational sections: why is nutrition important for the cancer survivor; how does cancer treatment impact eating patterns; strategies for managing eating problems during cancer treatment; maintaining a healthy weight during and after cancer treatment; healthy eating and active living after cancer treatment: nutrition recommendations for cancer survivors; frequently asked questions around healthy eating (this section was divided into 15 sections comprising: plant-based diet, fruits and vegetables, wholegrain and fiber, dairy, protein, animal-based protein, plant-based protein, fats, sugar and sugary drinks, sodium, drinks, nutrition labeling, supplements, fad diets, portion control); food safety; how to talk to your doctor about diet; how to evaluate nutrition information for cancer survivors and links to additional evidence-based resources. The oncology team followed up with a phone call within seven days of the baseline visit to reinforce the goals and to continue to champion and support the intervention. Participants were provided with a parking voucher and $25 gift card to compensate them for their time.

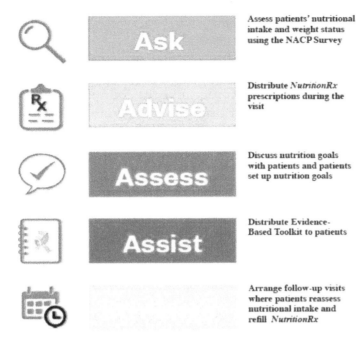

Figure 1. NutriCare Program Flowchart.

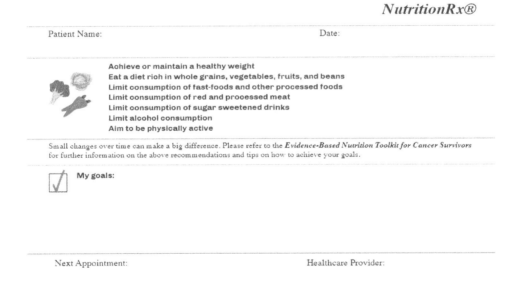

Figure 2. Nutrition Prescription Pad.

2.3. Intervention Measures

An information sheet was provided to all participants by the oncology team in Tufts Medical Centre prior to consent. All participants gave informed written consent before commencing any aspect of the study. The baseline visit coincided with a clinical visit to the Breast Clinic to make it more convenient for the participants. After consent, participants provided information on socioeconomic demographics as well as completing two quality of life questionnaires – the Patient-Reported Outcome Measurement Information System (PROMIS) -57 Profile v2.1 [17] and PROMIS Scale v1.2-Global Health [18]. They were also provided with unique login details to complete the National Institutes of Health Diet History Questionnaire (DHQ) III online [19]. This questionnaire asks participants to report their average consumption of a variety of foods in the last month. A unique identification number was given to all participants to maintain confidentiality. Height was self-reported while weight was measured as a standard part of care during the medical appointment, which coincided with the study's baseline visit and so this measurement was used.

Follow-up was six weeks after the in-person visit and consisted of a brief phone call and the mailing of the two quality of life questionnaires to be recompleted and new login details being provided to complete the DHQ III online again. The program's feasibility was assessed in a number of ways, including using participants' satisfaction ratings on an evaluation form provided at the six weeks follow-up, using the participants' ratings for understanding and ease of use of the provided resources, and the study's retention rates.

2.4. Data Analysis

The PROMIS -57 Profile v2.1 [17] and PROMIS Scale v1.2-Global Health [18] were both scored using the reference scoring manuals [20,21] to convert raw scores to T-scores ±SE.

For the components of the PROMIS -57 Profile v2.1 questionnaire, for the United States general population, a score of 50 is average with a standard deviation of 10. For concepts within this questionnaire that are positively worded, therefore, such as mobility, a T-score of 60 represents one standard deviation above average and a T-score of 40 represents one standard deviation below average. Conversely, with negatively worded concepts such as anxiety, a T-score of 60 represents one standard deviation below average, while a T-score of 40 represents one standard deviation above average [22].

The PROMIS Scale v1.2-Global Health gives values for both Global Mental and Global Physical Health. When reporting on Global Mental Health the cut-offs for poor, fair, good, very good and excellent are 29, 40, 48 and 56, respectively [23]. For Global Physical Health the cut-offs for poor, fair, good, very good and excellent are 35, 42, 50 and 58, respectively [23].

Dietary quality was assessed using the Healthy Eating Index (HEI)-2015 and its component score calculated by the Diet*Calc software developed by the National Cancer Institute [19], based on the dietary data collected in the DHQ III. The overall dietary quality uses a 100-point scale, with a higher score indicating a better dietary quality [24]. Thirteen components sum to make this total score of 100.

2.5. Statistical Analysis

Data were analyzed using SPSS version 24. Descriptive statistics were used to describe the demographic and health information and are presented as means, SDs, ranges, frequencies and percentages. The study was not powered to detect statistically significant differences, but pre-post intervention differences in dietary intake and quality of life measures were assessed using t-tests. Significance was set at $p < 0.05$.

2.6. Ethical Approval

This project was approved by the Institutional Review Board of Tufts University (Institutional Review Board Protocol No. 12954). The researchers obtained written informed consent from all study participants prior to enrolment in the study. All data was stored in password-protected computers and locked filing cabinets in Tufts University and only the first author and principal investigator had access to this data.

3. Results

3.1. Study Sample

Table 1 describes the characteristics of the individuals who took part in this pilot trial. Age ranged from 42 to 80 years of age with a mean (±SD) of 59.5 years (±9.9). 45% were within five years of diagnosis. The mean (±SD) of BMI was 30.2 kg/m^2 (±6.4). 30% of the cohort reported weight gain since diagnosis, and 15% reported weight loss in this timeframe. 80% previously underwent surgery, 75% underwent chemotherapy, and 75% underwent radiation therapy. 75% were receiving hormonal therapy at the time of the pilot. Additional characteristics can be found in Supplementary Table S1.

Table 1. Characteristics of the participants ($n = 20$) recruited into the NutriCare pilot trial.

	n (%) or Mean (SD)
Age, years, mean (SD)	59.5 (9.9)
BMI, mean (SD)	30.2 (6.4)
BMI classification, n (%)	
Underweight (<18.5 kg/m^2)	0 (0)
Healthy weight (18.5–24.99 kg/m^2)	6 (32)
Overweight (25–29.99 kg/m^2)	3 (15)
Obese (≥30 kg/m^2)	10 (53)
Weight gain, *since diagnosis*, n (%)	
Yes	6 (30)
No	14 (70)
Weight loss, *since diagnosis*, n (%)	
Yes	3 (15)
No	17 (85)
Diagnosis, *years since*, n (%)	
<5 years	9 (45)
5–10 years	7 (35)
10–15 years	1 (5)
15+ years	3 (15)
Breast cancer stage, n (%)	
1A	5 (25)
1B	0 (0)
2A	7 (35)
2B	3 (15)
3A	2 (10)
3B	1 (5)
3C	2 (10)
Hormonal Receptor Status, n (%)	
ER + PR + HER2-	10 (50)
ER-PR-HER2-	1 (5)
ER + PR + HER2 1 +	3 (15)
ER + PR + HER2 2 +	1 (5)
ER + PR + HER2 3 +	2 (10)
ER + PR + HER-	1 (5)
ER-PR-HER-	1 (5)
Previous Surgery, n (%)	
Yes	16 (80)
No	4 (20)
Previous Radiation, n (%)	
Yes	15 (75)
No	5 (25)
Years since radiation completion, mean(SD)	4.3 (4.1)
Previous Chemotherapy, n (%)	
Yes	15 (75)
No	5(25)
Years since chemotherapy completion, mean(SD)	6.5 (6.4)
Hormonal Therapy, n (%)	
Current	15 (75)
Previous	4 (20)
Never	1 (5)

Table 1. *Cont.*

	n (%) or Mean (SD)
Race/ethnicity, *n* (%)	
White Caucasian	18 (90)
Black/African American	1 (5)
Other	1 (5)
Education, *n* (%)	
High school	4 (20)
Associates degree	3 (15)
Some college	3 (15)
College	8 (40)
Graduate	2 (10)

3.2. Intervention

3.2.1. NACP Questionnaire

The results of the NACP questionnaires are outlined in Figure 3 and Supplementary Table S2. Fatigue (80%) and cravings (75%) were the most widely reported symptoms still experienced (Figure 3). The majority of participants (80%) were very willing to make changes to their current habits to improve their health (Supplementary Table S2).

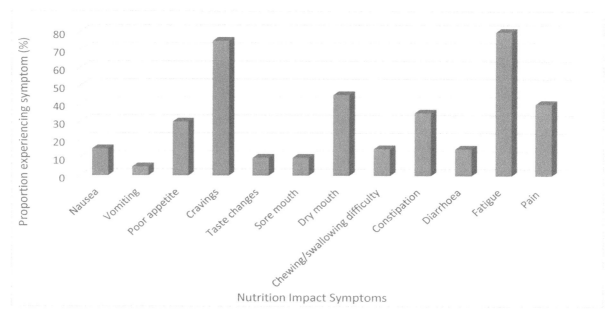

Figure 3. % of participants who reported experiencing nutrition impact symptoms.

3.2.2. Goals Chosen

The main goals chosen based on the results of the NACP (Figure 3 and Supplementary Table S2) and in consultation with the participants focused on tips to help manage fatigue (*n* = 8), increase vegetables by one portion on most days (*n* = 5), increase dairy by one portion on most days (*n* = 7), have breakfast (*n* = 6), include an extra portion of oily fish per week (*n* = 4), increase fruit by one portion on most days (*n* = 4) and increase fiber by introducing more wholegrains (*n* = 4).

3.3. Outcomes

Physical health scores ranged from 39.8 (fair) to 57.7 (very good) at baseline and from 39.8 (fair) to 67.7 (excellent) at follow-up. Mental health scores ranged from 31.3 (fair) to 67.7 (excellent) at baseline and from 33.8 (fair) to 67.7 (excellent) at follow-up (Table 2).

Table 2. Changes in quality of life and dietary quality after 6 weeks intervention.

	Baseline/Pre-Test Mean (SE)	Six Weeks/Post-Test Mean (SE)	Significance/*p*-Value
Quality of Life (PROMIS Scale v1.2-Global Health) [a]			
Physical	49.5 (6.0)	50.2 (6.7)	0.7
Mental	51.5 (9.4)	51.0 (7.4)	0.8
Quality of Life (PROMIS -57 Profile v2.1) [b,c]			
Physical Function	48.6 (7.4)	51.8 (7.9)	0.04
Anxiety	48.3 (9.3)	46.3 (9.4)	0.5
Depression	43.5 (8.9)	45.3 (8.5)	0.3
Fatigue	48.1 (8.4)	48.2 (7.7)	0.9
Sleep disturbance	49.8 (7.8)	49.6 (6.3)	0.9
Ability to participate	55.5 (7.4)	55.9 (8.1)	0.8
Pain interference	47.3 (7.8)	49.6 (7.5)	0.1
Pain intensity	2.3 (2.5)	2.2 (2.1)	0.8
	Baseline/pre-test Mean (SE)	Six weeks/post-test Mean (SE)	
Dietary quality (HEI-2015 component scores) [d]			
Total HEI-2015 score	74.3 (13.3)	74.3 (8.6)	1.0
Vegetables	4.5 (0.7)	4.4 (0.4)	0.9
Greens and beans	4.5 (1.3)	4.7 (0.8)	0.3
Total fruits	4.4 (1.2)	4.2 (1.4)	0.6
Whole fruits	4.5 (1.0)	4.7 (1.0)	0.6
Wholegrains	4.7 (2.6)	3.6 (2.0)	0.2
Dairy	6.0 (1.9)	6.7 (2.3)	0.3
Total protein foods	4.8 (0.6)	5.0 (1.4)	0.3
Seafood and plant proteins	4.7 (0.8)	4.8 (0.6)	0.3
Fatty acids	6.7 (2.8)	6.6 (2.8)	0.8
Sodium	4.7 (3.1)	4.9 (3.2)	0.9
Refined grains	9.6 (0.9)	9.5 (1.1)	0.7
Saturated fats	6.9 (3.7)	7.7 (2.5)	0.4
Added sugars	8.3 (2.0)	7.5 (1.7)	0.3
% calories from added sugars	9.2 (4.7)	10.8 (4.4)	0.4
% of calories from saturated fats	10.4 (3.2)	9.5 (2.4)	0.3

[a] Of participants enrolled in this trial (*n* = 20), these variables were available for 19 participants at pre-test, 18 at post-test and 17 for both time-points. [b] Of participants enrolled in this trial (*n* = 20), these variables were available for 20 participants at pre-test, 18 at post-test and 18 for both time-points. [c] The range of scores for physical function were 36.7 to 60.1 at baseline and 38.1 to 60.1 at follow-up, for anxiety 37.1 to 66.6 at baseline and 37.1 to 67.7 at follow-up, for depression 38.2 to 64.9 at baseline and 38.2 to 64.9 at follow-up, for fatigue 33.1 to 61.3 at baseline and 33.1 to 62.3 at follow-up, for sleep disturbance 30.5 to 59.1 at baseline and 35.3 to 59.1 at follow-up, ability to participate 41.1 to 65.4 at baseline and 44 to 65.4 at follow-up and pain interference 40.7 to 60.8 at baseline and 40.7 to 65.5 at follow-up. [d] Of participants enrolled in this trial (*n* = 20), these variables were available for 17 participants at pre-test, 12 at post-test and 11 for both time-points.

There was a statistically significant improvement in physical function over the course of the six-week intervention (*p* = 0.04). There were no additional statistically significant changes in quality of life or in overall dietary quality as measured by the HEI-2015 and its component scores from pre-test to post-test (Table 2).

3.4. Process Feasibility

3.4.1. Recruitment and Retention

A total of 46 participants were deemed eligible for inclusion by the oncology medical team. We were unable to make contact with 14 of these, 12 declined to participate citing time restraints and 20 agreed to participate (44% of those eligible) and were enrolled in the study. In all, 18 of these 20 participants (90%) completed post-testing.

3.4.2. Satisfaction and Acceptability

Participants were very positive about the NutriCare program (Table 3). They reported that goals were feasible (94.4%), that the program had a positive impact on their diet (77.8%), and over 80% reported that locating information was easy, the tips were practical and useful and that they would recommend the program to anyone with cancer. There was a strong commitment to continuing to use the toolkit provided (89%) and also a strong desire for the oncology team to continue to include nutrition as a topic during future consultations (83%).

Table 3. Participant Evaluation of the Six-Week Pilot of the NutriCare Program (*n* = 18).

Clinical Visit
Please Answer the Following Questions using the Scale Below

	Strongly Agree/Agree *n* (%)	Neutral *n* (%)	Disagree/Strongly Disagree *n* (%)
I think that nutrition is an important component of my care	17 (94.4)	1 (5.6)	0 (0)
The nutrition prescription was specific to me	11 (61.1)	7 (38.9)	0 (0)
The goals set were feasible to achieve	17 (94.4)	1 (5.6)	0 (0)
Overall, this program impacted my diet positively	14 (77.8)	4 (22.2)	0 (0)

Effectiveness and ease of use
Please answer the following questions on the toolkit provided to you during your visit using the scale below

The toolkit …	Strongly Agree/Agree *n* (%)	Neutral *n* (%)	Disagree/Strongly Disagree *n* (%)
Helped me to better understand the importance of nutrition in cancer care	17 (94.4)	1 (5.6)	0 (0)
Helped me to change my diet	17 (94.4)	1 (5.6)	0 (0)
Helped me to maintain/achieve a healthy weight	12 (66.7)	6 (33.3)	0 (0)
Locating information was easy	15 (83.3)	3 (16.7)	0 (0)
The tips provided were practical and useful	15 (83.3)	3 (16.7)	0 (0)
I would recommend the toolkit to anyone with cancer	16 (88.9)	2 (11.1)	0 (0)

Table 3. *Cont.*

Follow-up with oncology provider
Please answer the following questions using the scale below

	Yes *n* (%)	No *n* (%)	N/A *n* (%)
I received a follow-up phone call from my oncology provider	10 (55.6)	2 (11.1)	6 (33.3)
This call motivated me to achieve my dietary goals	7 (38.9)	1 (5.6)	10 (55.6)

Longer-term
Please answer the following questions using the scale below

	Strongly Agree/Agree *n* (%)	Neutral *n* (%)	Disagree/Strongly Disagree *n* (%)
I would like providers to continue the nutrition conversation at future visits	15 (83.3)	3 (16.7)	0 (0)
I will continue using the toolkit	16 (88.9)	2 (11.1)	0 (0)

3.5. Management Feasibility

Recruitment of participants occurred primarily by phone which proved difficult as not everyone could be reached or responded to phone messages. Focus groups to refine this program were carried out prior to implementation [10] and these highlighted the role of the doctor should be to champion this program. As such, the doctor introduced the program to all participants initially. Additionally, the oncology team followed up with phone calls to reiterate the importance of nutrition. These phone calls took approximately 10 min and feedback from the medical team reported that it was not feasible (logistic-wise) to reach patients by phone to discuss nutrition. The team only managed to contact over half (*n* = 10, 55.6%) of the enrolled participants by phone to follow-up (Table 3).

4. Discussion

The NutriCare program was well-received by breast cancer survivors in this study. There was an interest in continuing with the program and in receiving additional guidance from HCPs. There was a significant improvement (*p* = 0.04) in physical function over the six weeks; however no additional significant differences in quality of life or dietary quality were seen.

Enrollment in this study from a breast cancer clinic showed that about 44% of those eligible were contactable and willing to take part in this pilot intervention. Recruitment/response rates in previous studies with cancer survivors have not always been reported; however, where available they range from 3–81% [25–28]. The majority of interventions tend to focus disproportionately on breast cancer survivors [29,30]. While 90% of those enrolled completed this intervention, it was short in duration (six weeks) and recruited a highly motivated cohort. However, several previous studies have reported similar rates [25,26] for studies of longer duration (up to 12 months). Rates of attrition range from 0–50% in intervention studies with cancer survivors [29].

There was an interest in continuing to receive nutrition advice in the oncology setting and in continuing with the program. Cancer survivors have previously demonstrated an interest in modifying their dietary intake and physical activity levels in the hopes of preventing recurrence [31]. The involvement of the healthcare team, and in particular the oncologist in interventions, has been shown to influence the perceived behavioral control of the patient and to lead to improvements in the desired behavior [31]. Given the time and confidence in one's nutrition knowledge that inclusion of additional components into standard appointments can take [32,33] and the difficulty the medical team had in this study when trying to follow up with a phone call, it is worth considering how else this intervention could be delivered and supported by the oncology team. Interventions delivered online, particularly when supported with a variety of behavior change techniques have shown promise [34,35]. This would also help to address an additional barrier that has frequently been reported by cancer survivors, that of distance/traveling [29,36].

This pilot was not designed to test effectiveness but to demonstrate feasibility and acceptability and inform a future larger-scale trial. Still, our pilot data suggest an improvement in physical function after six weeks. A decline in physical functioning has been associated with loss of mobility, loss of independence, an increased risk of adverse outcomes, and mortality [37]. As cancer survivors are at an increased risk of losing physical functioning as they age [38–40], interventions that can improve this are needed. Typically, physical activity is recommended to prevent loss of physical function; however, given that only 30% of cancer survivors achieve recommended physical activity levels [41], it is important to consider the role of other lifestyle behaviors. A higher dietary quality (as seen in this group) has been strongly associated with better physical functioning and decreased odds of functional impairment [42].

Overall, the dietary quality of this group was good. Our findings are consistent with previous research that has shown dietary quality to be higher in well-educated cohorts of a high socioeconomic status compared to those who are less well educated and/or from a lower socioeconomic status [43–45]. However, it contrasts with a study of 1533 cancer survivors from the United States where overall dietary quality, as measured by HEI was shown to be 47.2 ($\pm$0.5) [6]. Assessing dietary quality proved challenging as using the Dietary Health Questionnaire, which is quite long had an impact on the number who were willing to complete it. Only 11 of the 20 completed this measure and so results should be interpreted with caution. There is also a chance that those who had a higher quality diet and overall better lifestyle behaviors were more likely to complete this measure [46].

Despite the fact that 55% of the cohort had been diagnosed greater than five years ago, fatigue and cravings were two nutrition impact symptoms that still affected the majority (80% and 75%, respectively). The impact that high levels of fatigue, as demonstrated in this group, could have on the ability to shop for and prepare food and therefore, overall dietary intake should not be ignored. A large meta-analysis of 12, 327 breast cancer survivors who had completed treatment reported that one in four suffered from severe fatigue post-treatment, with the prevalence reducing substantially in the first 6 months after treatment [47]. This is similar to previous work, which indicated that one-year post-treatment fatigue levels had returned to pre-treatment levels [48,49]. In contrast to this, prevalence rates of 38–66% have been reported in disease-free breast cancer survivors [50–52] with fatigue being reported in up to one-third of breast cancer survivors five to ten years after completion of treatment [53–55]. As the number of individuals surviving cancer increases, it is important to further improve our knowledge of the persistence of symptoms post-treatment. This information will help inform the development of nutrition guidelines and advice specific for cancer survivors (of specific cancer types), whose needs are quite different from those in the initial stages of treatment. One interesting area of exploration is the finding that diets high in fiber have been linked to reduced levels of fatigue in breast cancer survivors [56].

There were a number of limitations in the study. First, the survivors who enrolled in the study were highly educated, white, breast cancer survivors of high socioeconomic status and so the results of this pilot will not be applicable to broader cancer groups, cancer types or ethnic groups. This bias has been demonstrated regularly in previous work also [29,30]. In addition, the intervention took place over a short duration of time (six weeks). While this was designed to allow for the feasibility and acceptability of such a program to be determined, it meant that the impact of the program on dietary quality and quality of life, which are likely to take longer than six weeks, could not fully be determined. In addition, the use of a comprehensive online dietary food frequency questionnaire resulted in a lower number of responses being returned ($n = 11$) at the six-week follow-up. We also did not assess specific laboratory values, which could have served as risk surrogates indicating short-term changes and could also have acted as motivational tools.

5. Conclusions

In conclusion, cancer survivors were positive about the NutriCare program and its integration into practice. There was an interest in continuation with the program and additional guidance from HCPs. There is warrant in investigating the delivery of this program through different mediums, e.g., online, to ensure that patients and survivors who are attending centers that do not have the resources to run such a program will still be able to take part and get access to evidence-based nutrition guidance.

Author Contributions: Conceptualization, L.K. and F.F.Z.; data curation, L.K. and I.Y.; formal analysis, L.K.; funding acquisition, F.F.Z.; investigation, L.K. and F.F.Z.; methodology, L.K. and F.F.Z.; project administration, L.K. and I.Y.; resources, L.K.; supervision, F.F.Z.; visualization, L.K. and F.F.Z.; writing—original draft, L.K.; writing—review and editing, L.K., I.Y. and F.F.Z. All authors have read and agreed to the published version of the manuscript.

Acknowledgments: We would like to acknowledge all those who took the time to be part of this pilot as well as the oncology team, in particular John Erban and Cate Mullin, at Tufts Medical Centre for facilitating the study.

References

1. Barbera, L.; Seow, H.; Howell, D.; Sutradhar, R.; Earle, C.; Liu, Y.; Stitt, A.; Husain, A.; Sussman, J.; Dudgeon, D. Symptom Burden and Performance Status in a Population-Based Cohort of Ambulatory Cancer Patients. *Cancer* **2010**, *116*, 5767–5776. [PubMed]
2. Kubrak, C.; Olson, K.; Jha, N.; Jensen, L.; McCargar, L.; Seikaly, H.; Harris, J.; Scrimger, R.; Parliament, M.; Baracos, V.E. Nutrition impact symptoms: Key determinants of reduced dietary intake, weight loss, and reduced functional capacity of patients with head and neck cancer before treatment. *Head Neck* **2009**, *32*, 290–300.
3. Fearon, K.C.H.; Strasser, F.; Anker, S.D.; Bosaeus, I.; Bruera, E.; Fainsinger, R.L.; Jatoi, A.; Loprinzi, C.; Macdonald, N.; Mantovani, G.; et al. Definition and classification of cancer cachexia: An international consensus. *Lancet Oncol.* **2011**, *12*, 489–495. [PubMed]
4. Ryan, A.M.; Power, D.G.; Daly, L.; Cushen, S.J.; Bhuachalla, Ē.N.; Prado, C.M. Cancer-associated malnutrition, cachexia and sarcopenia: The skeleton in the hospital closet 40 years later. *Proc. Nutr. Soc.* **2016**, *75*, 199–211. [PubMed]
5. Van Veen, M.R.; Winkels, R.M.; Janssen, S.H.M.; Kampman, E.; Beijer, S. Nutritional Information Provision to Cancer Patients and Their Relatives Can Promote Dietary Behavior Changes Independent of Nutritional Information Needs. *Nutr. Cancer* **2018**, *70*, 483–489. [PubMed]
6. Zhang, F.F.; Liu, S.; John, E.M.; Must, A.; Demark-Wahnefried, W. Diet quality of cancer survivors and noncancer individuals: Results from a national survey. *Cancer* **2015**, *121*, 4212–4221.
7. Vance, V.; Hanning, R.M.; Mourtzakis, M.; McCargar, L. Weight gain in breast cancer survivors: Prevalence, pattern and health consequences. *Obes. Rev.* **2010**, *12*, 282–294. [PubMed]
8. Nardi, I.A.; Iakobishvili, Z. Cardiovascular Risk in Cancer Survivors. *Curr. Treat. Options Cardiovasc. Med.* **2018**, *20*, 47.
9. Jammu, A.; Chasen, M.; Van Heest, R.; Hollingshead, S.; Kaushik, D.; Gill, H.; Bhargava, R. Effects of a Cancer Survivorship Clinic—Preliminary results. *Support. Care Cancer* **2019**, *28*, 2381–2388. [CrossRef] [PubMed]
10. Keaver, L.; Yiannakou, I.; Folta, S.C.; Zhang, F.F. Perceptions of Oncology Providers and Cancer Survivors on the Role of Nutrition in Cancer Care and Their Views on the "NutriCare" Program. *Nutrients* **2020**, *12*, 1277.
11. Lawson, P.J.; Flocke, S.A.; Casucci, B. Development of an Instrument to Document the 5A's for Smoking Cessation. *Am. J. Prev. Med.* **2009**, *37*, 248–254. [PubMed]
12. Vallis, M.; Piccinini-Vallis, H.; Sharma, A.M.; Freedhoff, Y. Modified 5 As Minimal intervention for obesity counseling in primary care. *Can. Fam. Physician* **2013**, *59*, 27–31. [PubMed]
13. Lee, S.; Lim, H. Development of an Evidence-based Nutritional Intervention Protocol for Adolescent Athletes. *J. Exerc. Nutr. Biochem.* **2019**, *23*, 29–38. [CrossRef]
14. Coa, K.I.; Epstein, J.B.; Ettinger, D.; Jatoi, A.; McManus, K.; Platek, M.E.; Price, W.; Stewart, M.; Teknos, T.N.; Moskowitz, B. The Impact of Cancer Treatment on the Diets and Food Preferences of Patients Receiving Outpatient Treatment. *Nutr. Cancer* **2015**, *67*, 339–353. [PubMed]

15.   Gosain, R.; Miller, K. Symptoms and Symptom Management in Long-term Cancer Survivors. *Cancer J.* **2013**, *19*, 405–409. [PubMed]

16.   Gans, K.M.; Risica, P.M.; Wylie-Rosett, J.; Ross, E.M.; Strolla, L.O.; McMurray, J.; Eaton, C.B. Development and Evaluation of the Nutrition Component of the Rapid Eating and Activity Assessment for Patients (REAP): A New Tool for Primary Care Providers. *J. Nutr. Educ. Behav.* **2006**, *38*, 286–292. [PubMed]

17.   Promis Health Organisation (PHO). *Promis -57 Profile V2.1*; Northwestern University: Evanston, IL, USA, 2017.

18.   PROMIS Health Organization and PROMIS Cooperative Group. *Promis Scale V1.2-Global Health*; Northwestern University: Evanston, IL, USA, 2016.

19.   National Institutes of Health. *Diet History Questionnaire Iii*; U.S. Department of Health and Human Services: Washington, DC, USA, 2018.

20.   Healthmeasures. Promis Adult Profile Instruments. Northwestern University. Available online: http://www.healthmeasures.net/images/PROMIS/manuals/PROMIS_Adult_Profile_Scoring_Manual.pdf (accessed on 7 July 2018).

21.   Healthmeasures. Promis-Global Health. Northwestern University. Available online: http://www.healthmeasures.net/images/PROMIS/manuals/PROMIS_Global_Scoring_Manual.pdf (accessed on 7 July 2018).

22.   DeWitt, B.; Feeny, D.; Fischhoff, B.; Cella, D.; Hays, R.D.; Hess, R.; Pilkonis, P.A.; Revicki, D.A.; Roberts, M.S.; Tsevat, J.; et al. Estimation of a Preference-Based Summary Score for the Patient-Reported Outcomes Measurement Information System: The PROMIS®-Preference (PROPr) Scoring System. *Med Decis. Mak.* **2018**, *38*, 683–698.

23.   Hays, R.D.; Spritzer, K.L.; Thompson, W.W.; Cella, D.U.S. General Population Estimate for "Excellent" to "Poor" Self-Rated Health Item. *J. Gen. Intern. Med.* **2015**, *30*, 1511–1516.

24.   Krebs-Smith, S.M.; Pannucci, T.E.; Subar, A.F.; Kirkpatrick, S.I.; Lerman, J.L.; Tooze, J.A.; Wilson, M.M.; Reedy, J. Update of the Healthy Eating Index: HEI-2015. *J. Acad. Nutr. Diet.* **2018**, *118*, 1591–1602.

25.   Courneya, K.S.; Friedenreich, C.M.; Sela, R.A.; Quinney, H.A.; Rhodes, R.E.; Handman, M. The group psychotherapy and home-based physical exercise (group-hope) trial in cancer survivors: Physical fitness and quality of life outcomes. *Psycho Oncol.* **2003**, *12*, 357–374.

26.   Ohira, T.; Schmitz, K.H.; Ahmed, R.L.; Yee, D. Effects of weight training on quality of life in recent breast cancer survivors. *Cancer* **2006**, *106*, 2076–2083. [PubMed]

27.   Demark-Wahnefried, W.; Clipp, E.C.; Morey, M.C.; Pieper, C.F.; Sloane, R.; Snyder, D.C.; Cohen, H.J. Lifestyle Intervention Development Study to Improve Physical Function in Older Adults With Cancer: Outcomes From Project LEAD. *J. Clin. Oncol.* **2006**, *24*, 3465–3473. [PubMed]

28.   Demark-Wahnefried, W.; Jones, L.W.; Snyder, D.C.; Sloane, R.J.; Kimmick, G.G.; Hughes, D.C.; Badr, H.J.; Miller, P.E.; Burke, L.E.; Lipkus, I.M. Daughters and Mothers Against Breast Cancer (DAMES): Main outcomes of a randomized controlled trial of weight loss in overweight mothers with breast cancer and their overweight daughters. *Cancer* **2014**, *120*, 2522–2534. [PubMed]

29.   Stull, V.B.; Snyder, D.C.; Demark-Wahnefried, W. Lifestyle Interventions in Cancer Survivors: Designing Programs That Meet the Needs of This Vulnerable and Growing Population. *J. Nutr.* **2007**, *137*, 243S–248S.

30.   Burden, S.; Jones, D.J.; Sremanakova, J.; Sowerbutts, A.M.; Lal, S.; Pilling, M.; Todd, C. Dietary Interventions for Adult Cancer Survivors. *Cochrane Database Syst. Rev.* **2019**. [CrossRef]

31.   Demark-Wahnefried, W.; Peterson, B.; McBride, C.; Lipkus, I.; Clipp, E. Current health behaviors and readiness to pursue life-style changes among men and women diagnosed with early stage prostate and breast carcinomas. *Cancer* **2000**, *88*, 674–684.

32.   Kuhn, K.G.; Boesen, E.; Ross, L.; Johansen, C. Evaluation and outcome of behavioural changes in the rehabilitation of cancer patients: A review. *Eur. J. Cancer* **2005**, *41*, 216–224.

33.   Yarnall, K.S.H.; Pollak, K.I.; Østbye, T.; Krause, K.M.; Michener, J.L. Primary Care: Is There Enough Time for Prevention? *Am. J. Public Health* **2003**, *93*, 635–641.

34.   Murimi, M.W.; Nguyen, B.; Moyeda-Carabaza, A.F.; Lee, H.J.; Park, O.H. Factors That Contribute to Effective Online Nutrition Education Interventions: A Systematic Review. *Nutr. Rev.* **2019**, *77*, 663–690.

35.   Villinger, K.; Wahl, D.R.; Boeing, H.; Schupp, H.T.; Renner, B. The effectiveness of app-based mobile interventions on nutrition behaviours and nutrition-related health outcomes: A systematic review and meta-analysis. *Obes. Rev.* **2019** *20*, 1465–1484.

36. Wurz, A.; St-Aubin, A.; Brunet, J. Breast cancer survivors' barriers and motives for participating in a group-based physical activity program offered in the community. *Support. Care Cancer* **2015**, *23*, 2407–2416. [PubMed]

37. Gill, T.M.; Baker, D.I.; Gottschalk, M.; Peduzzi, P.N.; Allore, H.; Byers, A. A Program to Prevent Functional Decline in Physically Frail, Elderly Persons Who Live at Home. *N. Engl. J. Med.* **2002**, *347*, 1068–1074. [PubMed]

38. Rowland, J.H.; Bellizzi, K.M. Cancer Survivorship Issues: Life After Treatment and Implications for an Aging Population. *J. Clin. Oncol.* **2014**, *32*, 2662–2668. [PubMed]

39. Brown, J.C.; Harhay, O.M.; Harhay, M.N. Patient-reported versus objectively-measured physical function and mortality risk among cancer survivors. *J. Geriatr. Oncol.* **2016**, *7*, 108–115. [PubMed]

40. Hamaker, M.E.; Prins, M.C.; Schiphorst, A.H.; Van Tuyl, S.A.; Pronk, A.; Bos, F.V.D. Long-term changes in physical capacity after colorectal cancer treatment. *J. Geriatr. Oncol.* **2015**, *6*, 153–164.

41. Ballard-Barbash, R.; Friedenreich, C.M.; Courneya, K.S.; Siddiqi, S.M.; McTiernan, A.; Alfano, C.M. Physical Activity, Biomarkers, and Disease Outcomes in Cancer Survivors: A Systematic Review. *J. Natl. Cancer Inst.* **2012**, *104*, 815–840.

42. Hagan, K.A.; Grodstein, F. The Alternative Healthy Eating Index and Physical Function Impairment in Men. *J. Nutr. Health Aging* **2019**, *23*, 459–465.

43. U.S. Department of Agriculture, Food and Nutrition Service, Office of Research, Nutrition and Analysis. Diet Quality of Americans by Food Stamp Participation Status: Data from the National Health and Nutrition Examination Survey, 1999–2004, by Nancy Cole and Mary Kay Fox. Available online: https://fns-prod.azureedge.net/sites/default/files/NHANES-FSP.pdf (accessed on 6 October 2020).

44. Arabshahi, S.; Lahmann, P.H.; Williams, G.M.; Marks, G.C.; Van Der Pols, J. Longitudinal Change in Diet Quality in Australian Adults Varies by Demographic, Socio-Economic, and Lifestyle Characteristics. *J. Nutr.* **2011**, *141*, 1871–1879.

45. Harrington, J.M.; Dahly, D.L.; Fitzgerald, A.P.; Gilthorpe, M.S.; Perry, I.J. Capturing changes in dietary patterns among older adults: A latent class analysis of an ageing Irish cohort. *Public Health Nutr.* **2014**, *17*, 2674–2686.

46. Korkeila, K.; Suominen, S.; Ahvenainen, J.; Ojanlatva, A.; Rautava, P.; Helenius, H.; Koskenvuo, M. Non-response and related factors in a nation-wide health survey. *Eur. J. Epidemiol.* **2001**, *17*, 991–999.

47. Abrahams, H.J.G.; Gielissen, M.F.M.; Schmits, I.C.; Verhagen, C.A.H.H.V.M.; Rovers, M.M.; Knoop, H. Risk factors, prevalence, and course of severe fatigue after breast cancer treatment: A meta-analysis involving 12 327 breast cancer survivors. *Ann. Oncol.* **2016**, *27*, 965–974. [PubMed]

48. Curt, G.A. Impact of Fatigue on Quality of Life in Oncology Patients. *Semin. Hematol.* **2000**, *37*, 14–17. [PubMed]

49. De Jong, N.; Candel, M.J.J.M.; Schouten, H.C.; Abu-Saad, H.H.; Courtens, A.M. Prevalence and course of fatigue in breast cancer patients receiving adjuvant chemotherapy. *Ann. Oncol.* **2004**, *15*, 896–905. [PubMed]

50. Kim, S.H.; Son, B.H.; Hwang, S.Y.; Han, W.; Yang, J.-H.; Lee, S.; Yun, Y.H. Fatigue and Depression in Disease-Free Breast Cancer Survivors: Prevalence, Correlates, and Association with Quality of Life. *J. Pain Symptom Manag.* **2008**, *35*, 644–655.

51. Meeske, K.; Smith, A.W.; Alfano, C.M.; McGregor, B.A.; McTiernan, A.; Baumgartner, K.B.; Malone, K.E.; Reeve, B.B.; Ballard-Barbash, R.; Bernstein, L. Fatigue in breast cancer survivors two to five years post diagnosis: A HEAL Study report. *Qual. Life Res.* **2007**, *16*, 947–960. [PubMed]

52. Servaes, P.; Verhagen, S.; Bleijenberg, G. Determinants of chronic fatigue in disease-free breast cancer patients: A cross-sectional study. *Ann. Oncol.* **2002**, *13*, 589–598.

53. Minton, O.; Stone, P. How common is fatigue in disease-free breast cancer survivors? A systematic review of the literature. *Breast Cancer Res. Treat.* **2007**, *112*, 5–13.

54. Reinertsen, K.V.; Cvancarova, M.; Loge, J.H.; Edvardsen, H.; Wist, E.; Fosså, S.D. Predictors and course of chronic fatigue in long-term breast cancer survivors. *J. Cancer Surviv.* **2010**, *4*, 405–414.

55. Bower, J.E.; Ganz, P.A.; Desmond, K.A.; Bernaards, C.; Rowland, J.H.; Meyerowitz, B.E.; Belin, T.R. Fatigue in long-term breast carcinoma survivors. *Cancer* **2006**, *106*, 751–758.

56. Guest, D.D.; Evans, E.M.; Rogers, L.Q. Diet Components Associated with Perceived Fatigue in Breast Cancer Survivors. *Eur. J. Cancer Care* **2013**, *22*, 51–59.

Impact of Early Incorporation of Nutrition Interventions as a Component of Cancer Therapy in Adults

Julie Richards [1,*], Mary Beth Arensberg [2], Sara Thomas [2], Kirk W. Kerr [2], Refaat Hegazi [2] and Michael Bastasch [3]

[1]   Abbott Nutrition, Bob Evans Farms, Columbus, OH 43212, USA
[2]   Abbott Nutrition Division of Abbott, Columbus, OH 43219, USA; mary.arensberg@abbott.com (M.B.A.); sara.thomas@abbott.com (S.T.); kirk.kerr@abbott.com (K.W.K.); refaat.hegazi@abbott.com (R.H.)
[3]   Department of Medicine and Division of Radiation Oncology, University of Texas East Health, Athens, TX 75751, USA; bastaschmd@hotmail.com
*   Correspondence: julie.richards@abbott.com

Abstract: Malnutrition is prevalent among oncology patients and can adversely affect clinical outcomes, prognosis, quality of life, and survival. This review evaluates current trends in the literature and reported evidence around the timing and impact of specific nutrition interventions in oncology patients undergoing active cancer treatment. Previous research studies (published 1 January 2010–1 April 2020) were identified and selected using predefined search strategy and selection criteria. In total, 15 articles met inclusion criteria and 12/15 articles provided an early nutrition intervention. Identified studies examined the impacts of nutrition interventions (nutrition counseling, oral nutrition supplements, or combination of both) on a variety of cancer diagnoses. Nutrition interventions were found to improve body weight and body mass index, nutrition status, protein and energy intake, quality of life, and response to cancer treatments. However, the impacts of nutrition interventions on body composition, functional status, complications, unplanned hospital readmissions, and mortality and survival were inconclusive, mainly due to the limited number of studies evaluating these outcomes. Early nutrition interventions were found to improve health and nutrition outcomes in oncology patients. Future research is needed to further evaluate the impacts of early nutrition interventions on patients' outcomes and explore the optimal duration and timing of nutrition interventions.

Keywords: malnutrition; oncology; cancer care; nutrition interventions; early intervention; nutrition counseling; oral nutrition supplements; health outcomes

1. Introduction

Population aging and growth are driving the global burden of cancer, which is estimated to increase by more than 60% by 2040 and become the leading barrier to increasing life expectancy in this century [1]. At the same time, malnutrition persists as a growing crisis across the continuum of care. In the oncology population, the prevalence of malnourished patients or those at risk of malnutrition ranges from 25 to 70% [2–9]. Many patients with cancer are malnourished on diagnosis. Over the course of cancer and its treatment, malnutrition can also develop, continue, or worsen. However, malnutrition, particularly protein energy deficits and muscle loss, frequently remains underdiagnosed and undertreated among oncology patients [10]. This is a significant problem because malnutrition is related to multiple poor outcomes in patients with cancer. Indeed, malnutrition results in increased mortality rates, and 10–20% of deaths in cancer patients can be attributed to malnutrition vs. the malignancy itself [5,11,12].

Oncology patients can have complex nutrition problems, which often vary depending on the location and stage of the cancer. The side effects from cancer treatments can further exacerbate nutrition problems, including cancer cachexia. Cancer cachexia is characterized by a negative protein and energy intake combined with systemic inflammation and hyper-metabolism [13].

Thus, implementing nutrition interventions early is particularly critical for patients with cancer. Clinical guidelines, including those from the Academy of Nutrition and Dietetics (Academy) [14], the American Society for Parenteral and Enteral Nutrition (ASPEN) [15], and the European Society for Clinical Nutrition and Metabolism (ESPEN) [16], advocate for the importance of early nutrition screening and intervention in oncology patient populations.

Multiple nutrition interventions, including dietary counseling or advice, oral nutritional supplements (ONS), and enteral nutrition, have shown positive outcomes in malnourished hospitalized and community-dwelling adults with cancer [17–19]. Furthermore, systematic reviews have underscored the strength of evidence of such nutrition interventions on nutrition and health outcomes for oncology patients [20–24]. In addition to the positive effects of nutrition interventions on malnutrition, nutrition interventions have also been documented to improve outcomes such as quality of life (QoL) [18] and possibly survival [19] in cancer patients. However, it seems no previous review has evaluated the impact of early incorporation of nutrition interventions as a component of cancer therapy. The aim of this review was to evaluate the current evidence around the timing and impact of specific nutrition interventions in oncology patients undergoing active cancer treatment and to identify trends in the literature.

2. Materials and Methods

This study performed a basic review of the recent literature on specific nutrition interventions for oncology patients.

2.1. Search Strategy

A comprehensive electronic literature search was completed in April 2020 with a predefined search strategy. The databases that were searched included Allied and Complementary Medicine™ (EBSCO Information Services, Ipswich, MA, USA), BIOSIS Previews® (EBSCO Information Services, Ipswich, MA, USA), Embase® (Elsevier, Amsterdam, The Netherlands), EMCare® (Ovid, New York City, NY, USA), International Pharmaceutical Abstracts (EBSCO Information Services, Ipswich, MA, USA), MEDLINE® (Medical Literature Analysis and Retrieval System Online; National Library of Medicine, Bethesda, MD, USA), and ToxFile® (ProQuest Dialog, Ann Arbor, MI, USA). Key search terms are listed in Table 1, and the full electronic search strategy is included in Appendix A. Search results were limited to research in the adult population published from developed countries between 1 January 2010 and 1 April 2020 and written in the English language. This specific date range was chosen because past reviews [20–24] have already evaluated nutrition interventions from studies dated previously and because early nutrition intervention specifically is a more modern practice due to evidence-based position papers and clinical guidelines [14–16,25–27] that have raised awareness and provided guidance for nutrition interventions. Manual searches were also performed on existing systematic reviews and studies recommended for consideration from clinical nutrition experts.

The review focused on studies that investigated health and nutrition outcomes of specified nutrition interventions in adults diagnosed with any type of cancer who were receiving or planned to receive active treatment (other than surgery alone) for their cancer. Additionally, timing of nutrition intervention was of interest. Early intervention was defined as a specified nutrition intervention initiated within the first week of cancer treatment or before, while late intervention was identified as a specified nutrition intervention provided after the first week of cancer treatment. This cutoff for early nutrition intervention was chosen based on previous research, whereby early nutrition intervention was typically defined as being at the start of therapy or before [28,29]. Studies providing either early or late nutrition interventions were included in this review to compare outcomes. Studies evaluating nutrition intervention alone were included and studies with nutrition intervention along with other separate interventions (such as vitamin or mineral supplementation, exercise or physical activity, behavioral or mental health interventions, or alternative medicine) were excluded, since the focus of this review was on more general nutrition interventions vs. multicomponent therapies.

Table 1. Key search terms to identify studies involving early incorporation of nutrition interventions as a component of cancer therapy.

String	Terms
Cancer	Cancer, neoplasm, tumor, oncology, carcinoma, sarcoma
Treatment	Treatment, chemotherapy, radiation
Nutrition	Nutrition, food, diet
Intervention	Assessment, care plan, plan, planning, counsel, consult, diagnosis, education, evaluation, index, intervention, monitoring, screening, therapy, treatment, oral nutrition supplement (ONS), enteral, parenteral, intravenous, enteric, intragastric, intestinal, intraintestinal, tube, feeding, feeds

Health and nutrition outcomes of interest were anthropometric measures, nutritional and functional status, protein or energy intake, muscle strength, quality of life (QoL) measures, hospital readmissions or unplanned hospitalizations, response to treatment, emergency department (ED) visits, complications or morbidity, mortality, and healthcare costs. Mortality was generally defined as overall survival, rather than progression-free survival.

2.2. Inclusion and Exclusion Criteria

Studies identified through the electronic and manual searches were compared against the predetermined eligibility criteria, which were aligned with the population, intervention, comparison, outcome, time (PICOT) model, and are summarized in Table 2.

Table 2. Summary of inclusion and exclusion criteria to identify studies involving early incorporation of nutrition interventions as a component of cancer therapy.

	Inclusion Criteria	Exclusion Criteria
Population	Any setting (within last 10 years) ≥18 years of age Diagnosed with cancer Receiving or planning to receive active treatment for cancer diagnosis (unless receiving surgery only) Any nutritional status (well nourished, malnourished, or at-risk of malnutrition) Studies published within the last 10 years (January 2010 or later)	Animal studies <18 years of age No cancer diagnosis Not receiving or no plans to receive active treatment for cancer diagnosisOnly receiving surgery as a cancer treatment Pregnant or lactating females Studies published before January 2010
Intervention	Specified nutrition interventions (singly or in combination) for malnourished patients or those at-risk of malnutrition: - Oral nutritional supplements (ONS) - Enteral nutrition - Parenteral nutrition - Dietary counseling/dietary advice - Formalized nutrition discharge education - ONS coupons and literature on ONS-tailored nutritional care plans at discharge - Nutrition education, post-discharge phone calls - Home visits by registered dietitian nutritionist (RDN)	Nutrition interventions to prevent weight gain Non-commercially available or home-prepared ONS Any of the following (alone or in combination with any other interventions, including the specified nutrition interventions): - Vitamin or mineral supplementation or both - Exercise/physical activity - Behavioral/mental health interventions - Alternative medicine

Table 2. *Cont.*

	Inclusion Criteria	Exclusion Criteria
Comparison	Specified nutrition intervention(s) vs. no nutrition intervention(s) Specified nutrition intervention(s) vs. other specified nutrition intervention(s) Specified nutrition intervention(s) vs. standard of care Early specified nutrition intervention(s) vs. late intervention(s)	No comparison/control group
Duration of Intervention	>1 week	<1 week
Outcome	Anthropometrics - Body weight - Body mass index (BMI) Body composition - Muscle mass - Fat mass Nutritional status - Results of malnutrition screening/assesment - Energy intake - Protein intake Functional status - Muscle strength - Handgrip strength - Physical activity Quality of Life (QoL) Hospital readmissions/unplanned hospitalizations Response to treatment - Treatment tolerance - Treatment interruption - Full completion of treatment protocol Emergency Department (ED) visits Complications Morbidity Mortality Healthcare costs	Outcomes other than the specified health and nutrition outcomes

2.3. Data Extraction

Four reviewers (J.R., M.B.A., S.T., and K.W.K.) independently screened abstracts and assessed full-text articles for eligibility. Data were extracted per the PICOT framework and documented in Table 3. Reviewers met after the screening and full-text assessment steps to discuss all studies and reach an agreement on studies for final inclusion.

Table 3. Summary of studies included in review of incorporation of nutrition interventions as a component of cancer therapy

Study, Year	Design, Sample Size	Population, Country	Cancer Dx, Cancer Tx	Nutrition Status	Nutrition Intervention(s)	Early or Late Intervention(s), Duration	Outcomes of Nutrition Intervention(s)
Bourdel-Marchasson, 2014 [30]	RCT 341	Older adults (70+ years) France	Lymphoma or carcinoma CT	At risk for malnutrition	Counseling + ONS if needed (intervention group) vs. standard care	Early 3-6 months	↑ Energy intake *$^\phi$ No difference in weight loss $^\phi$ No difference in hospitalizations $^\phi$ No difference in response to cancer treatment $^\phi$ ↓ Complications (infections) *$^\phi$ No difference in mortality $^\phi$
Cereda, 2018 [31]	RCT 159	Any adults (18+ years) Italy	Head and neck cancer RT or RT plus systemic tx	Any nutrition status	Counseling + ONS (intervention group) vs. counseling only	Early Throughout RT, at 1 month and 3-month follow-up visits after end of RT	↓ Weight loss *$^\phi$ ↑ Energy intake *$^\phi$ ↑ Protein intake *$^\phi$ ↑ Handgrip strength $^\phi$ ↑ QoL *$^\phi$ ↑ Treatment tolerance $^\phi$
Kim, 2019 [32]	RCT 34	Any adults (20+ years) Korea	Pancreatic and bile duct cancers CT	Patients with a BMI > 30 kg/m² were excluded	Counseling + ONS (intervention group) vs. counseling only	Early for 61.8% of participants (initiated study participation in first cycle of CT) 8 weeks	↑ Nutrition status (measured by PG-SGA) *$^\natural$ No difference in weight loss $^{\phi\natural}$ No difference in skeletal muscle mass $^{\phi\natural}$ No difference in FFM $^{\phi\natural}$ ↑ Fat mass *$^{\phi\natural}$ ↑ Energy intake *$^\natural$ ↑ Protein intake *$^\natural$ ↑ QoL (fatigue symptoms) $^\natural$
Meng, 2019 [28]	Prospective cohort study 78	Adults 18-70 years China	Nasopharyngeal carcinoma CRT	Any nutrition status	Early nutrition intervention (intervention group) vs. late nutrition intervention Intervention for both groups was ONS + EN or PN if needed	Early for participants in the nutrition intervention group; late nutrition intervention group did not receive nutrition support until nutrition-related side effects from treatment developed Nutrition intervention lasted until 3 months after CRT	↓ Weight loss *$^\phi$ ↓ BMI change *$^\phi$ ↑ Treatment tolerance (lower incidence of mucositis) *$^\phi$ ↓ Treatment breaks (>3 days) *$^\phi$ ↓ Treatment delays for toxicity *$^\phi$ ↓ Unplanned hospitalizations *$^\phi$
Paccagnella, 2010 [29]	Retrospective cohort study 66	Any adults (18+ years) Italy	Head and neck cancer CRT	Any nutrition status	Individualized counseling + ONS/EN if needed (intervention group) vs. standard care	Early Nutrition intervention lasted until 6 months after CRT	↓ Weight loss *$^\phi$ ↑ Treatment tolerance *$^\phi$ ↓ Treatment delays *$^\phi$ ↓ Unplanned hospitalizations *$^\phi$
Poulsen, 2014 [33]	RCT 61	Any adults (18+ years) Denmark	GI gynecologic, or esophageal cancer CT and/or RT	Any nutrition status	Counseling + ONS-EPA if desired (intervention group) vs. standard care	Early Between 5–12 weeks, follow-up performed 3 months after treatment	↓ Weight loss *$^\phi$ ↑ Energy intake *$^\phi$ ↑ Protein intake *$^\phi$ No difference in change in FFM $^\phi$ No difference in change in fat mass $^\phi$ No difference in QoL $^\phi$
Ravasco, 2012 [34]	RCT 111	Any adults (18+ years) Portugal	Colorectal cancer RT followed by surgery + CT	Any nutrition status	Nutrition counseling and education using regular foods (group 1) vs. ONS + usual diet (group 2) vs. usual diet only (group 3)	Early 1.5 months	↑ Nutrition status (measured by PG-SGA; group 1) *$^\phi$ ↑ BMI (group 1) *$^\phi$ ↑ Energy intake (group 1) *$^\phi$ ↑ Protein intake (group 1) *$^\phi$ ↑ Treatment tolerance (measured by late radiotherapy toxicity; group 1) *$^\phi$ ↑ QoL (group 1) *$^\phi$ ↓ Mortality (group 1) *$^\phi$ *Results are from long-term follow-up (range = 4.9–8.2 years) and compared to groups 2 and 3*
Roca-Rodriguez, 2014 [35]	RCT 26	Adults 18–80 years Spain	ENT cancer RT, and CT if needed	Any nutrition status	ONS-EPA (intervention group) vs. isocaloric ONS	Late (14 days after start of RT) 76 days	↓ BMI decline $^\phi$
Sanchez-Lara, 2014 [36]	RCT 92	Adults 18–80 years Mexico	Non-small cell lung cancer CT	Any nutrition status	Diet plus ONS-EPA (intervention group) vs. isocaloric diet only Extra calories from ONS were subtracted from intervention group diet so both groups received an isocaloric diet	Early 8+ weeks	↓ Weight loss *$^\phi$ ↑ LBM *$^\phi$ ↑ Energy intake *$^{\phi\natural}$ ↑ Protein intake *$^{\phi\natural}$ ↑ QoL (increased global health status; $^\natural$ improved fatigue and loss of appetite $^{\natural\phi}$) * ↑ Treatment tolerance (less nausea, vomiting, and neuropathy) *$^\phi$ No difference in tumor response rate $^\phi$ No difference in overall survival $^\phi$ ↑ PFS $^\phi$

Table 3. *Cont.*

Study, Year	Design, Sample Size	Population, Country	Cancer Dx, Cancer Tx	Nutrition Status	Nutrition Intervention(s)	Early or Late Intervention(s), Duration	Outcomes of Nutrition Intervention(s)
Shirai, 2017 [37]	Retrospective cohort study 179	Adults 18–80 years Japan	GI cancer CT	>5% of pre-illness body weight	ONS-EPA (intervention group) vs. no additional nutritional treatment/placebo	Unknown 6 months	↑ Skeletal muscle mass and LBM *ᴨ No difference in overall survival ᵠ ↑ Treatment tolerance for patients with mGPS of 1 or 2 who received ONS-EPA ᵠ ↑ Prognosis for patients with mGPS of 1 or 2 who received ONS-EPA *ᵠ
Trabal, 2010 [38]	RCT 13	Any adults (18+ years) Spain	Colorectal cancer CT	Excluded patients with severe malnutrition (based on PG-SGA or BMI < 16.5 or >30 kg/m² Patients withdrawn if they developed malnutrition during the study	Counseling + ONS-EPA (intervention group) vs. counseling only	Early 12 weeks	↑ Weight *ᵠ ↑ Energy intake ᵠ ↑ Protein intake ᵠ ↑ QoL (improved fatigue, pain, physical function, social function) ᵠ ↑ Treatment tolerance ᵠ
van der Meij, 2010 [39]	RCT 40	Adults 18–80 years The Netherlands	Non-small cell lung cancer CRT	Any nutrition status	ONS-EPA (intervention group) vs. isocaloric ONS	Early 5 weeks	↓ Weight loss *ᵠ ↓ Loss of FFM *ᵠ No difference in energy intake ᵠ No difference in protein intake ᵠ
van der Meij, 2012 [40]	RCT 40	Adults 18–80 years The Netherlands	Non-small cell lung cancer CRT	Any nutrition status	ONS-EPA (intervention group) vs. isocaloric ONS	Early 5 weeks	↑ QoL (global health status, physical function, cognitive function, social function) *ᵠ ↑ Physical activity (during weeks 3 and 5) *ᵠ No difference in handgrip strength ᵠ ↑ Treatment tolerance (lower incidence of nausea/vomiting) *ᵠ No difference in treatment delays/dose reduction ᵠ No difference in unplanned hospital admissions ᵠ

Key: ↑ increased/higher; ↓ decreased/lower; * statistically significant ($p < 0.05$); ᵠ compared to control group/standard of care; ᴨ compared to baselin. **Abbreviations:** BMI, body mass index; CRT, chemoradiotherapy; CT, chemotherapy; Dx, diagnosis; EPA, eicosapentaenoic acid; EN, enteral nutrition; ENT, ear, nose and throat; FFM, fat free mass; GI, gastrointestinal; LBM, lean body mass; mGPS, modified Glasgow Prognostic Score; ONS, oral nutrition supplement; ONS-EPA, oral nutrition supplement containing eicosapentaenoic acid; PFS, progression-free survival; PG-SGA, Patient Generated Subjective Global Assessment; PN, parenteral nutrition; QOL, quality of life; RCT, randomized controlled trial; RT, radiotherapy; Tx, treatment.

3. Results

3.1. Literature Search

The literature search and selection steps are outlined in Figure 1. The electronic literature search resulted in 85 articles. In addition, 38 studies were recommended for consideration from clinical nutrition experts and manual search results, resulting in a total of 123 articles for consideration. After removal of duplicate publications, 118 articles were available for assessment. Only 15 studies met the predetermined eligibility criteria and were, thus, included in the final qualitative analysis.

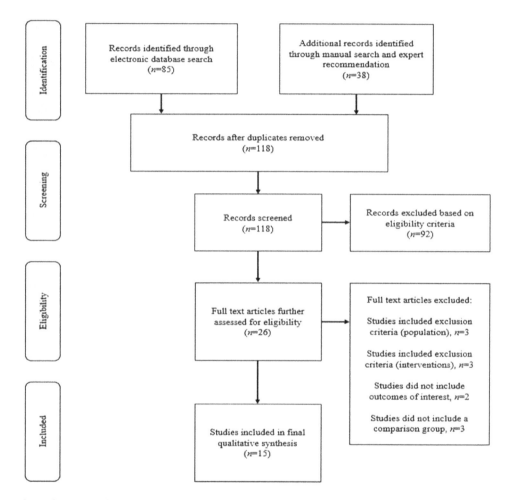

Figure 1. Flow diagram showing selection of studies for this review of early incorporation of nutrition interventions as a component of cancer therapy.

3.2. Study Characteristics

Specific characteristics of the 15 eligible studies [28–42] meeting the inclusion criteria, which included publication in the last 10 years, are detailed in Table 3. The key provided at the bottom of Table 3 provides further information on statistical significance and nutrition intervention group comparisons. Among the 15 included studies, 10 were randomized controlled trials (RCTs) [30–36,38–40,42]. Sample sizes ranged from 13 to 341 participants. Cancer diagnoses included from head and neck cancers (HNC) [28,29,31,35,42], non-small cell lung cancer [36,39–41], gastrointestinal (GI) cancers [33,34,37,38], gynecologic cancer [33], pancreatic or bile duct cancers [32], and lymphoma or carcinoma [30].

For over half (9/15) of the studies, nutrition counseling was a nutrition intervention strategy [29–34,38,41,42]. ONS was used in all 15 studies [28–42], although some studies (5/15) only provided ONS if identified as needed or desired [29,30,33,41,42]. Eight studies (8/15) used ONS containing eicosapentaenoic acid (ONS-EPA) [33,35–41]. Some of these studies compared counseling

+ ONS-EPA to standard care [33,41], or to nutrition counseling only [38], while others compared ONS-EPA to no nutrition treatment [10], an isocaloric diet [36], or an isocaloric ONS [35,39,40]. Only one study specifically compared the results of early vs. late nutrition intervention [28].

4. Outcomes

4.1. Anthropometrics, Body Composition, and Nutritional Status

Fourteen studies (14/15) evaluated the effects of nutrition interventions on anthropometric measures, including body weight, BMI, and body composition [28–39,41,42].

Seven (7/15) studies reported reduced weight loss in the intervention group, and these interventions included early counseling combined with ONS [29,31,33,42], providing ONS at the beginning of treatment [28], or providing ONS-EPA [36,39]. Tanaka et al. [41] and Trabal et al. [38] found that a nutrition prescription of ONS-EPA resulted in weight gain. Four studies reported on changes in BMI, with two studies finding an increase in BMI as a result of the nutrition interventions [34,41] and two finding a reduction in BMI decline after the nutrition intervention [28,35].

Five (5/15) studies evaluated the effects of nutrition interventions on body composition [32,33,36,37,39]. Sanchez-Lara et al. [36] and Shirai et al. [37] found significant increases in lean body mass (LBM) after providing nutrition interventions that included ONS-EPA compared to control groups, while van der Meij et al. [39] found significantly less loss of fat free mass (FFM) in the intervention group receiving ONS-EPA. However, Kim et al. and Poulsen et al. did not find a difference in FFM after providing the nutrition interventions, but Kim et al. did observe a significant increase in fat mass [32,33].

Three studies (3/15) evaluated nutritional status [32,34,42]. Two studies used the patient-generated subjective global assessment (PG-SGA) method and found significant improvements in nutritional status in the nutrition intervention groups, which received nutrition counseling with ONS [32] and nutrition counseling plus education [34]. Additionally, van der Berg et al. defined malnutrition as unintended weight loss $\geq$ 5% within 1 month and found a significant difference in malnutrition two weeks after the treatment between the nutrition intervention group receiving counseling plus ONS vs. the control group [42].

4.2. Nutritional Intake

Eight studies (8/15) evaluated energy intake [30–34,36,38,39], with six studies finding a significant increase in energy intake in the nutrition intervention groups [30–34,36] and one study finding an increased energy intake that was not significant [38]. Seven studies (7/15) evaluated protein intake [31–34,36,38,39], with five studies finding a significant increase in protein intake in the nutrition intervention groups [31–34,36] and one study finding an increased protein intake that was not significant [38]. Further, van der Meij et al. did not find a difference in energy or protein intake between groups; however, this study was comparing interventions of an ONS-EPA vs. an isocaloric ONS [39].

4.3. Functional Status

Three studies (3/15) evaluated functional status through physical activity, physical function, or handgrip strength [31,40,41]. Of these, van der Meij et al. found a significant increase in physical activity and physical function in the group provided ONS-EPA compared to controls provided with an isocaloric ONS [40]. Three studies used handgrip strength as a measure of functional status; Cereda et al. [31] saw an increase in handgrip strength after the nutrition intervention, while Tanaka et al. [41] saw a significant decrease and van der Meij et al. [40] did not find a difference.

4.4. QoL

Eight studies (8/15) evaluated QoL [31–34,36,38,40,41], with three studies reporting an overall improvement in QoL in the nutrition intervention groups compared to the control groups [31,34,41]. However, Poulsen et al. did not find a difference in QoL between the intervention and control groups [33].

Four studies (4/15) reported improvements in subscales of the QoL questionnaire [32,36,38,40]. Three studies reported improved fatigue in the nutrition intervention groups compared to control groups [32,36,38]. Two studies reported better physical and social function results in the intervention groups vs. the controls groups [38,40]. Improvements in appetite [36], global health status [36,40], and cognitive function [40] were also reported as a result of nutrition interventions. However, Trabel et al. found that loss of appetite worsened in the nutrition intervention group compared to the control group [38].

4.5. Response to Cancer Treatment

Ten studies (10/15) evaluated response to cancer treatment, including treatment tolerance or breaks or delays in treatment [28–31,34,36–38,40,41]. Five studies found a statistically significant improvement in treatment tolerance for those in the nutrition intervention groups vs. the control groups [28,29,34,36,40] and two other studies reported an improvement in treatment tolerance that was not significant [31,38]. Shirai et al. found an improved treatment tolerance in subjects who received ONS-EPA and had a modified Glasgow prognostic score (mGPS) of 1 or 2 compared to controls [37]. However, Tanaka et al. found no difference in treatment tolerance between the nutrition intervention group receiving counseling and ONS-EPA (as needed) and the control group receiving standard care [41].

Three studies reported on treatment breaks or delays [28,29,40]. Meng et al. found significantly fewer treatment delays for toxicity and significantly fewer CRT breaks (>3 days) in the early nutrition intervention group vs. the late nutrition intervention group [28], while Paccagnella et al. found significantly fewer treatment delays in the nutrition intervention group receiving counseling + ONS vs. the control group receiving standard care [29]. However, van der Meij et al. found no difference in treatment delays between the nutrition intervention group receiving ONS-EPA and the control group receiving isocaloric ONS [40].

Two studies reported on the results of cancer treatments. Bourdel-Marchasson et al. [30] did not observe a difference in full remission at the end of treatment between the nutrition intervention vs. control group, and Sanchez-Lara et al. [36] similarly did not observe a difference in overall tumor response rates between groups.

4.6. Complications and Unplanned Hospitalizations

One study (1/15) evaluated complications and found that the nutrition intervention group receiving counseling + ONS had significantly lower infections compared to the control group [30]. Three studies (3/15) evaluated unplanned hospitalizations [28,29,40]. Meng et al. [28] and Paccagnella et al. [29] found a statistically significant reduction in unplanned hospitalizations between nutrition intervention groups vs. control groups; however, van der Meij et al. [40] did not find a difference.

4.7. Mortality and Survival

Four studies (4/15) evaluated mortality and survival [30,34,36,37]. Ravasco et al. evaluated individualized nutrition counseling (group 1) vs. ONS with usual diet (group 2) vs. usual diet only (group 3) and found that the disease-specific survival time in group 3 < group 2 < group 1 ($p < 0.05$) [34]. However, three studies found no difference in mortality and survival between nutrition intervention groups and control groups [30,36,37].

When Sanchez-Lara et al. compared patients who consumed the complete dose of ONS-EPA (2 containers/day) vs. the control group, a trend was observed toward an increase in progression-free survival ($p = 0.07$) [36]. Additionally, Shirai et al. found a significantly better prognosis in subjects who received ONS-EPA and had a mGPS of 1 or 2 compared to controls [37].

4.8. Timing of Nutrition Intervention

The majority of the studies (12/15) provided an early nutrition intervention to the intervention groups [28–31,33,34,36,38–42]. Meng et al. specifically evaluated the impact of early vs. late nutrition interventions and found favorable outcomes for the early intervention group, including significantly reduced weight loss, significantly improved treatment tolerance, and significantly fewer unplanned hospitalizations [28]. Kim et al. provided early nutrition intervention to about 60% of subjects, since some subjects enrolled in the study were on later cycles of chemotherapy (CT) [32]. This study compared counseling plus ONS vs. counseling only. Since the different timing could have affected the results of the study, Kim et al. subdivided the subjects according to their cycle of CT. Body weight, skeletal muscle mass, and fat mass were increased significantly among subjects in their first cycle of CT who were receiving ONS, while only fat mass was increased among subjects in their second cycle or higher who were receiving ONS [32].

Roca-Rodriguez et al. evaluated ONS-EPA vs. standard ONS and provided these interventions 14 days after the start of RT, which in our review is categorized as a late nutrition intervention. Roca-Rodriguez reported a smaller decline in BMI for the ONS-EPA group vs. the standard ONS group, although this difference was not significant [35]. Shirai et al. did not specifically report when the nutrition intervention was initiated, so it is unclear if the intervention in their study was provided early or late [37].

5. Discussion

This review found that nutrition interventions had a positive impact on anthropometrics (body weight and BMI), nutrition status, protein and energy intake, QoL, and response to cancer treatments (treatment tolerance and treatment breaks/delays). The interventions used were ONS or ONS-EPA, nutrition counseling, or a combination of counseling and ONS. These results highlight the importance of early incorporation of nutrition interventions as a component of cancer therapy for the oncology patient population.

Inconclusive results were reported regarding body composition, functional status, complications, unplanned hospital readmissions, and mortality or survival. It is important to note that only a few studies focused on these measures and that these studies included small- to medium-sized samples. Additionally, the inconsistent and highly variable nutrition interventions and follow-up periods should be taken into consideration. Before conclusions can be drawn about the effects of nutrition interventions on these outcomes, further studies are necessary with larger sample sizes, consistent nutrition interventions of sufficient duration, and consistent timing of nutrition intervention and follow-up. Other outcomes of interest included in Table 2 but not addressed in the outcomes section were not reported in any of the identified studies.

Overall, the results of this review build upon the current body of evidence suggesting that nutrition interventions can result in improved outcomes for oncology patients. Other reviews of nutrition interventions for oncology patients have also shown positive results [21,22]. Due to the variations between study designs and interventions used in the studies we included, it is difficult to identify which nutrition intervention(s) led to the most beneficial outcomes. In the one long-term follow-up study included in our review by Ravasco et al. comparing individualized nutrition counseling and education (group 1), ONS plus usual diet (group 2), and usual diet only (group 3), it was found that group 1 had a significantly higher nutrition status, BMI, energy and protein intake, treatment tolerance, and QoL than group 2 and group 3 at the time of follow-up (4.9–8.2 years) [34]. Additionally, group 1 had significantly lower mortality [34]. These results support the long-term benefits of nutrition counseling for oncology patients and reinforce the Academy's Oncology Evidence-Based Nutrition Practice Guideline for Adults [14], which recommends oncology patients undergoing CT or radiation treatment should receive medical nutrition therapy (MNT) from Registered Dietitian Nutritionists (RDNs) based on strong, conditional evidence. As identified in a number of studies included in our review, ONS also helps to increase calorie and protein intake and can be particularly beneficial for patients before and while actively receiving cancer treatments who need more nutrition, have a loss of appetite, or are experiencing other treatment-related side effects. Moreover, to improve outcomes in oncology patients, dietary counseling that includes the use of ONS should be a first step toward increased energy and protein intake [14,16]. Indeed, many of the studies included in our review used counseling combined with ONS as the nutrition intervention [29–33,38,41,42].

Eight studies included in our review used ONS-EPA. Eicosapentaenoic acid (EPA) is a polyunsaturated long-chain omega-3 fatty acid. Its use has gained momentum in the oncology patient population due to its anti-inflammatory properties and evidence that it can prevent muscle loss [43], making EPA of particular interest for preventing and treating cancer cachexia. Previous systematic reviews have concluded there is insufficient evidence to support a recommendation that long-chain omega-3 fatty acids can treat cancer cachexia; however, these previous reviews did not include any studies published after June 2010 [44–46]. Nonetheless, evidence supports other benefits of long-chain omega-3 fatty acid use for oncology patients. Systematic reviews on the supplementation of long-chain omega-3 fatty acids in oncology patients found improved body weight, post-surgical morbidity, and QoL [47] and preserved body composition [48] as a result of supplementation. Similarly, the Academy's Oncology Evidence-Based Nutrition Practice Guideline for Adults [14] recommends, based on strong empirical evidence, the use of commercial supplements with EPA for patients with adequate dietary intake who are still experiencing weight or lean body mass loss. ESPEN's Guidelines on Nutrition in Cancer Patients [16] also recommend supplementation with long-chain N-3 fatty acids to stabilize or improve appetite, food intake, lean body mass, and body weight for patients with advanced cancer undergoing CT, but rated the level of evidence as low. Studies included in our review that evaluated a sole nutrition intervention of ONS-EPA vs. placebo, an isocaloric diet, or an isocaloric ONS found significantly reduced weight loss and loss of fat free mass, and significantly increased skeletal muscle mass and lean body mass, QoL, and treatment tolerance in the groups receiving ONS-EPA [35,37,39,40]. Because of its potential benefits, ONS-EPA should be considered for cancer patients with weight and lean body mass loss.

Most of the studies included in our review provided an early nutrition intervention, categorized as a nutrition intervention initiated within the first week of cancer treatment or before. The favorable outcomes reported across various studies demonstrate that early nutrition interventions can help improve patients' prognosis and outcomes. A definitive trial used to document the impact of early vs. late nutrition intervention could be difficult to undertake, since withholding needed nutrition care from patients could be considered unethical. However, a retrospective study or comparison of early nutrition intervention vs. standard care could provide further insights. The only study we identified that specifically examined the timing of nutrition interventions found that the early nutrition intervention group had significantly reduced weight loss, improved treatment tolerance, and fewer CRT breaks (>3 days), CRT delays for toxicity, and unplanned hospitalizations compared to the late nutrition intervention group [28]. Because the poor outcomes observed in the late nutrition intervention group can be detrimental to a patient's prognosis, early nutrition intervention may improve survival in oncology patients. This is supported by the long-term follow-up study by Ravasco et al., which provided early nutrition interventions and found that the disease-specific survival time in usual diet only (group 3) <ONS with usual diet (group 2) <individualized nutrition counseling (group 1) ($p < 0.05$) [34].

The positive outcomes seen in Meng et al. were also supported in the subset analysis by Kim et al. This analysis evaluated patients based on how far along they were in CT, since around 40% of patients started the study after CT was initiated. The effects of the nutrition intervention were greater in those who received the intervention early at the start of CT. Specifically, body weight, skeletal muscle mass, and fat mass were increased significantly among patients in their first cycle of CT who were receiving ONS, while only fat mass was increased among patients in their second cycle or higher who were receiving ONS [32]. Nonetheless, it is important to note that positive outcomes were also identified when late nutrition interventions were provided. Roca-Rodriguez et al. provided a late nutrition intervention fourteen days after the start of RT and reported a smaller decline in BMI for the intervention group vs. the control group [35]. In the study by Kim et al., providing a late nutrition intervention still resulted in increased fat mass for patients in their second cycle of CT or higher [32].

Our review documented the recent evidence supporting early incorporation of nutrition interventions as a component of cancer therapy for the oncology patient population. In the United States, 90% of cancer care is provided through outpatient cancer centers and clinics [49]. RDNs are uniquely trained to address malnutrition and can provide the individualized nutrition counseling and MNT needed, but they are inadequately staffed in cancer centers. A recent study found that the RDN-to-patient ratio in U.S. oncology centers is 1:2308 [50]. Indeed, only half (53.1%) of oncology centers screen for malnutrition, and a majority (76.8%) of these centers do not bill for nutrition services [50]. The recently introduced US Medical Nutrition Therapy Act of 2020 (H.R. 6971) could help change this and benefit patients by expanding Medicare Part B coverage for MNT for additional medical conditions, including cancer and malnutrition [51].

Individual teams and healthcare providers can also aim to fill existing gaps in malnutrition care and provide early nutrition interventions to improve oncology patients' outcomes. The recent ESPEN guidelines recommend: "Given the high incidence of nutritional deficits and metabolic derangements among cancer patients, it appears reasonable to monitor relevant parameters regularly in all cancer patients and to initiate interventions early and against all relevant impairments to prevent excessive deficits" [16]. Other professional organizations, such as ASPEN, have not recently published new guidelines on nutrition care for oncology patients. Thus, ESPEN's recommendation on the implementation of early nutrition interventions and the findings of reviews such as this one can help encourage organizations to consider updating their professional and clinical guidelines to recommend early nutrition interventions. One way to help achieve the recommendations in ESPEN's guidelines and improve outcomes is through the implementation of a nutrition-focused quality improvement program (QIP). While to date the development and implementation of nutrition-focused QIPs in cancer care appears to be limited [52], several QIPs that included oncology patient populations have illustrated how a nutrition-focused QIP can both improve health and provide economic benefits [53]. Moving forward, nutrition-focused QIPs engaging a multidisciplinary team could be executed in cancer centers to improve nutrition care processes and deliver early malnutrition care.

Our review had several limitations. First, the effects of nutrition interventions in the diverse oncology patient population can be difficult to study and may potentially limit the sample size, number of RCTs, and other research studies performed. Second, our PICOT criteria, electronic search strategy, and databases searched may have excluded studies. For example, our review did not include any studies evaluating enteral or parenteral nutrition as intervention methods. Third, although strict inclusion criteria were applied in our review to minimize the heterogeneity of the studies evaluated, the different study designs and settings, variable nutrition intervention and comparison groups, and the inconsistency of the methods used assess results among the studies likely influenced the findings. Fourth, the accuracy of the results reported from each study cannot be guaranteed, since no original data were accessed. Fifth, we did not complete a formal systematic review or meta-analysis, and thus did not address risk of bias, effect size, or clinical significance. While it has limitations, our review, along with new studies evaluating the benefits of comprehensive nutrition care in patients receiving cancer treatments, could be utilized to help develop nutrition care guidelines, optimize patient-centered care, and subsequently help improve patient outcomes.

6. Conclusions

Patients with cancer are at a high risk of malnutrition. This review showed that nutrition interventions in oncology patients receiving active cancer treatment helped improve body weight and BMI, nutrition status, protein and energy intake, QoL, and response to cancer treatments. The reported evidence is limited by the heterogeneity of study designs, small- to medium-sized samples, inconsistent and highly variable nutrition interventions and follow-up periods, and lack of standardized measurements for assessing reported outcomes. Further research is needed to better understand the impact of early nutrition interventions on patients' outcomes. The optimal duration and timing of nutrition interventions should also be explored. Additionally, future research should investigate the results of implementing a nutrition-focused QIP in cancer centers to improve nutrition care processes and early malnutrition care. This review may help inform the design of quality and comprehensive early nutrition care programs.

Author Contributions: Conceptualization, J.R., M.B.A., and K.W.K.; methodology, J.R., M.B.A., S.T. K.W.K., R.H., and M.B.; formal analysis, J.R., M.B.A., S.T., and K.W.K.; resources, J.R., M.B.A., S.T., K.W.K., R.H., and M.B.; Writing—original draft preparation, J.R.; writing—Review and editing, M.B.A., S.T., K.W.K., R.H., and M.B.; All authors have read and agreed to the published version of the manuscript.

Acknowledgments: We would like to thank Sherri Ho for assisting us with the literature search.

Appendix A

Table A1. Full electronic search strategy.

Search Strategy
(Ti,ab((cancer[*1] OR neoplas* OR tumor[*1] OR tumour[*1] OR *carcinoma* OR *sarcoma* OR oncolog*) n/10 (treatment* OR treat* OR chemothera* OR chemo-therap* OR radiat*) n/3 (((diet* OR food OR nutrition*) n/3 (assessment[*1] OR (care n/3 plan) OR plans OR planning OR plan OR counsel* OR council OR diagnos* OR consult* OR (discharg* n/1 education*) OR education* OR evaluation[*1] OR index OR indices OR intervention[*1] OR monitoring[*1] OR "ONS" OR screening[*1] OR therap* OR treatment[*1] OR supplement* OR enteral* OR parental*)) OR "oral nutritional supplement*" OR (parenteral n/1 fluid*) OR ((enteral* OR parenteral* OR intravenous* OR enteric* OR intragastric* OR intestinal* OR intraintestinal* OR tube* OR force*) n/3 (feed OR feeding* OR feeds OR alimentation* OR hyperalimentation*)))) AND ti,ab(((nutrition OR early OR late) n/3 intervention*) OR (standard* n/3 care*)) AND ti,ab,mesh,emb,su,if,au,low,loc,cnt,rg(Australia OR Australian OR Austria OR Austrian OR Belgium OR Belgian OR Bulgaria OR Bulgarian OR Canada OR Canadian OR Croatia OR Croatian OR Cyprus OR Cyprian OR "Czech Republic" OR Czech OR Denmark OR Danish OR Estonia OR Estonian OR "EU-15" OR Finland OR Finnish OR France OR French OR Germany OR German OR Greece OR Greek OR Hungary OR Hungarian OR Iceland OR Icelandic OR Ireland OR Irish OR Italy OR Italian OR Japan OR Japanese OR Latvia OR Latvian OR Lithuania OR Lithuanian OR Luxembourg OR Luxembourgian OR Malta OR Maltese OR Netherlands OR Dutch OR "New Zealand" OR Norway OR Norwegian OR Poland OR Polish OR Portugal OR Portuguese OR Romania OR Romanian OR Slovakia OR Slovakian OR Slovenia OR Slovene OR Spain OR Spanish OR Sweden OR Swedish OR Switzerland OR Swiss OR "United Kingdom" OR British OR "UK" OR "U.K." OR "United States" OR "US" OR "U.S." OR "USA" OR "U.S.A." OR American) AND YR(>=2010) AND la(English)) NOT (dog OR dogs OR cat OR cats OR canine* OR feline* OR porcine* OR pig OR pigs OR piglet* OR cow OR cows OR mice OR mouse OR rat OR rats OR cattle OR veterinar* OR monkey* OR rabbit* OR horse OR horses OR equine* OR zoo OR zoological OR zoology OR zoos OR (animal* n/3 stud*) OR bovine OR geese OR goose OR estuary* OR rodent* OR fish OR fishes OR marine OR dolphin* OR chick OR chicks OR goat OR goats OR ecolog* OR bird* OR sheep* OR zebrafish* OR hamster* OR bat OR bats OR (alternat* n/3 (medicat* OR medicine*)) OR pregnan* OR lactate* OR lactating* OR child* OR adolescen* OR infant* OR infancy OR newborn* OR neonat* OR baby OR babies OR preschool* OR teenage* OR toddler* OR juvenile* OR boy OR boys OR girl* OR pediatric* OR paediatric* OR ("pre" p/0 school*) OR suckling* OR youth OR schoolchild* OR preadolescen* OR ((vitamin* OR mineral*) n/3 supplement*) OR exercis* OR (physical n/3 activ*) OR ((behavior* OR mental*) n/3 health*) OR hospice[*1] OR (palliative n/1 (care OR nursing)))

References

1.   The American Cancer Society. The Burden of Cancer. 2019. Available online: https://canceratlas.cancer.org/wp-content/uploads/2019/09/CA3_TheBurdenofCancer.pdf (accessed on 31 August 2020).

2.   Muscaritoli, M.; Lucia, S.; Farcomeni, A.; Lorusso, V.; Saracino, V.; Barone, C.; Plastino, F.; Gori, S.; Magarotto, R.; Carteni, G.; et al. Prevalence of malnutrition in patients at first medical oncology visit: The PreMiO study. *Oncotarget* **2017**, *8*, 79884–79896. [CrossRef]

3.   Attar, A.; Malka, D.; Sabaté, J.M.; Bonnetain, F.; LeComte, T.; Aparicio, T.; Locher, C.; Laharie, D.; Ezenfis, J.; Taïeb, J. Malnutrition is high and underestimated during chemotherapy in gastrointestinal cancer: An AGEO prospective cross-sectional multicenter study. *Nutr. Cancer* **2012**, *64*, 535–542. [CrossRef]

4. Hébuterne, X.; Lemarié, E.; Michallet, M.; de Montreuil, C.B.; Schneider, S.M.; Goldwasser, F. Prevalence of malnutrition and current use of nutrition support in patients with cancer. *J. Parenter. Enter. Nutr.* **2014**, *38*, 196–204. [CrossRef]

5. Pressoir, M.; Desné, S.; Berchery, D.; Rossignol, G.; Poiree, B.; Meslier, M.; Traversier, S.; Vittot, M.; Simon, M.I.S.D.S.; Gekiere, J.P.; et al. Prevalence, risk factors and clinical implications of malnutrition in French Comprehensive Cancer Centres. *Br. J. Cancer* **2010**, *102*, 966–971. [CrossRef]

6. Silva, F.R.; de Oliveira, M.G.; Souza, A.S.; Figueroa, J.N.; Santos, C.S. Factors associated with malnutrition in hospitalized cancer patients: A croos-sectional study. *Nutr. J.* **2015**, *14*, 123. [CrossRef]

7. Maasberg, S.; Knappe-Drzikova, B.; Vonderbeck, D.; Jann, H.; Weylandt, K.-H.; Grieser, C.; Pascher, A.; Schefold, J.C.; Pavel, M.; Wiedenmann, B.; et al. Malnutrition Predicts Clinical Outcome in Patients with Neuroendocrine Neoplasia. *Neuroendocrinology* **2017**, *104*, 11–25. [CrossRef]

8. Planas, M.; Álvarez-Hernández, J.; León-Sanz, M.; Celaya-Pérez, S.; Araujo, K.; de Lorenzo, A.G. Prevalence of hospital malnutrition in cancer patients: A sub-analysis of the PREDyCES® study. *Support. Care Cancer* **2016**, *24*, 429–435. [CrossRef]

9. Platek, M.E.; Popp, J.V.; Possinger, C.S.; Denysschen, C.A.; Horvath, P.; Brown, J.K. Comparison of the prevalence of malnutrition diagnosis in head and neck, gastrointestinal, and lung cancer patients by 3 classification methods. *Cancer Nurs.* **2011**, *34*, 410–416. [CrossRef]

10. Williams, D.G.A.; Ohnuma, T.; Krishnamoorthy, V.; Raghunathan, K.; Sulo, S.; Cassady, B.A.; Hegazi, R.; Wischmeyer, P.E. Postoperative Utilization of Oral Nutritional Supplements in Surgical Patients in US Hospitals. *J. Parenter. Enter. Nutr.* **2020**. [CrossRef]

11. Wie, G.A.; Cho, Y.A.; Kim, S.Y.; Kim, S.M.; Bae, J.M.; Joung, H. Prevalence and risk factors of malnutrition among cancer patients according to tumor location and stage in the National Cancer Center in Korea. *Nutrition* **2010**, *26*, 263–268. [CrossRef]

12. Sesterhenn, A.M.; Szalay, A.; Zimmermann, A.P.; Werner, J.A.; Barth, P.J.; Wiegand, S. Significance of autopsy in patients with head and neck cancer. *Laryngo-Rhino-Otologie* **2012**, *91*, 375–380.

13. Kim, D.H. Nutritional issues in patients with cancer. *Intest. Res.* **2019**, *17*, 455–462. [CrossRef] [PubMed]

14. Thompson, K.L.; Elliott, L.; Fuchs-Tarlovsky, V.; Levin, R.M.; Voss, A.C.; Piemonte, T. Oncology Evidence-Based Nutrition Practice Guideline for Adults. *J. Acad. Nutr. Diet.* **2017**, *117*, 297.e247–310.e247. [CrossRef]

15. August, D.A.; Huhmann, M.B. ASPEN clinical guidelines: Nutrition support therapy during adult anticancer treatment and in hematopoietic cell transplantation. *J. Parenter. Enter. Nutr.* **2009**, *33*, 472–500. [CrossRef]

16. Arends, J.J.; Bachmann, P.P.; Baracos, V.V.; Barthelemy, N.N.; Bertz, H.H.; Bozzetti, F.; Fearon, K.C.; Hütterer, E.E.; Isenring, E.E.; Kaasa, S.; et al. ESPEN guidelines on nutrition in cancer patients. *Clin. Nutr.* **2017**, *36*, 11–48. [CrossRef]

17. Sauer, A.C.; Li, J.; Partridge, J.; Sulo, S. Assessing the impact of nutrition interventions on health and nutrition outcomes of community-dwelling adults: A systematic review. *Nutr. Diet. Suppl.* **2018**, *10*, 45–57. [CrossRef]

18. Baldwin, C.; Spiro, A.; Ahern, R.; Emery, P.W. Oral nutritional interventions in malnourished patients with cancer: A systematic review and meta-analysis. *J. Natl. Cancer Inst.* **2012**, *104*, 371–385. [CrossRef]

19. Elia, M.; Van Bokhorst-de van der Schueren, M.A.; Garvey, J.; Goedhart, A.; Lundholm, K.; Nitenberg, G.; Stratton, R. Enteral (oral or tube administration) nutritional support and eicosapentaenoic acid in patients with cancer: A systematic review. *Int. J. Oncol.* **2006**, *28*, 5–23. [CrossRef]

20. Blackwood, H.A.; Hall, C.C.; Balstad, T.R.; Solheim, T.S.; Fallon, M.; Haraldsdottir, E.; Laird, B.J. A systematic review examining nutrition support interventions in patients with incurable cancer. *Support. Care Cancer* **2020**, *28*, 1877–1889. [CrossRef]

21. de van der Schueren, M.A.E.; Laviano, A.; Blanchard, H.; Jourdan, M.; Arends, J.; Baracos, V.E. Systematic review and meta-analysis of the evidence for oral nutritional intervention on nutritional and clinical outcomes during chemo(radio)therapy: Current evidence and guidance for design of future trials. *Ann. Oncol.* **2018**, *29*, 1141–1153. [CrossRef] [PubMed]

22. Lee, J.L.C.; Leong, L.P.; Lim, S.L. Nutrition intervention approaches to reduce malnutrition in oncology patients: A systematic review. *Support. Care Cancer* **2016**, *24*, 469–480. [CrossRef]

23. Rinninella, E.; Fagotti, A.; Cintoni, M.; Raoul, P.; Scaletta, G.; Quagliozzi, L.; Miggiano, G.A.D.; Scambia, G.; Gasbarrini, A.; Mele, M.C. Nutritional Interventions to Improve Clinical Outcomes in Ovarian Cancer: A Systematic Review of Randomized Controlled Trials. *Nutrients* **2019**, *11*, 1404. [CrossRef]

24. Kiss, N.K.; Krishnasamy, M.; Isenring, E.A. The effect of nutrition intervention in lung cancer patients undergoing chemotherapy and/or radiotherapy: A systematic review. *Nutr. Cancer* **2014**, *66*, 47–56. [CrossRef]

25. Caccialanza, R.; Pedrazzoli, P.; Cereda, E.; Gavazzi, C.; Pinto, C.; Paccagnella, A.; Beretta, G.D.; Nardi, M.; Laviano, A.; Zagonel, V. Nutritional Support in Cancer Patients: A Position Paper from the Italian Society of Medical Oncology (AIOM) and the Italian Society of Artificial Nutrition and Metabolism (SINPE). *J. Cancer* **2016**, *7*, 131–135. [CrossRef]

26. Aapro, M.; Arends, J.; Bozzetti, F.; Fearon, K.; Grunberg, S.M.; Herrstedt, J.; Hopkinson, J.; Jacquelin-Ravel, N.; Jatoi, A.; Kaasa, S.; et al. Early recognition of malnutrition and cachexia in the cancer patient: A position paper of a European School of Oncology Task Force. *Ann. Oncol.* **2014**, *25*, 1492–1499. [CrossRef]

27. Arends, J.J.; Baracos, V.V.; Bertz, H.H.; Bozzetti, F.; Calder, P.P.; Deutz, N.; Erickson, N.N.; Laviano, A.A.; Lisanti, M.M.; Lobo, D.N.D.; et al. ESPEN expert group recommendations for action against cancer-related malnutrition. *Clin. Nutr.* **2017**, *36*, 1187–1196. [CrossRef] [PubMed]

28. Meng, L.; Wei, J.; Ji, R.; Wang, B.; Xu, X.; Xin, Y.; Jiang, X. Effect of Early Nutrition Intervention on Advanced Nasopharyngeal Carcinoma Patients Receiving Chemoradiotherapy. *J. Cancer* **2019**, *10*, 3650–3656. [CrossRef] [PubMed]

29. Paccagnella, A.; Morello, M.; Da Mosto, M.C.; Baruffi, C.; Marcon, M.L.; Gava, A.; Baggio, V.; Lamon, S.; Babare, R.; Rosti, G.; et al. Early nutritional intervention improves treatment tolerance and outcomes in head and neck cancer patients undergoing concurrent chemoradiotherapy. *Support. Care Cancer* **2010**, *18*, 837–845. [CrossRef]

30. Bourdel-Marchasson, I.; Blanc-Bisson, C.; Doussau, A.; Germain, C.; Blanc, J.-F.; Dauba, J.; Lahmar, C.; Terrebonne, E.; Lecaille, C.; Ceccaldi, J.; et al. Nutritional advice in older patients at risk of malnutrition during treatment for chemotherapy: A two-year randomized controlled trial. *PLoS ONE* **2014**, *9*, e108687. [CrossRef]

31. Cereda, E.; Cappello, S.; Colombo, S.; Klersy, C.; Imarisio, I.; Turri, A.; Caraccia, M.; Borioli, V.; Monaco, T.; Benazzo, M.; et al. Nutritional counseling with or without systematic use of oral nutritional supplements in head and neck cancer patients undergoing radiotherapy. *Radiother. Oncol.* **2018**, *126*, 81–88. [CrossRef]

32. Kim, S.H.; Lee, S.M.; Jeung, H.C.; Lee, I.J.; Park, J.S.; Song, M.; Lee, D.K.; Lee, S.-M. The Effect of Nutrition Intervention with Oral Nutritional Supplements on Pancreatic and Bile Duct Cancer Patients Undergoing Chemotherapy. *Nutrients* **2019**, *11*, 1145. [CrossRef]

33. Poulsen, G.M.; Pedersen, L.L.; Østerlind, K.; Bæksgaard, L.; Andersen, J.R. Randomized trial of the effects of individual nutritional counseling in cancer patients. *Clin. Nutr.* **2014**, *33*, 749–753. [CrossRef]

34. Ravasco, P.; Monteiro-Grillo, I.; Camilo, M. Individualized nutrition intervention is of major benefit to colorectal cancer patients: Long-term follow-up of a randomized controlled trial of nutritional therapy. *Am. J. Clin. Nutr.* **2012**, *96*, 1346–1353. [CrossRef]

35. Roca-Rodríguez, M.M.; García-Almeida, J.M.; Lupiañez-Pérez, Y.; Rico, J.M.; Toledo, M.; Alcaide-Torres, J.; Cardona, F.; Medina, J.A.; Tinahones, F.J. Effect of a specific supplement enriched with n-3 polyunsaturated fatty acids on markers of inflammation, oxidative stress and metabolic status of ear, nose and throat cancer patients. *Oncol. Rep.* **2014**, *31*, 405–414. [CrossRef]

36. Sánchez-Lara, K.; Turcott, J.G.; Juárez-Hernández, E.; Nuñez-Valencia, C.; Villanueva, G.; Guevara, P.; De La Torre-Vallejo, M.; Mohar, A.; Arrieta, O. Effects of an oral nutritional supplement containing eicosapentaenoic acid on nutritional and clinical outcomes in patients with advanced non-small cell lung cancer: Randomised trial. *Clin. Nutr.* **2014**, *33*, 1017–1023. [CrossRef]

37. Shirai, Y.; Okugawa, Y.; Hishida, A.; Ogawa, A.; Okamoto, K.; Shintani, M.; Morimoto, Y.; Nishikawa, R.; Yokoe, T.; Tanaka, K.; et al. Fish oil-enriched nutrition combined with systemic chemotherapy for gastrointestinal cancer patients with cancer cachexia. *Sci. Rep.* **2017**, *7*, 4826. [CrossRef] [PubMed]

38. Trabal, J.; Leyes, P.; Forga, M.; Maurel, J. Potential usefulness of an EPA-enriched nutritional supplement on chemotherapy tolerability in cancer patients without overt malnutrition. *Nutr. Hosp.* **2010**, *25*, 736–740.

39. van der Meij, B.S.; Langius, J.A.E.; Smit, E.F.; Spreeuwenberg, M.D.; Von Blomberg, B.M.E.; Heijboer, A.C.; Paul, M.A.; Van Leeuwen, P.A.M. Oral nutritional supplements containing (n-3) polyunsaturated fatty acids affect the nutritional status of patients with stage III non-small cell lung cancer during multimodality treatment. *J. Nutr.* **2010**, *140*, 1774–1780. [CrossRef]

40. van der Meij, B.S.; Langius, J.A.; Spreeuwenberg, M.D.; Slootmaker, S.M.; Paul, M.A.; Smit, E.F.; Van Leeuwen, P.A.M. Oral nutritional supplements containing n-3 polyunsaturated fatty acids affect quality of

life and functional status in lung cancer patients during multimodality treatment: An RCT. *Eur. J. Clin. Nutr.* **2012**, *66*, 399–404. [CrossRef]

41. Tanaka, N.; Takeda, K.; Kawasaki, Y.; Yamane, K.; Teruya, Y.; Kodani, M.; Igishi, T.; Yamasaki, A. Early Intensive Nutrition Intervention with Dietary Counseling and Oral Nutrition Supplement Prevents Weight Loss in Patients with Advanced Lung Cancer Receiving Chemotherapy: A Clinical Prospective Study. *Yonago Acta Med.* **2018**, *61*, 204–212. [CrossRef]

42. van den Berg, M.G.; Rasmussen-Conrad, E.L.; Wei, K.H.; Lintz-Luidens, H.; Kaanders, J.H.; Merkx, M.A. Comparison of the effect of individual dietary counselling and of standard nutritional care on weight loss in patients with head and neck cancer undergoing radiotherapy. *Br. J. Nutr.* **2010**, *104*, 872–877. [CrossRef]

43. Murphy, R.A.; Yeung, E.; Mazurak, V.C.; Mourtzakis, M. Influence of eicosapentaenoic acid supplementation on lean body mass in cancer cachexia. *Br. J. Nutr.* **2011**, *105*, 1469–1473. [CrossRef]

44. Dewey, A.; Baughan, C.; Dean, T.; Higgins, B.; Johnson, I. Eicosapentaenoic acid (EPA, an omega-3 fatty acid from fish oils) for the treatment of cancer cachexia. *Cochrane Database Syst. Rev.* **2007**, *2007*, Cd004597. [CrossRef] [PubMed]

45. Ries, A.; Trottenberg, P.; Elsner, F.; Stiel, S.; Haugen, D.F.; Kaasa, S.; Radbruch, L. A systematic review on the role of fish oil for the treatment of cachexia in advanced cancer: An EPCRC cachexia guidelines project. *Palliat Med.* **2012**, *26*, 294–304. [CrossRef]

46. Mazzotta, P.; Jeney, C.M. Anorexia-cachexia syndrome: A systematic review of the role of dietary polyunsaturated Fatty acids in the management of symptoms, survival, and quality of life. *J. Pain Symptom Manag.* **2009**, *37*, 1069–1077. [CrossRef]

47. Colomer, R.; Moreno-Nogueira, J.M.; García-Luna, P.P.; García-Peris, P.; García-De-Lorenzo, A.; Zarazaga, A.; Quecedo, L.; Del Llano, J.; Usán, L.; Casimiro, C. N-3 fatty acids, cancer and cachexia: A systematic review of the literature. *Br. J. Nutr.* **2007**, *97*, 823–831. [CrossRef]

48. de Aguiar Pastore Silva, J.; Emilia de Souza Fabre, M.; Waitzberg, D.L. Omega-3 supplements for patients in chemotherapy and/or radiotherapy: A systematic review. *Clin. Nutr.* **2015**, *34*, 359–366. [CrossRef]

49. Halpern, M.T.; Yabroff, K.R. Prevalence of outpatient cancer treatment in the United States: Estimates from the Medical Panel Expenditures Survey (MEPS). *Cancer Investig.* **2008**, *26*, 647–651. [CrossRef]

50. Trujillo, E.B.C.K.; Dixon, S.W.; Hill, E.B.; Braun, A.; Lipinski, E.; Platek, M.E.; Vergo, M.T.; Spees, C. Inadequate Nutrition Coverage in Outpatient Cancer Centers: Results of a National Survey. *J. Oncol.* **2019**, *2019*, 7462940. [CrossRef]

51. Congress.gov. H.R.6971—Medical Nutrition Therapy Act of 2020. 2020. Availabl online: https://www.congress.gov/bill/116th-congress/house-bill/6971?q=%7B%22search%22%3A%5B%22H.R. +6971%22%5D%7D&s=1&r=1 (accessed on 31 August 2020).

52. Arensberg, M.; Richards, J.; Benjamin, J.; Kerr, K.; Hegazi, R. Opportunities for Quality Improvement Programs (QIPs) in the Nutrition Support of Patients with Cancer. *Healthcare* **2020**, *8*, 227. [CrossRef]

53. Arensberg, M.B.; Sulo, S.; Drawert, S. Addressing Malnutrition in Cancer Care with Nutrition-Focused Quality Improvement Programs (QIPs) that Support Value-based Payment in the United States. *J. Clin. Nutr. Food Sci.* **2020**, *3*, 48–55.

3

Nutritional Status of Pediatric Cancer Patients at Diagnosis and Correlations with Treatment, Clinical Outcome and the Long-Term Growth and Health of Survivors

Vassiliki Diakatou [1,2] **and Tonia Vassilakou** [2,]*

[1] Children's & Adolescents' Oncology Radiotherapy Department, Athens General Children's Hospital "Pan. & Aglaia Kyriakou", GR-11527 Athens, Greece; vdiakatou@hotmail.com

[2] Department of Public Health Policy, School of Public Health, University of West Attica, Athens University Campus, 196 Alexandras Avenue, GR-11521 Athens, Greece

* Correspondence: tvasilakou@uniwa.gr

Abstract: Malnutrition is caused either by cancer itself or by its treatment, and affects the clinical outcome, the quality of life (QOL), and the overall survival (OS) of the patient. However, malnutrition in children with cancer should not be accepted or tolerated as an inevitable procedure at any stage of the disease. A review of the international literature from 2014 to 2019 was performed. Despite the difficulty of accurately assessing the prevalence of malnutrition, poor nutritional status has adverse effects from diagnosis to subsequent survival. Nutritional status (NS) at diagnosis relates to undernutrition, while correlations with clinical outcome are still unclear. Malnutrition adversely affects health-related quality of life (HRQOL) in children with cancer and collective evidence constantly shows poor nutritional quality in childhood cancer survivors (CCSs). Nutritional assessment and early intervention in pediatric cancer patients could minimize the side effects of treatment, improve their survival, and reduce the risk of nutritional morbidity with a positive impact on QOL, in view of the potentially manageable nature of this risk factor.

Keywords: childhood cancer; pediatric oncology; nutritional status; malnutrition

1. Introduction

The importance of nutrition in children with cancer is indisputable [1]. Nutrition influences most cancer control parameters in pediatric oncology, including prevention, epidemiology, biology, treatment, supportive care, recuperation, and survival [2]. It is widely recognized that the nutritional status (NS) of children diagnosed with and treated for cancer will be probably affected during the course of the disease.

NS of pediatric cancer patients has been researched for a lengthy time and nutritional problems have long-been recognized [3–8]. Indeed, publications on childhood cancer related undernutrition have appeared since the 1970s [9], however its management remains variable [1,4,10], with many undernourished children not timely recognized and therefore not treated [11].

The importance of NS in childhood cancer patients concerns its potential impact on disease progression and survival [1]. The NS at the time of diagnosis can affect outcomes in terms of morbidity and mortality [12]. Additionally, nutrition related problems can affect the quality of life (QOL) of survivors, as well as predispose them to other chronic diseases [2]. This fact highlights the need for scientific management and nutritional support for this population.

At the same time, the available data regarding the prevalence of poor nutritional status are derived at different phases of the disease and are highly variable among diagnostic groups, as well as between developed and developing countries [1,13–15]. The heterogeneity of diagnoses, the different stages of treatment and the followed treatment protocols complicate any straightforward comparison among studies. Moreover, the variety of definitions for malnutrition, the methodology used to assess the NS—in terms of anthropometric measurements—as well as criteria and cut-off points, make an accurate estimation of the prevalence of cancer related malnutrition very difficult.

This review aims to identify NS alterations that occur during the management of childhood cancer. The purpose of the study is to investigate how neoplastic diseases affect the NS of children and adolescents, as well as how the nutritional profile affects treatment response, clinical outcome and long-term growth and health of survivors. By investigating the multifactorial components of nutrition in childhood cancer morbidity, this work aims to be the trigger to recognize the importance of nutrition in order to become an integral part of cancer treatment in children and adolescents in Greece.

2. Materials and Methods

An electronic search of the international literature was performed, using the Cochrane Library, MEDLINE, SCOPUS, and PUBMED to identify systematic reviews, meta-analyses, randomized controlled trials and observational studies published during the period 2014–2019. The search strategy identified the following keywords and medical subject heading searches (MeSH): "childhood cancer", "pediatric oncology", "nutritional status", and "malnutrition". The reference list of all relevant articles was also examined, and possibly relevant corresponding articles were hand-searched. Particular attention has been paid to most recent articles, meta-analyses and systematic reviews conducted in countries with different socioeconomic status in order to identify possible influence. Studies involving adult patients were excluded.

3. Results

3.1. Nutritional Status at Diagnosis

Many former and recent studies have investigated the issue of weight changes in children diagnosed with cancer. Pediatric cancer includes a heterogeneous group of diagnoses, while the repercussions, prognosis and the therapeutic planning differ according to tumor location, histological type, nature as well as biological behavior and age of incidence [16]. Such differences also influence the NS, in a way that some patients present with weight loss at diagnosis, thus being at higher risk for suboptimal NS during the anticancer treatment [17,18]. NS at the time of the diagnosis is an important factor which influences the response to the treatment as well as the possibility of recovery [1].

In the cross-sectional observational study of Maia Lemos et al. [16], the authors assessed the NS of 1154 children and adolescents with malignant neoplasms in Brazil at the time of diagnosis. At that time point, 67.63% of patients presented adequate body mass index (BMI). The overall prevalence of undernutrition was 10.8%, 27.3%, 24.5% and 13.6%, based on BMI, triceps skinfold thickness (TSFT), mid-upper arm circumference (MUAC), and arm muscle circumference (AMC), respectively [16].

Villanueva et al. [19] studied the NS of 1060 patients diagnosed with cancer in Guatemala. NS was evaluated by MUAC, TSFT, and serum albumin (ALB) levels. Children were nutritionally classified as adequately nourished, moderately depleted, and severely depleted. With regard to diagnoses, leukemia accounted for 51% of all diagnoses, followed by solid tumors (33%), lymphomas (11%), and brain tumors (BT) (5%). At diagnosis, 47% ($n = 495$) of patients were severely nutritionally depleted, 19% ($n = 207$) were moderately depleted, and 34% ($n = 358$) were adequately nourished.

In total, 74 pediatric oncology patients newly diagnosed with hematological malignancies ($n = 56$) or solid tumors ($n = 18$), were included in a prospective observational cohort study conducted in Istanbul [20]. Anthropometric measurements included body weight, height, BMI, BMI for age percentile, MUAC, TSFT as well as z-scores for weight for age (WFA), height for age (HFA), BMI for age, weight for height for age, MUAC for age, and TSFT for age. At diagnosis, undernutrition (BMI for age z<−2 standard deviation (SD)) was evident in nine (12.3%) of 74 patients, including six (10.9%) patients with hematological malignancies and three (16.7%) patients with solid tumors, whereas undernutrition (BMI<5th age percentile) was evident in 10 (13.7%) of 74 patients, including six (10.9%) patients with hematological malignancies and four (22.2%) patients with solid tumors. In addition, increased body weight (BMI for age z > 2 SD) was evident in five (6.8%) patients.

Pribnow et al. [21] conducted a retrospective review of newly diagnosed patients with acute lymphoblastic leukemia (ALL), acute myeloid leukemia (AML), Wilms tumor, Hodgkin lymphoma (HL), or Burkitt lymphoma (BL) in Nicaragua. A total of 473 patients were assessed and 282 patients were recruited in the study. At diagnosis weight, height or length measurements were recorded and NS assessment included BMI, MUAC, TSFT, and levels of serum albumin. At diagnosis, on the basis of NS categories, 67% of patients were undernourished, 19.1% suffered from moderate undernutrition and 47.9% were severely undernourished. Undernutrition rates were higher in patients with Wilms tumor (85.7%) and BL (75%) and lower in those with HL (58.3%). Patients with high-risk malignancies were inclined to have inferior NS regardless diagnosis, when comparing adequately nourished (37.3% of patients with high-risk disease) to severely undernourished (62.7% of those with high-risk disease) groups ($p = 0.08$). Similar trends are also observed in high-income countries (HICs) and can be attributed to disease burden.

In the same country, a cohort of 104 patients was screened for NS at diagnosis [22]. The NS assessment was based on weight, height or length and the anthropometric measures of MUAC and TSFT. Thirty-four patients were affected by ALL, five by AML, 13 by lymphomas and 52 by solid tumors, including BT ($n = 20$), retinoblastoma ($n = 3$), bone and soft-tissue sarcoma ($n = 15$), Wilms' tumor ($n = 7$) and others ($n = 7$). Yet, diseases were clustered in two groups—leukemia/lymphomas and solid tumors—for further analyses. According to their anthropometric measurements, patients were overall classified as 65.4% severely depleted, 13.5% moderately depleted, and 21.1% borderline/adequately nourished, that is considered at risk of developing undernutrition during treatment.

In the largest study so far from India, a total of 1693 new patients were enrolled, of whom 1187 had all anthropometric measurements performed [23]. The prevalence of undernutrition—defined by World Health Organization (WHO) criteria—at the time of diagnosis was very high ranging from 40–80% depending on the method used for assessment, being higher with MUAC and lowest with BMI. Specifically, the prevalence of undernutrition was 38%, 57%, 76%, 69%, and 81% on the basis of BMI, TSFT, MUAC, AMC, and arm TSFT + MUAC, respectively. Addition of BMI and serum albumin to arm anthropometry increased the proportion classified as severely nutritionally depleted by a mere 2% and 1.5% respectively. Among disease groups, no considerable differences were found in undernutrition rates, consistent with findings of a similar large study published at that time [24]. On the other extreme, only 14 (0.8%) of children in this study were obese among the whole group, much lower than the 14% rate of obesity in a recent large study from the United States of America (USA), reflecting the socio-economic influence on NS [25].

Another study conducted in India, analyzed retrospectively weight records collected at diagnosis for patients with ALL, AML, solid tumors, and lymphomas [26]. A total of 295 pediatric patients were enrolled in the analysis. Patients' weight was plotted on WFA growth charts of Center for Disease Control and Prevention (CDC) [27]. At diagnosis, 153 out of 295 (52%) of patients had WFA between 3rd and 97th centile and were therefore considered to be well-nourished, 130 out of 295 (44%) patients were undernourished and 12/295 (4%) patients were obese. The prevalence of undernutrition at admission among males and females was 44% and 42%, respectively. As regards the diagnosis, there was no significant difference in NS at diagnosis between hematological malignancies and solid tumors ($p = 0.8$).

NS at the time of cancer diagnosis is dependent on a cancer type, its localization and clinical stage of the disease [1]. In addition, prevalence rates of malnutrition depend not only on methods and criteria used to assess NS, timing of assessment and composition of the study population—in terms of types of malignancies—, but also on socio-economic status [3]. Studies carried out in countries with better socio-economic conditions showed different results from the above mentioned. Moreover, other factors such as poverty, lack of adequate education and health support can aggravate nutritional risk especially in developing countries [16]. In general, undernutrition rates have been found much higher in low- or low-middle-income countries (LMICs) (40–90%) in comparison to countries with high or medium income (0–30%) [4,24,28–30].

In the USA, a cohort of 2,008 children treated for high-risk ALL enrolled in Children's Oncology Group study CCG–1961 (Children's Cancer Group) [25]. Weight status by z-score and percentile was determined as per guidelines from the CDC using BMI for children age 2–20 years and Weight for Length (WFL) for those age <2 years [31,32]. Of the 2.008 evaluable children, 279 (14%) were obese and 117 (6%) 17 were underweight at diagnosis.

In Italy, 126 newly diagnosed pediatric cancer patients were included in the study of Triarico et al. [33]. For each patient, nutritional risk has been assessed with STRONGKids—a quick, reliable, and practical screening tool—to identify patients with risk of undernutrition [34,35]. Subsequently, anthropometric measurements—such as weight, height, BMI z-scores—were evaluated. The analysis showed a 100% rate of patients at risk of undernutrition at diagnosis. Respectively at diagnosis 90 patients (71.4%) presented a moderate risk of undernutrition (STRONGkids 2 or 3), whereas the other 36 (28.6%) were at high risk of undernutrition (STRONGkids 4 or 5). Sixteen patients (12.7%) presented mild undernutrition (BMI z-score from (−1)–(−1.9)), two patients (1.6%) presented moderate undernutrition (BMI z-score from (−2)–(−2.9)) and four patients (3.1%) showed severe undernutrition (BMI z-score ≤ −3).

In Poland, the authors of [36] studied the frequency of undernutrition and obesity at diagnosis. A study group of 734 patients with various diagnoses was enrolled. Patients were divided into groups depending on the type of neoplasms: ALL, acute non-lymphoblastic leukemia (ANLL), HL, non-Hodgkin lymphoma (NHL), neuroblastoma (NB), Wilms' tumor, and mesenchymal malignant tumor (MMT). Body weight and height were measured, and BMI was calculated at the time of diagnosis. At cancer diagnosis moment, 21.5% (158) of patients were undernourished, 64.7% (475) weighed properly and 13.8% (101) were overweight. Height deficiency was observed in 8% (57) of the patients, of whom 10% (34) were boys and 9% (23) were girls. Both underweight and short stature were found in 2% (15) of the patients. Among diagnoses, there were no notable difference considering height deficiencies. Patients in the ALL group were overweight more often than the rest of the study group (Risk Ratio (RR) = 1.82, Confidence Interval (CI) 95% 1.26–2.63, $p = 0.002$)—18.6% of them were overweight. However, children with MMT were less susceptible to overweight than the rest of the patients (RR = 0.36, CI 95% 0.15–0.87, $p = 0.021$)—only 5.4% of them were overweight. Girls with ALL were undernourished more often than other patients (RR = 1.72, CI 95% 1.08–2.75, $p = 0.03$). There were no significant differences in the undernutrition/obesity frequency in other neoplasms groups.

In Australia, Small et al. [37] retrospectively reviewed the growth and NS—assessed by BMI—of children diagnosed with NB. One hundred fifty-four children were diagnosed with NB, while only 129 of them had length/height and weight measurements recorded at diagnosis. At that moment, almost a quarter—31 children—(24.0%) were classified as underweight indicating a high incidence of undernutrition, while the percentage of overweight patients was 11.6% ($n = 15$). There was no noteworthy difference in gender, age, or disease stage at diagnosis across children who were classified as underweight, normoweight or overweight.

It is therefore understood that weight and height are important measurements for assessing a child's NS. According to Brinksma et al. [38], the evaluation of weight and height at the time of diagnosis in comparison with the measurements prior to diagnosis is particularly important in children who have recently been diagnosed with cancer. However, children who suffer from severe weight loss or lack of linear growth, but have what is considered appropriate weight and height parameters—between −2 and +2 standard deviation scores (SDS)—, may also be poorly nourished [38]. The authors studied a group of 95 patients, 45 (47%) of which were females. Children were diagnosed with hematological malignancies (57%), solid (26%) and brain (17%) tumors. At diagnosis, weight and height measurements were recorded and compared with the child's own growth potential—authors used data collected in Primary Health Care Corporation (PHCC). Undernutrition was observed in 2% (2 out of 95), 4% (4 out of 95), and 7% (7 out of 95) of the children according to zWFA<-2 SDS, zHFA<-2 SDS, and z-scores for weight for height (WFH) <-2 SDS, respectively. However, when compared to their growth curves another 20–24% of children lost more than 0.5 SDS in WFA, HFA, and WFH z-score. In conclusion comparison of weight and height at diagnosis with data from growth curves indicated that—on average—children's z-scores of weight and height at diagnosis were lower than predicted from their growth curves. Actually, more children were poorly nourished than weight and height at diagnosis indicated [38].

In the same country, Loeffen et al. [39] studied—amongst others—malnutrition at diagnosis within a heterogeneous childhood cancer population. The study sample consisted of 269 children with cancer, receiving treatment for various malignancies. BMI z-scores were used as indicator of NS. At the time of diagnosis, 14 children (5.2%) were classified as undernourished (BMI z-score < −2), 229 children (56.9%) were adequately nourished while 19 (7.1%) were over-nourished (BMI z-score > 2). Undernourished children showed poorer survival versus adequately nourished (hazard ratio (HR) = 3.63, 95% confidence interval (CI) = 1.52–8.70, $p = 0.004$).

According to published studies, the majority of data on NS of children with cancer at the time of diagnosis relates to undernutrition. Numerous studies include diverse measures and assessment methods, leading to a highly variable prevalence of undernutrition at diagnosis [1]. Table 1 summarizes the characteristics of eligible studies that assess nutritional status at the time of diagnosis.

The reported differences between studies are due to the fact that nutrition related problems—particularly the prevalence of undernutrition—depend on factors such as the timing of nutritional assessment. Nutritional assessment at diagnosis is often postponed in the context of many other procedures that may have a higher priority, some of which may even affect it [40]. In addition, there is no clinical "gold standard" to assess the NS [1]. The methods used make the criteria of malnutrition heterogeneous, as the process depends on the sensitivity and specificity of the parameters [8]. Furthermore, the time of cancer development is not the same for all diagnoses. If cancer develops more rapidly—e.g., hematological malignancies against solid tumors—the shortage of weight is lower, as there is not enough time to develop severe nutrition deficiencies [36]. Moreover, the reported differences as regards the prevalence of undernutrition are due to the composition of each study population regarding the types of malignancies. In the majority of studies, patients are categorized into hematologic, solid, and brain malignancies [3].

Nutritional assessment at the time of diagnosis, is probably the most appropriate time to prevent the deterioration of NS. Undernutrition worsens as the disease progresses, meaning that the longer the diagnosis is delayed, the higher the risk of undernutrition [41]. Therefore, the early diagnosis of undernutrition and early intervention should be a priority in all interdisciplinary oncological teams in an effort to solve at least part of the problem [24].

Table 1. Characteristics of listed studies that assess NS at diagnosis.

Author, Year (Location)	Study Design	Patients (N)	Diagnosis	Assessment Method	Nutritional Related Problems
Maia Lemos et al., 2016 [16] (Brazil)	Cross-sectional observational study	1154	Various diagnoses	BMI [1], TSFT [2], MUAC [3], AMC [4]	Undernutrition
Villanueva et al., 2019 [19] (Guatemala)	Retrospective cohort study	1060	Hematological Malignancies Solid tumors Brain tumors	TSFT, MUAC, ALB [5] levels	Undernutrition
Yoruk et al., 2018 [20] (Istanbul)	Prospective observational cohort study	74	Hematological malignances Solid tumors	BMI, TSFT, MUAC, WFA [6], HFA [7]	Malnutrition
Pribnow et al., 2017 [21] (Nicaragua)	Retrospective study	282	ALL [8], AML [9], HL [10], BL [11], Wilms tumors	BMI, TSFT, MUAC, ALB levels	Undernutrition
Peccatori et al., 2018 [22] (Nicaragua)	Intervention study	104	Hematological malignancies Solid tumors	TSFT, MUAC, Height, Weight	Undernutrition
Shah et al., 2014 [23] (India)	Retrospective observational study	1693	Various diagnoses	BMI, TSFT, MUAC, ALB levels	Malnutrition
Radhakrishnan et al., 2015 [26] (India)	Retrospective study	295	Various diagnoses	WFA	Malnutrition
Orgel et al., 2014 [25] (USA)	Retrospective cohort study	2008	High-risk ALL	BMI	Malnutrition
Triarico et al., 2019 [33] (Italy)	Retrospective study	126	Hematological malignances Solid tumors CNS [12] tumors,	STRONG$_{Kids}$ score	Undernutrition
Połubok et al., 2017 [36] (Poland)	Retrospective cohort study	734	ALL, ANLL [13], HL, NHL [14], NB [15], MMT [16], Wilms tumors	BMI	Malnutrition
Small et al., 2015 [37] (Australia)	Retrospective review	154	NB	Height, Weight, BMI	Malnutrition
Brinksma et al., 2015 [38] (The Netherlands)	Retrospective study	95	Hematological Malignancies Solid tumors Brain tumors	Height, Weight	Growth alterations
Loeffen et al., 2015 [39] (The Netherlands)	Retrospective study	269	Hematological Malignancies Solid tumors Brain tumors	BMI	Malnutrition

[1] Body Mass Index (BMI), [2] Triceps Skinfold Thickness (TSFT), [3] Mid–Upper Arm Circumference (MUAC), [4] Arm Muscle Circumference (AMC), [5] Serum albumin (ALB), [6] Weight for Age (WFA), [7] Height for Age (HFA), [8] Acute Lymphoblastic Leukemia (ALL), [9] Acute Myeloid Leukemia (AML), [10] Hodgkin Lymphoma (HL), [11] Burkitt Lymphoma (BL), [12] Central Nervous System (CNS), [13] Acute Non–Lymphoblastic Leukemia (ANLL), [14] Non–Hodgkin Lymphoma (NHL), [15] Neuroblastoma (NB), [16] Mesenchymal Malignant Tumor (MMT).

3.2. Nutritional Status during Treatment

NS at the time of diagnosis is an important factor which influences the response to the treatment, as well as the possibility of recovery [1]. However, malnutrition in pediatric patients with cancer is dynamic and development of impaired NS is commonly seen during subsequent treatment [42]. The adverse effects of nutritional problems during treatment, such as reduced tolerance of chemotherapy, alterations in drug metabolism, reduced immunity, increased risk of infection, and compromised QOL, have been established, however the quality of the evidence supporting each of these effects is variable [43].

Previous reports addressing the impact of weight on treatment-related toxicity (TRT) and event-free survival (EFS) in acute leukemia were limited by taking into account patient's weight only at diagnosis [44–46]. As weight varies significantly during the treatment course of pediatric ALL [47], Orgel et al. [25] evaluated the effect of weight alterations on EFS and development of TRT, all along the treatment period in contrast to weight at diagnosis. A multitudinous group of children diagnosed with and treated for high-risk ALL was enrolled in the analysis. Orgel et al. [25] observed that only those children with constant underweight or obese status across intensive phases of treatment for high-risk ALL were at substantially higher risk for TRT occurrence, relapse, or death. Furthermore, for patients whose NS status-either obesity or underweight-was constant for > half of pre-maintenance therapy, the risk for future relapse or death was up to double compared with patients who remained normoweight during the treatment course. Contrarily, the risk of patients who began treatment obese or underweight and subsequently ended up normoweight/overweight, decreased to become comparable to being normoweight throughout. In addition, obese or underweight children were facing greater risk for specific toxicity profiles, an essential independent issue in efforts to decrease morbidity resulting from effective but toxic treatment protocols.

Paciarotti et al. [48] performed a prospective cohort study, aiming to determine both the prevalence of undernutrition and over-nutrition—overweight and obesity—and to detect critical changes in NS with reference to tumor type, treatments, and nutritional interventions. NS assessment combined several parameters—dietary intake, BMI centile, TSFT and MUAC—and was performed at diagnosis and at three months after treatment initiation. In terms of diagnosis, cohort was grouped in children with leukemia and in children with other types of cancer. Undernutrition prevalence—determined by BMI centiles—was highest among the "other cancers" group at diagnosis. The low BMI centiles were correlated with a higher prevalence rate of undernourished children in comparison to the anticipated undernutrition rate for the UK population [28]. On the other hand, the "leukemia" group, demonstrated excess BMI centiles at both time points and the prevalence of obesity was greater than the expected for the UK population. The BMI alterations, as time went on, followed the anthropometric variations. The "leukemia" patients had excess fat reserves during treatment course—measured by Upper Arm Fat Area (UAFA)—being 130% of standard at three-month time. The "other cancers" group had depleted fat stores, with UAFA values getting lower from 78% at diagnosis to 70% of standard at three months of treatment, suggesting a negative energy status existing prior to diagnosis. Consequently, both undernutrition and obesity are frequent disorders during the first phase of treatment for pediatric cancer with clear differences among cancer diagnoses.

There are several studies that present data on malnutrition in children with cancer, however little is known about the timing of under- and over-nutrition onset, as well as their respective causes. Brinksma et al. [49] intended to determine in which treatment phase NS deterioration occurred, and which factors lead to these alterations. A prospective cohort study of 133 newly diagnosed cancer patients with hematological malignancies, solid and brain tumors was performed. Anthropometric measurements and related date were recorded at admission and at three, six and 12 months after diagnosis. Despite initial weight loss at the beginning of treatment in patients with hematological and solid malignancies, BMI, and fat mass (FM) increased within three months by 0.13 SDS ($p < 0.001$) and 0.05 SDS ($p = 0.021$) respectively. Increase continued during the following months and resulted in a doubling of the number of over-nourished patients. Fat-free mass (FFM)—which was already low at diagnosis—remained low. During the entire study period about 17% of the patients were undernourished on the basis of low FFM. The most important changes took place within three months after diagnosis. Particularly WFA and BMI decreased at first, in patients with hematological malignancies and solid tumors, while tended to increase in patients with brain tumors. In a three–month period both WFA and BMI increased in all diagnoses, compared to the time of diagnosis. Furthermore, HFA decreased in all diagnostic groups, whereas MUAC increased. TSFT, % FM, and FM were higher, especially for patients with BT. FFM was constant and values were lower in patients with brain tumors in comparison to children with hematological malignancies and solid tumors. Furthermore, stagnation of growth in terms of height contributed to increase in BMI. Consequently, it is imperative for clinicians to comprehend that in order to prevent increase in BMI during treatment, weight should remain stable until growth in height continues.

Iniesta et al. [50] performed a prospective cohort study to examine the prevalence of malnutrition, NS alterations and factors contributing to nutritional disorders in Scottish pediatric cancer patients aged < 18 years. Clinical and nutritional data, as well as anthropometric measurements—MUAC and TSFT—were recorded at specific periods up until 36 months after diagnosis. The study population was grouped conforming to the wider definition of solid and brain tumors, hematologic malignancies, and other associated diagnoses. The prevalence of malnutrition—undernutrition, overweight and obesity—differed at various time points and among the anthropometric measurements. Overall, undernutrition was higher at diagnosis than at any other time whereas no patient was undernourished at the end, i.e., 30 and 36 months. In contrast, overnutrition increased over time. Particularly overweight was highest at 36 months and obesity was most prevalent at 30 months. As to diagnoses, patients with brain tumors and other associated diagnoses had the highest prevalence of overweight and obesity, even at the start of treatment. Contrarily, children diagnosed with solid tumors had the highest prevalence of undernutrition, followed by brain tumors and hematological malignancies during the first stages of treatment. In conclusion, the study highlights that children diagnosed with and treated for cancer are at high risk of undernutrition—notably during the first three months of treatment—and of over-nutrition at later stages. The most significant component contributing to undernutrition during the first three months of treatment was high treatment risk.

With regard to solid tumors, NB is one of the most common solid tumors in children [51]. Small et al. [37] wanted to examine retrospectively the BMI status of children treated for NB. One hundred and twenty-nine children diagnosed with NB were recruited in the study. Anthropometric measurements were collected at diagnosis as well as at various time points, up until five years after diagnosis. At diagnosis 24% of children were classified as undernourished and 11.6% were overweight. At six months after diagnosis, children in almost all disease stages showed a significant decrease in age and sex adjusted BMI. Subsequently, weight z-scores began to increase so that at 12 months' time higher BMI z-scores were observed in children in all disease stages. Over the following four years, BMI z-scores either gradually changed or stabilized depending on the stage of the disease. Almost five years after diagnosis, the proportion of underweight children decreased to 8.7% while the proportion of children who were classified as overweight doubled to 28%. Even though low BMI values are common in children with NB—particularly at diagnosis and during treatment—the authors did not find any association between BMI and survival rates. Yet, the high proportion of overweight children at follow-up underscores the importance of nutritional interventions [37].

In India, Radhakrishnan et al. [26] conducted a study to look at the prevalence of malnutrition and to assess the impact of treatment on NS of pediatric cancer patients. A total of 295 pediatric patients were enrolled in the analysis. They were provided all meals and nutritional supplements by the hospital during their treatment duration. Data on WFA were available for 295 patients at diagnosis, 282 patients at midway through treatment, and 152 patients at the end of treatment. At diagnosis, undernutrition was seen in 44% patients, which increased to 46% midway during treatment, and decreased to 27% at the end of treatment ($p = 0.0005$). Even though undernutrition is a common problem in patients in resource-poor countries such as India, this study highlights that active nutritional intervention and education were able to significantly reduce the prevalence of undernutrition in patients at the end of treatment.

Nutritional support aims to reverse undernutrition seen at diagnosis, prevent undernutrition associated with treatment and promote weight and growth. There is no doubt that a poor nutritional state is a clear prognostic factor for treatment response and has an effect on the outcome of children with cancer [42].

3.3. Nutritional Status and Clinical Outcome

The presence of undernutrition correlates with a greater number of complications and relapses, as well as with decreased level of recovery [1,52]. Undernutrition can adversely affect the overall survival (OS), because it may reduce the tolerance to chemotherapy, increasing treatment-related morbidity (TRM) and decreasing EFS [21,39,53].

According to Barr et al. [43], two landmark retrospective studies were performed in the (CCG). Lange [54] conducted a study which included 768 children and adolescents with AML. Eighty-four patients (10.9%) of the study population underwent weight loss and 114 (14.8%) were overweight or obese, defined by BMI (≤10th percentile and ≥95th percentile respectively). Children with abnormal weight had remarkably worse survival than normoweight because of higher TRM rates.

Butturini et al. conducted the subsequent report, regarding >4000 children and adolescents with ALL. The CCG researchers focused on the effect of obesity, again as defined by BMI. The five-year EFS was poorer and the relapse rate higher in obese (n = 343,8%) compared to non-obese patients, but only in those aged 10 years and older. After these two landmark studies in pediatric leukemia, multiple analyses from international research centers have since described inconsistent associations between obesity and leukemia survival [25,45,55–58], raising uncertainty as to whether such a relation exists and, if so, to what extent.

Amankwah et al. [59] performed a meta-analysis which further complicated data interpretation through inclusion of a wide variety of leukemia types, therapeutic modalities, and differences in baseline survival rates between high- and low-income countries (LICs) [60,61]. The authors aimed to evaluate the association between BMI at diagnosis and pediatric acute leukemia mortality and relapse. An increased risk of mortality with a high BMI at diagnosis was observed (OS: HR = 1.30, 95% CI = 1.16–1.46 and EFS: HR = 1.46, 95% CI = 1.29–1.64). Sub-group analysis for ALL, the most prevalent form of pediatric acute leukemia, revealed a stronger association for both OS (HR = 2.25, 95% CI = 1.33–3.82, p = 0.002) and EFS (HR = 1.49, 95% CI = 1.30–1.71, p < 0.001). Overall a high BMI at diagnosis was associated with poor OS and EFS among pediatric acute leukemia patients [59].

In contrast to the previous review [59], Orgel et al. [62] included in their analysis a relatively uniform population from HICs in order to determine whether a higher BMI at diagnosis of pediatric ALL or AML is associated with worse EFS, OS, and cumulative incidence of relapse (CIR). As regards ALL, the authors observed poorer EFS in children with a higher BMI (RR = 1.35, 95% CI = 1.20–1.51) than in those with a lower BMI. A higher BMI was associated with significantly increased mortality (RR = 1.31, 95% CI = 1.09–1.58) and a statistically nonsignificant trend toward greater risk of relapse (RR = 1.17, 95% CI = 0.99–1.38) compared with a lower BMI. In AML, a higher BMI was significantly associated with poorer EFS and OS (RR = 1.36, 95% CI = 1.16–1.60 and RR = 1.56, 95% CI = 1.32–1.86, respectively) than was a lower BMI. However, other studies have reported different outcomes.

In the recent retrospective analysis, Saenz et al. [63] evaluated the association between overweight/obesity (BMI ≥ 85th percentile) at pediatric leukemia diagnosis and relapse or mortality. The study included 181 pediatric patients diagnosed with ALL, AML, and chronic myeloid leukemia (CML). The authors observed a statistically significant association between mortality and obesity status in unadjusted models that disappeared in both age- and sex-adjusted and multivariable-adjusted analysis. Analysis limited to ALL patients—the most common type of leukemia—showed no association between relapse or mortality and obesity status. As expected, analysis based on the small number of AML cases only, did not show any statistically significant association for relapse (HR = 3.93,

95% CI = 0.71–21.82, $p = 0.12$) or mortality (HR = 1.39, 95% CI = 0.31–6.27, $p = 0.67$) either. A meta–analysis combining these findings with those of previous studies was also performed. Concerning ALL overweight/obese patients, the meta-analysis revealed an increased mortality and relapse risk (HR = 1.79, 95% CI = 1.03–3.10) and (HR = 1.28, 95% CI = 1.04–1.57) respectively. Similarly, an association between obesity and increased risk of mortality was observed for AML patients (HR = 1.64, 95% CI = 1.32–2.04) [63].

Aldhafiri et al. [55] conducted a study in the UK, on a cohort of 1,033 patients. The authors found no evidence to support the association between overweight/obesity at diagnosis and childhood leukemia relapse [55]. These findings are consistent with previous studies as well. In the UK, Weir et al. [64] examined the effects of BMI at diagnosis on leukemia relapse in children ($n = 1,025$) and found no statistically significant association between obesity and relapse. Two more studies in the US [57,65] also failed to detect an association between obesity at diagnosis and risk of relapse in children with ALL. In Turkey, Karakurt et al. [66] did not observe any difference between mean BMI at diagnosis and relapsed or non-relapsed patients. The authors of [67] did not find any association between BMI at diagnosis and prognosis for children aged 2–9 years, but they observed a trend for improved outcome in overweight patients aged 10–17 years.

So far, data have been related to hematological malignancies, while studies evaluating the role of NS in pediatric solid tumors are lacking. Joffe et al. [68] conducted a study aiming to summarize data reporting on the association of NS and treatment-related outcomes—TRT, EFS, CIR and OS—in children and adolescents diagnosed with a solid tumor. Finally, 10 reports met the criteria and were included in the review. Up to 62% of patients were over- or undernourished at diagnosis [69]. Four out of 10 included studies identify abnormal BMI as a poor prognostic indicator in this group of patients [70–73]. Abnormal BMI was associated with worse OS in Ewing sarcoma (HR = 3.46, $p = 0.022$), osteosarcoma (HR = 1.6, $p < 0.005$), and there was a trend toward poorer OS in rhabdomyosarcoma (HR = 1.70, $p = 0.0596$). High BMI in osteosarcoma was associated with increased nephrotoxicity and postoperative complications. Regarding other included disease categories, NS was not a significant predictor of outcomes.

Iniesta et al. [74] aimed to evaluate the primary research on the prevalence of malnutrition in children with cancer and determine whether there are correlations between malnutrition and clinical outcomes. According to the authors [74], correlations between undernutrition and clinical outcomes remain unclear, with some researchers arguing that undernutrition is associated with worse outcomes [8,75–77] and others claiming that there are no such associations [64,78]. Undernutrition may be associated with higher mortality [8,77]. Yet, both studies referred to developing countries, so findings may have been affected by other factors regarding mortality. As regards undernutrition and relapse, two large studies [8,64] found no associations. Obesity in children with ALL was not associated with a decrease in EFS, when obese children were compared with normoweight children [65]. On the contrary, Butturini et al. [44] found that obesity at diagnosis independently predicted the likelihood of relapse in pre-teenagers and adolescents with ALL.

Moreover, the majority of research studies regarding the effect of malnutrition on infections and mortality have been conducted in homogenous populations including patients with one diagnosis. Loeffen et al. [39] investigated whether malnutrition is a prognostic factor for infection rates and survival, within a heterogeneous childhood cancer population. The authors of [39] showed the strong association between rapid weight reduction within the first three months of treatment and increased rate of Febrile Neutropenia (FN) episodes. A group 269 children diagnosed with and treated for cancer were enrolled in the analysis. During the first year after diagnosis, 332 admissions for FN were recorded. As regards the incidence of these episodes, there were no statistically remarkable difference between patients who were adequately nourished at diagnosis and patients who were under- or over-nourished. Nevertheless, BMI z-score decrease >1.0 ($n = 13$) and weight loss >5% of the initial body weight within the first three months after diagnosis, were strongly associated with FN episodes occurrence—($p = 0.010$) and ($p = 0.004$) respectively. Regarding NS, survival was notably worse ($p = 0.01$) for undernourished children at diagnosis ($n = 14$) than for those who were adequately and over-nourished ($n = 248$).

Pribnow et al. [21] examined the correlations between NS and cancer type, TRM and EFS. A total of 282 patients diagnosed with Wilms tumor, ALL, AML, HL or BL were included in the study. Children diagnosed with Wilms tumor had the highest prevalence of undernutrition (85.7%), followed by children with BL (75%) and AML (74.3%). As regards TRM, 92.2% of patients experienced morbidity during the first three months of treatment whereas 84% of patients experienced severe morbidity. TRM in pediatric patients with cancer was associated with NS, as morbidity was greater in children with severe undernutrition than in those with adequate nutrition ($p = 0.023$). Another crucial finding in this study was the association between NS and severe infection, as infection is a major cause of mortality and was the second leading cause of death during the study period (22.9%). Particularly undernutrition was associated with severe infection ($p = 0.033$). In addition, undernourished patients had inferior median EFS ($p = 0.049$) and abandoned therapy more frequently ($p = 0.015$).

With regard to the increased risk of infections and their incidence, Triarico et al. [33] recently confirmed their association with nutrition related problems. In their retrospective study 126 newly diagnosed children 3–18 years old were included. Overall, 298 admissions for FN occurred during the first year after diagnosis. On average, children had two admissions for FN while 54 patients (42.9%) had ≥3 admissions for FN during the first year after diagnosis. A number of hospitalization for FN ≥3 was found in children moderately to severely undernourished at three and six months after diagnosis, in patients with weight loss ≥5% at three months, in the case of a weight loss ≥10% at six months and finally in patients with a BMI z-score decrease ≥1 at six months. Analyses of weight loss and BMI z-score decrease demonstrate that in a period of three and six months from diagnosis there was a three-fold increase of the rate of at least moderate undernutrition, from 4.7% to 14.3% and 13.5% respectively. Indeed, at three months 58 children (46%) underwent weight loss ≥5%. At six months, they were 63 (50%), while 28 of them (22.2%) had lost ≥10% of their body weight. Furthermore, weight loss ≥5% at three months and weight loss ≥10% at six months after diagnosis were remarkably associated with higher mortality. Mortality risk increased by 294% in patients who lost ≥5% of weight in a three-month period after diagnosis and by 110% in patients who reported weight loss ≥10% at six-month time.

Given the high prevalence of nutrition related problems during childhood cancer treatment and their impact on clinical outcomes, nutritional assessment should be mandatory from diagnosis and during treatment, in view of the possible manageable nature of this risk factor. Early adaptation of the NS screening for pediatric cancer patients could not only improve their survival, but also their QOL [33].

3.4. Nutritional Status and Health-Related Quality of Life

Malnutrition during treatment for childhood cancer has not only substantial clinical implications, but may also adversely affect a child's QOL [79]. Until recently, QOL in children with cancer was unexplored [80]. In recent decades, cancer survival rates have increased thus emphasizing the importance of children's personal needs. As a result, health-related quality of life (HRQOL) in childhood cancer patients has become a crucial issue in clinical practice [79]. HRQOL of children and adolescents is complex as children grow and develop. On the other hand, multimodal therapy that combines intensive chemotherapeutic protocols, surgery and radiotherapy induces many side effects which adversely affect children's HRQOL [81].

Tsiros et al. [82] conducted a literature review on HRQOL in healthy, though obese children and adolescents. Findings support that being overweight/obese has an unfavorable impact on social and emotional functioning. In addition, other previous studies [83–86] have found that children diagnosed with and treated for malignancies had the lowest HRQOL, in comparison to healthy peers or children with other diseases. Broadly, it is considered that HRQOL in undernourished patients is lower when compared with adequately nourished patients [87] and that NS amelioration will lead to better HRQOL.

However, the correlation between NS and HRQOL in childhood cancer patients had not been examined until 2015.

Brinksma et al. are the first to examine the association between NS and HRQOL across childhood cancer patients. Notably, they studied the association of undernutrition, over-nutrition, weight loss, weight gain with HRQOL in a heterogeneous group of children with cancer one year after diagnosis. In total, 104 patients (aged 2–18 years) diagnosed with hematological (43%), solid (33%), or brain malignancies (24%) participated in the study. Weight, height, and BMI were assessed and expressed as SDS. Furthermore, FFM and FM were calculated based on bioelectrical impedance analysis (BIA). The child- and parent-report versions of the PedsQL 4.0 Generic scale [86,88] and the PedsQL 3.0 Cancer Module [89] were used in order to measure generic and cancer-specific HRQOL. According to Brinksma et al. [79] nutrition related problems adversely affect HRQOL in childhood cancer patients. Undernourished as well as over-nourished children experienced poorer QOL than children who were well-nourished. Similarly, both noteworthy weight loss and weight gain led to worse HRQOL. Actually, impaired physical functioning prevailed in undernourished patients and in patients with weight loss. It is widely known that undernutrition and weight loss are associated with muscle mass deficit and muscle deficiency, resulting in fatigue [90]. Therefore, undernourished children did not have the vitality and muscle strength needed to involve themselves in physical activities. Furthermore, undernutrition adversely affected children's social functioning. This finding can be justified by the pain, nausea, and tiredness these children encounter, which impair their ability to sufficiently participate in physical and social activities with their peers. As regards the psychosocial field, both over-nourished children and children with weight gain showed impaired functioning—when compared to adequately nourished patients—particularly in the emotional and cognitive sphere. They were more susceptible to feelings of fear, sorrow, and anger. Hence, they experienced more difficulties in interacting with others and they struggled to perform cognitive tasks—compared to adequately nourished patients with cancer.

These results have implications in clinical practice as they indicate the significance of adequate NS in children with cancer. Although the study could not demonstrate a causal relationship between nutrition related problems and HRQOL, undernourished and over-nourished patients experienced the lowest HRQOL across all cancer patients.

3.5. Nutritional Status during Survivorship

Advances in treatment have resulted in considerable improvements in survival rates of pediatric cancer. This success translates into a growing population of long-term survivors [91]. However, almost two-third of childhood cancer survivors (CCSs) will encounter at least one late effect while 40% of them are vulnerable to experience a disabling or potentially fatal condition even 30 years after diagnosis [92]. Even though late effects and chronic health conditions may be largely attributed to cancer and its treatment [93], the effects of NS that extend into survivorship put survivors at risk for numerous nutrition-related morbidities considering the pre-existing risk factors CCSs are facing [94]. There is a significant body of literature on NS among cancer survivors in childhood and adolescence after completion of treatment in HICs [43]. Special attention has been paid to ALL diagnosis, given its dominant prevalence in this age group worldwide [95] (Table 2).

Zhang et al. [96] performed a meta-analysis on the prevalence of obesity in pediatric ALL survivors in order to evaluate whether survivors are more likely to be obese than a reference population. Forty-seven studies met the inclusion criteria reporting on 9223 pediatric ALL survivors. Even though there was significant heterogeneity among studies, pediatric ALL survivors had considerably higher BMI than the reference population. There was a consistently high prevalence of overweight/obesity in both recent and long-term survivors regardless of patient- and treatment-related characteristics.

Table 2. Characteristics of listed studies that assess NS in CCSs.

Author, Year (Location)	Study Design	Survivors, N/(Control)	Diagnosis	Assessment Criteria	Nutritional Related Problems
Zhang et al., 2014 [96] (USA)	Systematic Review and Meta-analysis	9223	ALL	BMI	Overweight/obesity
Zhang et al., 2014 [97] (USA)	Retrospective cohort study	83	ALL	BMI	Overweight/obesity
Zhang et al., 2015 [98] (USA)	Systematic Review and Meta-analysis	1791	ALL	BMI	Overweight/obesity
Collins et al., 2017 [99] (Canada)	Cross-sectional cohort study	75	ALL	BMI Arm anthropometry	Malnutrition
Karlage et al., 2015 [100] (USA)	Longitudinal cohort study	1361	Various diagnoses	BMI DXA [1] Anthropometry	Overweight/obesity
Marriott et al., 2018 [101] (Canada)	Cross-sectional study	75	ALL	LBM [2] FM [3] Whole-body BMC [4]	Overweight/obesity Sarcopenic obesity
Molinari et al., 2017 [102] (Brazil)	Cross-sectional study	101	ALL	Bone densitometry Anthropometry	Overweight/obesity BMD [5]
Wang et al., 2018 [103] (Canada)	Systematic Review and Meta-analysis	2032	BT [6]	BMI FM	Overweight/obesity
Warner et al., 2014 [104] (USA)	Population-based study	1060/(5410)	Various diagnoses	BMI	Malnutrition
Prasad et al., 2015 [105] (India)	Retrospective cohort study	648	Various diagnoses	BMI	Malnutrition MS [7]

[1] Dual-energy X-ray Absorptiometry (DXA), [2] Lean Body Mass (LBM), [3] Fat Mass, [4] Bone Mineral Content (BMC), [5] Bone Mineral Density (BMD), [6] Brain Tumors, [7] Metabolic Syndrome (MS).

Although many studies have focused on obesity and the consequences of being overweight, it was unclear at which time period survivors experienced excessive weight gain. Zhang et al. [97] performed a retrospective cohort study of 83 children with ALL. BMI status was examined at various time points during and after treatment, as well as annually up to five years after treatment. The percentage of patients who were overweight or obese (BMI ≥ 85th percentile) doubled from 20% at diagnosis to about 40% after treatment completion [97]. Particularly, 26.7% of normoweight children became overweight/obese at the end of treatment and 36.1% were overweight/obese five years post-treatment. Among those who were overweight/obese at diagnosis, 81.3% and 66.7% remained overweight/obese at the end of treatment and five years post-treatment, respectively. The overall increase in BMI z-score from diagnosis to the end of treatment was associated with a more than threefold increased risk of being overweight/obese five years after treatment. The study reveals that patients with pediatric ALL were at risk of becoming overweight or obese early during treatment, while these changes in weight status remained throughout treatment and after treatment completion.

Zhang et al. [98] conducted a subsequent meta-analysis and come to similar conclusions. Findings demonstrated significant increase in mean BMI z-score and weight during treatment that persisted beyond treatment completion. Actually, unsound weight gain was prevalent in pediatric ALL patients regardless of receipt of cranial irradiation therapy (CRT), sex, and weight status [98].

Collins et al. [99] performed arm anthropometry to assess the NS in long-term survivors of ALL in childhood and adolescence, as BMI does not distinguish muscle from adipose tissue [106]. Seventy-five patients diagnosed with ALL at least before a decade, were enrolled in the study. According to BMI values only six survivors were undernourished and none of them severely. Twenty-five survivors were overweight/obese, while only six (8%) were actually obese. However, 15 (20%) survivors were obese—assessed by TSFT—and only 3% suffered from sarcopenia according to MUAC. As it results, malnutrition rates varied according to assessment methods performed.

Karlage et al. [100] reported similar inconsistencies regarding BMI and anthropometric measurements of body composition. Obesity rates varied between 40% determined by BMI, 62% by three site skinfolds and 85% by Dual-energy X-ray Absorptiometry (DXA). Even though skinfolds undervalued the percent body fat of CCSs when compared with DXA, they indicated higher sensitivity than BMI when used to assort survivors as obese or not obese. Particularly nearly 47% of males and 53% of females of the study population were misclassified as non-obese when assessed by BMI, which may result in CCSs not receiving appropriate nutritional support and guidance.

As regards to body composition, Marriott et al. [101] conducted a study focusing on skeletal muscle mass (SMM) alterations. The study included 75 long-term survivors—37 male and 38 female—diagnosed with ALL at least before a decade. Whole-body DXA scans were obtained, as well as measures of lean body mass (LBM), FM, and whole-body bone mineral content (BMC). According to fat mass index (FMI), the majority of females and two-thirds of males were overweight/obese—12% and 18% were obese respectively. On the basis of BMI, the percentages of overweight/obese became 35.3% for females and 31.3% for males—5.9% and 9.8% were obese respectively. The analysis of appendicular lean mass (ALM) showed that 50% of survivors ≤18 years old suffered from SMM deficit. Thirty-two survivors (43%) were identified with positive z-scores for FMI and negative scores for appendicular lean mass index (ALMI). Consequently, sarcopenic obesity prevails in long-term survivors of ALL, which puts them at risk of both excess body fat and insufficient SMM.

Apart from body composition alterations, changes in bone metabolism constitute extensive adverse late effects of cancer treatment. They represent a major cause of morbidity in the CCSs population through pain, fractures, decrease of BMD and chronic deterioration of bone function [107,108]. Molinari et al. [102] evaluated BMD and body composition in 101 patients treated for ALL, using bone densitometry and anthropometric data. As regards to NS, 22.8% of survivors were overweight and 15.8% were obese. As to body composition the LBM levels and BMC were higher in males, while FM levels and fat percentages were higher in females. The more time had passed from treatment completion until the time of the study, the higher the values of LBM, FM, percentage of fat and BMC. Among children and adolescents <20 years old (n = 79), three survivors (2.9%) had low BMD and 16 (15.8%) were classified as at risk for low BMD. Among survivors aged >20 years old, eight (7.9%) had osteopenia and none of them had osteoporosis. In comparison to the reference population most of the survivors had normal BMD values. However, the risk group—considered by the literature as with normal BMD—actually presented significantly lower bone mass values. Eventually, ALL survivors can regain lost bone mass during the post-treatment period. Yet, some of them will never achieve their higher BMD acquisition potential, presenting considerable bone deficit [109].

So far, most publications on the NS of CCSs focus on ALL. Wang et al. [103] systematically reviewed the prevalence of overweight and obesity of CCSs diagnosed with BT. As it emerges, evidence for weight gain and obesity among survivors of childhood brain tumors (SCBT) varies. Some studies report an increase [110,111], whereas others have shown no significant differences compared to healthy controls [112,113]. Among participants, survivors diagnosed with brain tumors other than craniopharyngioma and craniopharyngioma survivors were analyzed in separate groups in order not to overrate the prevalence of obesity in overall SCBT population, as patients diagnosed with craniopharyngioma are known to be at high risk of developing obesity [114,115]. According to BMI measures, overweight and obesity rates were similar for SCBT and general population—rate of combined overweight and obesity 42.6% and 40.4%, respectively. Yet, survivors had higher adiposity. As regards to craniopharyngioma, the participants had higher prevalence of obesity and combined overweight and obesity than SCBT and healthy controls. Specifically, overweight and obesity affected almost two-thirds of patients with craniopharyngioma.

Warner et al. [104] conducted a population-based study in order to evaluate the prevalence of undernutrition and overweight/obesity among 1060 adult CCSs of various diagnoses. The most prevalent diagnoses among female survivors were epithelial cancer (26.1%) and lymphoma (17.4%), while for males were lymphoma (23.8%) and central nervous system (CNS) tumors (16.3%). Considering all diagnoses, there were no differences between female or male survivors versus the age- and sex-matched comparison population, regarding the risk of being underweight or overweight/obese. However, according to BMI values 36% of females and 61% of male survivors were classified as overweight/obese. When further analyzed by cancer diagnosis, female epithelial survivors were less likely to be overweight or obese than the comparison population and only male CNS survivors had a slightly higher risk of being overweight or obese than the reference cohort.

Even though overweight, obesity, and MS have been broadly reported in the Western literature, data from developing countries are lacking. Prasad et al. [105] conducted a retrospective study and NS was assessed in a cohort of 648 Indian CCSs. At the time of the study 471 survivors were <18 years—child and adolescent survivors (CASs)—and 177 were 18 years or older. The prevalence of obesity, overweight, normal NS and undernutrition was 2.6%, 10.8%, 62.7%, and 28.8% for CASs while 0%, 8.5%, 62.7% and 28.8% for adult survivors, respectively. Regarding adult survivors, those >30 years old had higher prevalence of overweight compared to those <30 years old (22.2% vs. 6.9%, p = 0.004). None of them fit the strict criteria of MS, though 17 (9.6%) fit the lenient criteria which included overweight survivors as well as obese. As to CASs none participant fit the strict criteria for MS. However, 11 (2.4%) survivors had features of MS when the weight criteria were lenient. There was a higher prevalence of overweight/obesity between those diagnosed with ALL or BT (16.5% and 20.7%, respectively, p = 0.07) and the rest of survivors (13.6%). Overall the prevalence of obesity/overweight was lower in this cohort when compared to western literature. Yet, it is unclear whether these rates reflect the underlying undernutrition in developing countries such as India or the CCSs population of this study differ from their western counterparts. Despite the lower prevalence of overweight/obesity and MS in this cohort of survivors, CCSs remain at high risk for cardiometabolic complications.

Some of the risk factors for overweight, obesity and MS are modifiable and in the hands of CCSs themselves. There are guidelines for promoting health in cancer survivors, including encouraging healthy nutrition, physical exercise and avoiding high-risk behaviors [116,117]. Yet, dietary guidelines developed for cancer survivors—such as those developed by the American Cancer Society [118] and the World Cancer Research Fund/the American Institute for Cancer Research (WCRF/AICR) [119]—do not elaborate on CCSs. Furthermore, the long-term follow-up guidelines for CCS developed by the Children's Oncology Group (COG) do not include cancer- and treatment-specific guidelines on nutrition [120].

Nevertheless, according to Brinkman et al. [121] healthy diet and physical exercise can moderate several late effects of cancer treatment, including obesity, hyperlipidemia, diabetes mellitus, cardiovascular disease, hypertension, and osteoporosis. Unfortunately, many CCSs do not meet the recommended dietary guidelines, with 54% of them exceeding their daily caloric requirements [122]. According to Zhang et al. [123], only 4%, 19%, 24%, and 29% of survivors follow the guidelines for vitamin D, sodium, calcium, and saturated fat intake, respectively. Nevertheless, nutritional intake in CCS has not been adequately studied [123]. Even though there are a few existing studies providing evidence that current dietary guidelines are not met [124–127], data are mainly derived from small groups of survivors or focus on specific cancer diagnoses—such as pediatric lymphoblastic leukemia. Zhang et al. [128] aimed to evaluate diet quality and dietary intake in a large cohort of 2570 adult CCSs. As regards diagnoses, leukemia was the most prevalent followed by lymphoma, embryonal tumor, sarcoma, and CNS tumor. The overall evidence emerges poor diet quality in CCSs, while older survivors had better diet quality than younger survivors did.

Unhealthy dietary behaviors have been associated with increased risk for health threatening conditions [94]. In addition, according to preliminary studies among CCSs, better quality diets may conduce to improved long-term health outcomes. There is developing evidence indicating that healthy dietary behaviors may reduce the risk of nutrition-related chronic conditions [94], thus it becomes essential to incorporate nutrition interventions and particularly dietary counseling into the clinical framework of survivorship care.

4. Discussion

Childhood cancer is an illness related to severe morbidity and mortality. The malignancy itself remains the main cause of death among childhood cancer patients [129,130]. Concurrently nutrition is a fundamental part of the pediatric cancer patients' care. Adequate and appropriate nutrition is required to maintain optimal growth and development. Furthermore, adequate nutrition is likely to enhance survival outcome, reduce toxicity and improve QOL [53].

It has been widely recognized in literature that the NS of children diagnosed with and treated for cancer is likely to be affected at some point during the disease trajectory. Actually, for many childhood cancer patients, the early progression of the disease and the commencement of antineoplastic therapies can affect the NS, leading to malnutrition with many adverse consequences [8,74,131].

One of the most important findings of this review—that focuses on NS alterations that occur during the management of childhood cancer—is that the reported prevalence of malnutrition—undernutrition, overweight and obesity—varies between different types of cancer, different stages of the disease, type of treatment, as well as among studies, highlighting the complexity and diversity of this population. Children diagnosed with specific cancer types develop nutrition related problems more often than others. For instance, at diagnosis prevalence of undernutrition is higher in patients with solid tumors—especially Wilms tumor or neuroblastoma—and much lower in children with ALL and HL [4,11,14,21]. At the same time patients with brain tumors demonstrate high prevalence of overweight and obesity [50]. During treatment, children with solid tumors are more frequently nutritionally depleted, followed by brain tumors and hematological malignancies [49,74]. The detected differences in malnutrition among various diagnoses are inconsistent in LMICs, as delays in diagnosis and limited access to healthcare may lead to higher undernutrition rates, regardless of cancer type [21]. In addition, undernutrition is more often observed in high-risk diseases across all cancer types [21].

The majority of data that focus on NS of children with cancer at the time of diagnosis relates to undernutrition, the prevalence of which ranges from 10.8% [16] to 76% [23]. These reported differences between studies are due both to the stage of the disease at diagnosis and the parameters used to assess NS [8]. To date, there is a lack of consensus on the definition of malnutrition [1,28]. In addition, the criteria for NS assessment are heterogeneous [1,8,28]. Nutritional assessment is a process that depends on the sensitivity and specificity of the parameters performed [8]. Unfortunately, this procedure is often postponed in the context of many other procedures that may have a higher priority, some of which may even affect it [40]. Most studies refer to BMI as, it is widely used in clinical practice. Yet, it is not the most appropriate method for NS assessment because it does not measure body fat directly. Even though every method for clinical assessment of NS has restrictions, indicators such as MUAC, TSFT, and BIA provide more information regarding body composition changes that occur in paediatric cancer patients. Nonetheless, the diversity among different indicators of NS does not allow any straightforward comparisons among them. The prevalence of nutrition related problems depends not only on the methods and criteria used to assess the NS [8], the timing of the assessment [40] and the composition of the study population [3]—in terms of types of malignancies—but also on the socio-economic status. In general, undernutrition rates were much higher in LICs than in HICs [3,23,25].

Clearly, the NS at the time of diagnosis is an important prognostic factor that affects treatment response as well as the possibility of recovery [1]. However, nutrition related problems in pediatric cancer patients are dynamic and their development is usually observed during subsequent treatment.

Currently, the most relevant research is retrospective or cross-sectional. The few prospectively designed studies that have been published principally concern children diagnosed with hematological malignancies while most of them do not refer to the NS at all stages of treatment [74]. In addition, research has focused on the study of undernutrition during cancer treatment, while excessive energy intake or poor diet quality is being overlooked [74]. The adverse effects of undernutrition during treatment have been established [43]. Among others these include reduced tolerance to chemotherapy, changes in the metabolism of medicinal products, reduced immunity, increased risk of infections and degraded QOL [43]. However, the quality of data supporting each of these results varies.

Studies that investigate the association between NS at diagnosis and clinical outcome suggest that NS may affect cancer prognosis in children with cancer. Particularly, observed inferior survival was generally stable among studies [59]. The presence of undernutrition was associated with a large number of complications and relapses, as well as a reduced level of recovery [1,52,68]. On the other hand, excess weight gain and obesity negatively affected the response to treatment and led to reduced cure rates [1,4,52,53]. Yet, the correlations between nutrition related problems and clinical outcomes remain unclear, with some researchers claiming that they are associated to worse outcomes and others claiming that there are no such associations [53,74].

The NS status of children with cancer has not only significant clinical implications, but also can adversely affect the long–term development and health of survivors, including children's QOL which as shown by the review remains underestimated [79]. There is a significant body of research on the NS of childhood and adolescent cancer survivors. Most studies focus on children with hematological malignancies—mainly in HICs—taking into account their predominant prevalence [43]. Furthermore, many reports confirm the impact of low or excessive body weight on survival, while collective evidence consistently shows poor diet quality in CCSs [128].

The lack of standard protocols and algorithms for assessment and treatment of nutritional problems, as well as limited in time dietary interventions are important factors that contribute to significant rates of malnutrition according to the literature. Meanwhile there is a lack of international specific dietary guidelines for children with cancer. Future scientific research should emphasize on proposing certain criteria that could assist the establishment of dietary instructions, such as cancer type, NS at diagnosis, treatment protocol, as well as children's gender and age.

Nutritional assessment should be mandatory from diagnosis and during treatment, in view of the possible manageable nature of this risk factor [33]. Therefore, early assessment of NS and timely intervention should be a priority in all interdisciplinary oncology teams, in order to integrate nutritional counseling into the clinical framework of care in an effort to address at least part of the problem [24].

5. Conclusions

NS of pediatric cancer patients plays a crucial role during the disease trajectory. The malignancy itself and the progression of the disease cause NS alterations, leading to malnutrition. In addition, the commencement of antineoplastic therapies affects energy balance with many negative consequences.

Malnutrition—undernutrition, overweight, and obesity—is linked to adverse outcomes from diagnosis to long-term survivorship. NS at the time of diagnosis is an important prognostic factor that affects treatment response and the possibility of recovery. The impact of impaired NS on clinical outcome and cancer prognosis is related to treatment intolerance due to nutrient deficiency and immune incompetence. Increased risk of infection and alterations in drug metabolism lead to delays and treatment cessation that result in higher relapse rates and lower survival rates. In addition, undernutrition during treatment correlates to a greater number of complications, increasing TRM and decreasing EFS. Yet, correlations between NS alterations and clinical outcomes remain unclear. Nutrition related problems can also adversely affect the long-term health of survivors, including children's HRQOL. The effects of NS that extend into survivorship put survivors at risk for numerous nutrition-related morbidities.

Given the high prevalence of malnutrition during childhood cancer and as NS represents a modifiable risk factor, nutritional assessment should be mandatory from diagnosis, during treatment and subsequently. There are several methods for the clinical assessment of NS and each one of them has limitations and constraints. Among those performed in clinical practice MUAC, TSFT and BIA provide more information concerning body composition changes than BMI does. Nonetheless, the diversity among different indicators of NS prevents us from extracting safe results regarding the most suitable one. Ideally, the most appropriate indicator is the one that would not allow a malnourished child to remain underdiagnosed.

As regards pediatric oncology, advances in treatment and follow-up care are significant. However, there is still a lack of international specific dietary guidelines for children with cancer. Hopefully, future scientific research should emphasize establishing cancer- and treatment-specific guidelines for nutrition. Early monitoring and adaptation of pediatric cancer patients' NS as well as timely nutritional intervention could improve their treatment response, their clinical outcome, their survival, but also their QOL.

Author Contributions: Conceptualization, V.D. and T.V.; methodology, V.D. and T.V.; investigation, V.D.; writing–original draft preparation, V.D.; writing–review and editing, V.D. and T.V.; visualization, V.D.; supervision, T.V. All authors have read and agreed to the published version of the manuscript.

Acknowledgments: The authors wish to thank Elena Vlastou, medical physicist, for her constructive advice and general support.

References

1. Sala, A.; Pencharz, P.; Barr, R.D. Children, Cancer, and Nutrition—A Dynamic Triangle in Review. *Cancer* **2004**, *100*, 677–687. [CrossRef]
2. Rogers, P.C. Importance of Nutrition in Pediatric Oncology. *Indian J. Cancer* **2015**, *52*, 176. [CrossRef]
3. Antillon, F.; Rossi, E.; Molina, A.L.; Sala, A.; Pencharz, P.; Valsecchi, M.G.; Barr, R. Nutritional Status of Children during Treatment for Acute Lymphoblastic Leukemia in Guatemala. *Pediatr. Blood Cancer* **2013**, *60*, 911–915. [CrossRef] [PubMed]
4. Brinksma, A.; Huizinga, G.; Sulkers, E.; Kamps, W.; Roodbol, P.; Tissing, W. Malnutrition in Childhood Cancer Patients: A Review on Its Prevalence and Possible Causes. *Crit. Rev. Oncol. Hematol.* **2012**, *83*, 249–275. [CrossRef] [PubMed]

5.   Jaime-Pérez, J.C.; González-Llano, O.; Herrera-Garza, J.L.; Gutiérrez-Aguirre, H.; Vázquez-Garza, E.; Gómez-Almaguer, D. Assessment of Nutritional Status in Children with Acute Lymphoblastic Leukemia in Northern México: A 5-Year Experience. *Pediatr. Blood Cancer* **2008**, *50*, 506–508. [CrossRef] [PubMed]

6.   Odame, I.; Reilly, J.J.; Gibson, B.E.S.; Donaldson, M.D.C. Patterns of Obesity in Boys and Girls after Treatment for Acute Lymphoblastic Leukaemia. *Arch. Dis. Child.* **1994**, *71*, 147–149. [CrossRef] [PubMed]

7.   Reilly, J.J. Obesity during and after Treatment for Childhood Cancer. *Endocr. Dev.* **2009**, *15*, 40–58.

8.   Sala, A.; Rossi, E.; Antillon, F.; Molina, A.L.; de Maselli, T.; Bonilla, M.; Hernandez, A.; Ortiz, R.; Pacheco, C.; Nieves, R.; et al. Nutritional Status at Diagnosis Is Related to Clinical Outcomes in Children and Adolescents with Cancer: A Perspective from Central America. *Eur. J. Cancer* **2012**, *48*, 243–252. [CrossRef]

9.   Van Eys, J. Malnutrition in Children with Cancer: Incidence and Consequence. *Cancer* **1979**, *43*, 2030–2035.

10. Reilly, J.J.; Dorosty, A.R.; Emmett, P.M. Prevalence of Overweight and Obesity in British Children: Cohort Study. *BMJ* **1999**, *319*, 1039. [CrossRef]

11. Antillon, F.; de Maselli, T.; Garcia, T.; Rossi, E.; Sala, A. Nutritional Status of Children during Treatment for Acute Lymphoblastic Leukemia in the Central American Pediatric Hematology Oncology Association (AHOPCA): Preliminary Data from Guatemala. *Pediatr. Blood Cancer* **2008**, *50*, 502–505. [CrossRef] [PubMed]

12. Barr, R.D. Nutritional Status in Children with Cancer: Before, during and after Therapy. *Indian J. Cancer* **2015**, *52*, 173. [CrossRef] [PubMed]

13. Barr, R.; Atkinson, S.; Pencharz, P.; Arguelles, G.R. Nutrition and Cancer in Children. *Pediatr. Blood Cancer* **2008**, *50*, 437. [CrossRef]

14. Sala, A.; Rossi, E.; Antillon, F. Nutritional Status at Diagnosis in Children and Adolescents with Cancer in the Asociacion de Hemato-Oncologia Pediatrica de Centro America (AHOPCA) Countries: Preliminary Results from Guatemala. *Pediatr. Blood Cancer* **2008**, *50*, 499–501. [CrossRef]

15. Sala, A.; Antillon, F.; Pencharz, P.; Barr, R.; AHOPCA Consortium. Nutritional Status in Children with Cancer: A Report from the AHOPCA Workshop Held in Guatemala City, August 31-September 5, 2004. *Pediatr. Blood Cancer* **2005**, *45*, 230–236. [CrossRef] [PubMed]

16. Dos Maia Lemos, P.S.; Ceragioli Oliveira, F.L.; Monteiro-Caran, E.M. Nutritional Status at Diagnosis in Children with Cancer in Brazil. *Pediatr. Ther.* **2016**, *6*. [CrossRef]

17. Ladas, E.J.; Sacks, N.; Brophy, P.; Rogers, P.C. Standards of Nutritional Care in Pediatric Oncology: Results from a Nationwide Survey on the Standards of Practice in Pediatric Oncology. A Children's Oncology Group Study. *Pediatr. Blood Cancer* **2006**, *46*, 339–344. [CrossRef]

18. Rogers, P.C.; Melnick, S.J.; Ladas, E.J.; Halton, J.; Baillargeon, J.; Sacks, N. Children's Oncology Group (COG) Nutrition Committee. *Pediatr. Blood Cancer* **2008**, *50*, 447–450. [CrossRef]

19. Villanueva, G.; Blanco, J.; Rivas, S.; Molina, A.L.; Lopez, N.; Fuentes, A.L.; Muller, L.; Caceres, A.; Antillon, F.; Ladas, E.; et al. Nutritional Status at Diagnosis of Cancer in Children and Adolescents in Guatemala and Its Relationship to Socioeconomic Disadvantage: A Retrospective Cohort Study. *Pediatr. Blood Cancer* **2019**, *66*, e27647. [CrossRef]

20. Yoruk, M.A.; Durakbasa, C.U.; Timur, C.; Sahin, S.S.; Taskin, E.C. Assessment of Nutritional Status and Malnutrition Risk at Diagnosis and Over a 6-Month Treatment Period in Pediatric Oncology Patients with Hematologic Malignancies and Solid Tumors. *J. Pediatr. Hematol. Oncol.* **2018**, *41*, e308–e321. [CrossRef]

21. Pribnow, A.K.; Ortiz, R.; Báez, L.F.; Mendieta, L.; Luna-Fineman, S. Effects of Malnutrition on Treatment-Related Morbidity and Survival of Children with Cancer in Nicaragua. *Pediatr. Blood Cancer* **2017**, *64*, e26590. [CrossRef]

22. Peccatori, N.; Ortiz, R.; Rossi, E.; Calderon, P.; Conter, V.; Garcia, Y.; Biondi, A.; Espinoza, D.; Ceppi, F.; Mendieta, L.; et al. Oral/Enteral Nutritional Supplementation In Children Treated For Cancer In Low-Middle-Income Countries Is Feasible And Effective: The Experience Of The Children's Hospital Manuel De Jesus Rivera "La Mascota" In Nicaragua. *Mediterr. J. Hematol. Infect. Dis.* **2018**, *10*, e2018038. [CrossRef] [PubMed]

23. Shah, P.; Jhaveri, U.; Idhate, T.B.; Dhingra, S.; Arolkar, P.; Arora, B. Nutritional Status at Presentation, Comparison of Assessment Tools, and Importance of Arm Anthropometry in Children with Cancer in India. *Indian J. Cancer* **2015**, *52*, 210–215.

24. Dos Lemos, P.S.M.; de Oliveira, F.L.C.; Caran, E.M.M. Nutritional Status of Children and Adolescents at Diagnosis of Hematological and Solid Malignancies. *Rev. Bras. Hematol. E Hemoter.* **2014**, *36*, 420–423. [CrossRef]

25. Orgel, E.; Sposto, R.; Malvar, J.; Seibel, N.L.; Ladas, E.; Gaynon, P.S.; Freyer, D.R. Impact on Survival and Toxicity by Duration of Weight Extremes During Treatment for Pediatric Acute Lymphoblastic Leukemia: A Report From the Children's Oncology Group. *J. Clin. Oncol.* **2014**, *32*, 1331–1337. [CrossRef]
26. Radhakrishnan, V.; Ganesan, P.; Rajendranath, R.; Ganesan, T.S.; Sagar, T.G. Nutritional Profile of Pediatric Cancer Patients at Cancer Institute, Chennai. *Indian J. Cancer* **2015**, *52*, 207. [CrossRef]
27. CDC Growth Charts. Available online: http://www.cdc.gov/growthcharts/ (accessed on 4 August 2020).
28. Garófolo, A.; Lopez, F.A.; Petrilli, A.S. High Prevalence of Malnutrition among Patients with Solid Non-Hematological Tumors as Found by Using Skinfold and Circumference Measurements. *Sao Paulo Med. J.* **2005**, *123*, 277–281. [CrossRef]
29. Smith, D.E.; Stevens, M.C.G.; Booth, I.W. Malnutrition at Diagnosis of Malignancy in Childhood: Common but Mostly Missed. *Eur. J. Pediatr.* **1991**, *150*, 318–322. [CrossRef]
30. Tazi, I.; Hidane, Z.; Zafad, S.; Harif, M.; Benchekroun, S.; Ribeiro, R. Nutritional Status at Diagnosis of Children with Malignancies in Casablanca. *Pediatr. Blood Cancer* **2008**, *51*, 495–498. [CrossRef]
31. Kuczmarski, R.J.; Ogden, C.L.; Grummer-Strawn, L.M.; Flegal, K.M.; Guo, S.S.; Wei, R.; Mei, Z.; Curtin, L.R.; Roche, A.F.; Johnson, C.L. CDC Growth Charts: United States. *Adv. Data* **2000**, *314*, 1–27.
32. Mei, Z.; Grummer-Strawn, L.M.; Pietrobelli, A.; Goulding, A.; Goran, M.I.; Dietz, W.H. Validity of Body Mass Index Compared with Other Body-Composition Screening Indexes for the Assessment of Body Fatness in Children and Adolescents. *Am. J. Clin. Nutr.* **2002**, *75*, 978–985. [CrossRef] [PubMed]
33. Triarico, S.; Rinninella, E.; Cintoni, M.; Capozza, M.A.; Mastrangelo, S.; Mele, M.C.; Ruggiero, A. Impact of Malnutrition on Survival and Infections among Pediatric Patients with Cancer: A Retrospective Study. *Eur. Rev. Med. Pharmacol. Sci.* **2019**, *23*, 1165–1175. [PubMed]
34. Huysentruyt, K.; Alliet, P.; Muyshont, L.; Rossignol, R.; Devreker, T.; Bontems, P.; Dejonckheere, J.; Vandenplas, Y.; De Schepper, J. The STRONG(Kids) Nutritional Screening Tool in Hospitalized Children: A Validation Study. *Nutr.* **2013**, *29*, 1356–1361. [CrossRef]
35. Joosten, K.F.M.; Hulst, J.M. Nutritional Screening Tools for Hospitalized Children: Methodological Considerations. *Clin. Nutr.* **2014**, *33*, 1–5. [CrossRef]
36. Połubok, J.; Malczewska, A.; Rąpała, M.; Szymocha, J.; Kozicka, M.; Dubieńska, K.; Duczek, M.; Kazanowska, B.; Barg, E. Nutritional Status at the Moment of Diagnosis in Childhood Cancer Patients. *Pediatr. Endocrinol. Diabetes Metab.* **2017**, *23*, 77–82. [CrossRef]
37. Small, A.G.; Thwe, L.M.; Byrne, J.A.; Lau, L.; Chan, A.; Craig, M.E.; Cowell, C.T.; Garnett, S.P. Neuroblastoma, Body Mass Index, and Survival: A Retrospective Analysis. *Medicine.* **2015**, *94*, e713. [CrossRef] [PubMed]
38. Brinksma, A.; Roodbol, P.F.; Sulkers, E.; Hooimeijer, H.L.; Sauer, P.J.J.; van Sonderen, E.; de Bont, E.S.J.M.; Tissing, W.J.E. Weight and Height in Children Newly Diagnosed with Cancer: Weight and Height in Children With Cancer. *Pediatr. Blood Cancer* **2015**, *62*, 269–273. [CrossRef]
39. Loeffen, E.A.H.; Brinksma, A.; Miedema, K.G.E.; de Bock, G.H.; Tissing, W.J.E. Clinical Implications of Malnutrition in Childhood Cancer Patients—Infections and Mortality. *Support. Care Cancer* **2015**, *23*, 143–150. [CrossRef]
40. Collins, L.; Nayiager, T.; Doring, N.; Kennedy, C.; Webber, C.; Halton, J.; Walker, S.; Sala, A.; Barr, R.D. Nutritional Status at Diagnosis in Children with Cancer, I. An Assessment by Dietary Recall—Compared with Body Mass Index and Body Composition Measured by Dual Energy X-ray Absorptiometry. *J. Pediatr. Hematol. Oncol.* **2010**, *32*, e299–e303. [CrossRef]
41. Eys, J.V. Benefits of Nutritional Intervention on Nutritional Status, Quality of Life and Survival. *Int. J. Cancer* **1998**, *78*, 66–68.
42. Gaynor, E.P.T.; Sullivan, P.B. Nutritional Status and Nutritional Management in Children with Cancer. *Arch. Dis. Child.* **2015**, *100*, 1169–1172. [CrossRef] [PubMed]
43. Barr, R.D.; Gomez-Almaguer, D.; Jaime-Perez, J.C.; Ruiz-Argüelles, G.J. Importance of Nutrition in the Treatment of Leukemia in Children and Adolescents. *Arch. Med. Res.* **2016**, *47*, 585–592. [CrossRef] [PubMed]
44. Butturini, A.M.; Dorey, F.J.; Lange, B.J.; Henry, D.W.; Gaynon, P.S.; Fu, C.; Franklin, J.; Siegel, S.E.; Seibel, N.L.; Rogers, P.C.; et al. Obesity and Outcome in Pediatric Acute Lymphoblastic Leukemia. *J. Clin. Oncol..* **2007**, *25*, 2063–2069. [CrossRef]
45. Ethier, M.-C.; Alexander, S.; Abla, O.; Green, G.; Lam, R.; Sung, L. Association between Obesity at Diagnosis and Weight Change during Induction and Survival in Pediatric Acute Lymphoblastic Leukemia. *Leuk. Lymphoma* **2012**, *53*, 1677–1681. [CrossRef] [PubMed]

46. Reilly, J.J.; Odame, I.; McColl, J.H.; McAllister, P.J.; Gibson, B.E.; Wharton, B.A. Does Weight for Height Have Prognostic Significance in Children with Acute Lymphoblastic Leukemia? *Am. J. Pediatr. Hematol. Oncol.* **1994**, *16*, 225–230. [CrossRef]

47. Withycombe, J.S.; Post-White, J.E.; Meza, J.L.; Hawks, R.G.; Smith, L.M.; Sacks, N.; Seibel, N.L. Weight Patterns in Children With Higher Risk ALL: A Report From the Children's Oncology Group (COG) for CCG 1961. *Pediatr. Blood Cancer* **2009**, *53*, 1249–1254. [CrossRef] [PubMed]

48. Paciarotti, I.; McKenzie, J.M.; Davidson, I.; Edgar, A.B.; Brougham, M.; Wilson, D.C. Short Term Effects of Childhood Cancer and Its Treatments on Nutritional Status: A Prospective Cohort Study. *EC Nutr.* **2015**, *3*, 528–540.

49. Brinksma, A.; Roodbol, P.F.; Sulkers, E.; Kamps, W.A.; de Bont, E.S.J.M.; Boot, A.M.; Burgerhof, J.G.M.; Tamminga, R.Y.J.; Tissing, W.J.E. Changes in Nutritional Status in Childhood Cancer Patients: A Prospective Cohort Study. *Clin. Nutr.* **2015**, *34*, 66–73. [CrossRef]

50. Revuelta Iniesta, R.; Paciarotti, I.; Davidson, I.; McKenzie, J.M.; Brougham, M.F.H.; Wilson, D.C. Nutritional Status of Children and Adolescents with Cancer in Scotland: A Prospective Cohort Study. *Clin. Nutr. ESPEN* **2019**, *32*, 96–106. [CrossRef]

51. Schleiermacher, G.; Janoueix-Lerosey, I.; Delattre, O. Recent Insights into the Biology of Neuroblastoma: Biology of Neuroblastoma. *Int. J. Cancer* **2014**, *135*, 2249–2261. [CrossRef]

52. Gómez-Almaguer, D.; Ruiz-Argüelles, G.J.; Ponce-de-León, S. Nutritional Status and Socio-Economic Conditions as Prognostic Factors in the Outcome of Therapy in Childhood Acute Lymphoblastic Leukemia. *Int. J. Cancer* **1998**, *78*, 52–55. [CrossRef]

53. Rogers, P.C. Nutritional Status as a Prognostic Indicator for Pediatric Malignancies. *J. Clin. Oncol.* **2014**, *32*, 1293–1294. [CrossRef]

54. Lange, B.J. Mortality in Overweight and Underweight Children with Acute Myeloid Leukemia. *JAMA* **2005**, *293*, 203. [CrossRef] [PubMed]

55. Aldhafiri, F.K.; McColl, J.H.; Reilly, J.J. Prognostic Significance of Being Overweight and Obese at Diagnosis in Children with Acute Lymphoblastic Leukemia. *J. Pediatr. Hematol. Oncol.* **2014**, *36*, 234–236. [CrossRef]

56. Canner, J.; Alonzo, T.A.; Franklin, J.; Freyer, D.R.; Gamis, A.; Gerbing, R.B.; Lange, B.J.; Meshinchi, S.; Woods, W.G.; Perentesis, J.; et al. Differences in Outcomes of Newly Diagnosed Acute Myeloid Leukemia for Adolescent/Young Adult and Younger Patients: A Report from the Children's Oncology Group. *Cancer* **2013**, *119*, 4162–4169. [CrossRef]

57. Hijiya, N.; Panetta, J.C.; Zhou, Y.; Kyzer, E.P.; Howard, S.C.; Jeha, S.; Razzouk, B.I.; Ribeiro, R.C.; Rubnitz, J.E.; Hudson, M.M.; et al. Body Mass Index Does Not Influence Pharmacokinetics or Outcome of Treatment in Children with Acute Lymphoblastic Leukemia. *Blood* **2006**, *108*, 3997–4002. [CrossRef]

58. Inaba, H.; Surprise, H.C.; Pounds, S.; Cao, X.; Howard, S.C.; Ringwald-Smith, K.; Buaboonnam, J.; Dahl, G.; Bowman, W.P.; Taub, J.W.; et al. Effect of Body Mass Index on the Outcome of Children with Acute Myeloid Leukemia. *Cancer* **2012**, *118*, 5989–5996. [CrossRef] [PubMed]

59. Amankwah, E.K.; Saenz, A.M.; Hale, G.A.; Brown, P.A. Association between Body Mass Index at Diagnosis and Pediatric Leukemia Mortality and Relapse: A Systematic Review and Meta-Analysis. *Leuk. Lymphoma* **2016**, *57*, 1140–1148. [CrossRef]

60. Hunger, S.P.; Sung, L.; Howard, S.C. Treatment Strategies and Regimens of Graduated Intensity for Childhood Acute Lymphoblastic Leukemia in Low-Income Countries: A Proposal. *Pediatr. Blood Cancer* **2009**, *52*, 559–565. [CrossRef]

61. Murphy, A.J.; Mosby, T.T.; Rogers, P.C.; Cohen, J.; Ladas, E.J. An International Survey of Nutritional Practices in Low- and Middle-Income Countries: A Report from the International Society of Pediatric Oncology (SIOP) PODC Nutrition Working Group. *Eur. J. Clin. Nutr.* **2014**, *68*, 1341–1345. [CrossRef]

62. Orgel, E.; Genkinger, J.M.; Aggarwal, D.; Sung, L.; Nieder, M.; Ladas, E.J. Association of Body Mass Index and Survival in Pediatric Leukemia: A Meta-Analysis. *Am. J. Clin. Nutr.* **2016**, *103*, 808–817. [CrossRef]

63. Saenz, A.M.; Stapleton, S.; Hernandez, R.G.; Hale, G.A.; Goldenberg, N.A.; Schwartz, S.; Amankwah, E.K. Body Mass Index at Pediatric Leukemia Diagnosis and the Risks of Relapse and Mortality: Findings from a Single Institution and Meta-Analysis. *J. Obes.* **2018**, *2018*, 1–8. [CrossRef]

64. Weir, J.; Reilly, J.J.; McColl, J.H.; Gibson, B.E.S. No Evidence for an Effect of Nutritional Status at Diagnosis on Prognosis in Children with Acute Lymphoblastic Leukemia. *J. Pediatr. Hematol. Oncol.* **1998**, *20*, 534–538. [CrossRef]

65. Baillargeon, J.; Langevin, A.M.; Lewis, M.; Estrada, J.; Mullins, J.; Pitney, A.; Ma, J.Z.; Chisholm, G.B.; Pollock, B.H. Obesity and Survival in a Cohort of Predominantly Hispanic Children with Acute Lymphoblastic Leukemia. *J. Pediatr. Hematol. Oncol.* **2006**, *28*, 575–578. [CrossRef]

66. Karakurt, H.; Sarper, N.; Kılıç, S.Ç.; Gelen, S.A.; Zengin, E. Screening Survivors of Childhood Acute Lymphoblastic Leukemia for Obesity, Metabolic Syndrome, and Insulin Resistance. *Pediatr. Hematol. Oncol.* **2012**, *29*, 551–561. [CrossRef]

67. Løhmann, D.J.A.; Abrahamsson, J.; Ha, S.-Y.; Jónsson, Ó.G.; Koskenvuo, M.; Lausen, B.; Palle, J.; Zeller, B.; Hasle, H. Effect of Age and Body Weight on Toxicity and Survival in Pediatric Acute Myeloid Leukemia: Results from NOPHO-AML 2004. *Haematologica* **2016**, *101*, 1359–1367. [CrossRef]

68. Joffe, L.; Dwyer, S.; Glade Bender, J.L.; Frazier, A.L.; Ladas, E.J. Nutritional Status and Clinical Outcomes in Pediatric Patients with Solid Tumors: A Systematic Review of the Literature. *Semin. Oncol.* **2019**, *46*, 48–56. [CrossRef]

69. Brown, T.R.; Vijarnsorn, C.; Potts, J.; Milner, R.; Sandor, G.G.S.; Fryer, C. Anthracycline Induced Cardiac Toxicity in Pediatric Ewing Sarcoma: A Longitudinal Study. *Pediatr. Blood Cancer* **2013**, *60*, 842–848. [CrossRef]

70. Altaf, S.; Enders, F.; Jeavons, E.; Krailo, M.; Barkauskas, D.A.; Meyers, P.; Arndt, C. High-BMI at Diagnosis Is Associated with Inferior Survival in Patients with Osteosarcoma: A Report from the Children's Oncology Group. *Pediatr. Blood Cancer* **2013**, *60*, 2042–2046. [CrossRef]

71. Goldstein, G.; Shemesh, E.; Frenkel, T.; Jacobson, J.M.; Toren, A. Abnormal Body Mass Index at Diagnosis in Patients with Ewing Sarcoma Is Associated with Inferior Tumor Necrosis. *Pediatr. Blood Cancer* **2015**, *62*, 1892–1896. [CrossRef] [PubMed]

72. Hingorani, P.; Seidel, K.; Krailo, M.; Mascarenhas, L.; Meyers, P.; Marina, N.; Conrad, E.U.; Hawkins, D.S. Body Mass Index (BMI) at Diagnosis Is Associated with Surgical Wound Complications in Patients with Localized Osteosarcoma: A Report from the Children's Oncology Group. *Pediatr. Blood Cancer* **2011**, *57*, 939–942. [CrossRef] [PubMed]

73. Rodeberg, D.A.; Stoner, J.A.; Garcia-Henriquez, N.; Randall, R.L.; Spunt, S.L.; Arndt, C.A.; Kao, S.; Paidas, C.N.; Million, L.; Hawkins, D.S. Tumor Volume and Patient Weight as Predictors of Outcome in Children with Intermediate Risk Rhabdomyosarcoma: A Report from the Children's Oncology Group. *Cancer* **2011**, *117*, 2541–2550. [CrossRef] [PubMed]

74. Iniesta, R.R.; Paciarotti, I.; Brougham, M.F.H.; McKenzie, J.M.; Wilson, D.C. Effects of Pediatric Cancer and Its Treatment on Nutritional Status: A Systematic Review. *Nutr. Rev.* **2015**, *73*, 276–295. [CrossRef]

75. Donaldson, S.S.; Wesley, M.N.; DeWys, W.D.; Suskind, R.M.; Jaffe, N.; vanEys, J. A Study of the Nutritional Status of Pediatric Cancer Patients. *Am. J. Dis. Child.* **1981**, *135*, 1107–1112. [CrossRef]

76. Lobato-Mendizábal, E.; Ruiz-Argüelles, G.J.; Marín-López, A. Leukaemia and Nutrition I: Malnutrition Is an Adverse Prognostic Factor in the Outcome of Treatment of Patients with Standard-Risk Acute Lymphoblastic Leukaemia. *Leuk. Res.* **1989**, *13*, 899–906. [CrossRef]

77. Mejía-Aranguré, J.M.; Fajardo-Gutiérrez, A.; Reyes-Ruíz, N.I.; Bernáldez-Ríos, R.; Mejía-Domínguez, A.M.; Navarrete-Navarro, S.; Martínez-García, M.C. Malnutrition in Childhood Lymphoblastic Leukemia: A Predictor of Early Mortality during the Induction-to-Remission Phase of the Treatment. *Arch. Med. Res.* **1999**, *30*, 150–153. [CrossRef]

78. Pedrosa, F.; Bonilla, M.; Liu, A.; Smith, K.; Davis, D.; Ribeiro, R.C.; Wilimas, J.A. Effect of Malnutrition at the Time of Diagnosis on the Survival of Children Treated for Cancer in El Salvador and Northern Brazil. *J. Pediatr. Hematol. Oncol.* **2000**, *22*, 502–505. [CrossRef]

79. Brinksma, A.; Sanderman, R.; Roodbol, P.F.; Sulkers, E.; Burgerhof, J.G.M.; de Bont, E.S.J.M.; Tissing, W.J.E. Malnutrition Is Associated with Worse Health-Related Quality of Life in Children with Cancer. *Support. Care Cancer* **2015**, *23*, 3043–3052. [CrossRef]

80. Malihi, Z.; Kandiah, M.; Chan, Y.M.; Hosseinzadeh, M.; Sohanaki Azad, M.; Zarif Yeganeh, M. Nutritional Status and Quality of Life in Patients with Acute Leukaemia Prior to and after Induction Chemotherapy in Three Hospitals in Tehran, Iran: A Prospective Study. *J. Hum. Nutr. Diet.* **2013**, *26* (Suppl. 1), 123–131. [CrossRef]

81. Nathan, P.C.; Furlong, W.; Barr, R.D. Challenges to the Measurement of Health-Related Quality of Life in Children Receiving Cancer Therapy. *Pediatr. Blood Cancer* **2004**, *43*, 215–223. [CrossRef]

82. Tsiros, M.D.; Olds, T.; Buckley, J.D.; Grimshaw, P.; Brennan, L.; Walkley, J.; Hills, A.P.; Howe, P.R.C.; Coates, A.M. Health-Related Quality of Life in Obese Children and Adolescents. *Int. J. Obes.* **2009**, *33*, 387–400. [CrossRef] [PubMed]

83. Varni, J.W.; Limbers, C.; Burwinkle, T.M. Literature Review: Health-Related Quality of Life Measurement in Pediatric Oncology: Hearing the Voices of the Children. *J. Pediatr. Psychol.* **2007**, *32*, 1151–1163. [CrossRef] [PubMed]

84. Varni, J.W.; Burwinkle, T.M.; Jacobs, J.R.; Gottschalk, M.; Kaufman, F.; Jones, K.L. The PedsQL in Type 1 and Type 2 Diabetes: Reliability and Validity of the Pediatric Quality of Life Inventory Generic Core Scales and Type 1 Diabetes Module. *Diabetes Care* **2003**, *26*, 631–637. [CrossRef]

85. Varni, J.W.; Seid, M.; Smith Knight, T.; Burwinkle, T.; Brown, J.; Szer, I.S. The PedsQL in Pediatric Rheumatology: Reliability, Validity, and Responsiveness of the Pediatric Quality of Life Inventory Generic Core Scales and Rheumatology Module. *Arthritis Rheum.* **2002**, *46*, 714–725. [CrossRef]

86. Varni, J.W.; Seid, M.; Kurtin, P.S. PedsQL™ 4.0: Reliability and Validity of the Pediatric Quality of Life Inventory™ Version 4.0 Generic Core Scales in Healthy and Patient Populations. *Med. Care* **2001**, *39*, 800–812. [CrossRef]

87. Ladas, E.J.; Sacks, N.; Meacham, L.; Henry, D.; Enriquez, L.; Lowry, G.; Hawkes, R.; Dadd, G.; Rogers, P. A Multidisciplinary Review of Nutrition Considerations in the Pediatric Oncology Population: A Perspective from Children's Oncology Group. *Nutr. Clin. Pract.* **2005**, *20*, 377–393. [CrossRef]

88. Varni, J.W.; Limbers, C.A.; Burwinkle, T.M. Parent Proxy-Report of Their Children's Health-Related Quality of Life: An Analysis of 13,878 Parents' Reliability and Validity across Age Subgroups Using the PedsQL™ 4.0 Generic Core Scales. *Health Qual. Life Outcomes* **2007**, *5*. [CrossRef]

89. Varni, J.W.; Burwinkle, T.M.; Katz, E.R.; Meeske, K.; Dickinson, P. The PedsQL in Pediatric Cancer: Reliability and Validity of the Pediatric Quality of Life Inventory Generic Core Scales, Multidimensional Fatigue Scale, and Cancer Module. *Cancer* **2002**, *94*, 2090–2106. [CrossRef]

90. Evans, W.J.; Lambert, C.P. Physiological Basis of Fatigue. *Am. J. Phys. Med. Rehabil.* **2007**, *86*, S29–S46. [CrossRef] [PubMed]

91. Mariotto, A.B.; Rowland, J.H.; Yabroff, K.R.; Scoppa, S.; Hachey, M.; Ries, L.; Feuer, E.J. Long-Term Survivors of Childhood Cancers in the United States. *Cancer Epidemiol. Prev. Biomark.* **2009**, *18*, 1033–1040. [CrossRef]

92. Hudson, M.M.; Oeffinger, K.C.; Jones, K.; Brinkman, T.M.; Krull, K.R.; Mulrooney, D.A.; Mertens, A.; Castellino, S.M.; Casillas, J.; Gurney, J.G.; et al. Age-Dependent Changes in Health Status in the Childhood Cancer Survivor Cohort. *J. Clin. Oncol.* **2015**, *33*, 479–491. [CrossRef]

93. Oeffinger, K.C.; Mertens, A.C.; Sklar, C.A.; Kawashima, T.; Hudson, M.M.; Meadows, A.T.; Friedman, D.L.; Marina, N.; Hobbie, W.; Kadan-Lottick, N.S.; et al. Childhood Cancer Survivor Study. Chronic Health Conditions in Adult Survivors of Childhood Cancer. *N. Engl. J. Med.* **2006**, *355*, 1572–1582. [CrossRef] [PubMed]

94. Ladas, E. Nutritional Counseling in Survivors of Childhood Cancer: An Essential Component of Survivorship Care. *Children* **2014**, *1*, 107–118. [CrossRef] [PubMed]

95. Ferlay, J.; Soerjomataram, I.; Dikshit, R.; Eser, S.; Mathers, C.; Rebelo, M.; Parkin, D.M.; Forman, D.; Bray, F. Cancer Incidence and Mortality Worldwide: Sources, Methods and Major Patterns in GLOBOCAN 2012. *Int. J. Cancer* **2015**, *136*, 359–386. [CrossRef]

96. Zhang, F.F.; Kelly, M.J.; Saltzman, E.; Must, A.; Roberts, S.B.; Parsons, S.K. Obesity in Pediatric ALL Survivors: A Meta-Analysis. *Pediatrics* **2014**, *133*, e704–e715. [CrossRef] [PubMed]

97. Zhang, F.F.; Rodday, A.M.; Kelly, M.J.; Must, A.; MacPherson, C.; Roberts, S.B.; Saltzman, E.; Parsons, S.K. Predictors of Being Overweight or Obese in Survivors of Pediatric Acute Lymphoblastic Leukemia (ALL): Predictors of Obesity in ALL Survivors. *Pediatr. Blood Cancer* **2014**, *61*, 1263–1269. [CrossRef]

98. Zhang, F.F.; Liu, S.; Chung, M.; Kelly, M.J. Growth Patterns during and after Treatment in Patients with Pediatric ALL: A Meta-Analysis: Growth Patterns During in Patients with Pediatic All. *Pediatr. Blood Cancer* **2015**, *62*, 1452–1460. [CrossRef]

99. Collins, L.; Beaumont, L.; Cranston, A.; Savoie, S.; Nayiager, T.; Barr, R. Anthropometry in Long-Term Survivors of Acute Lymphoblastic Leukemia in Childhood and Adolescence. *J. Adolesc. Young Adult Oncol.* **2017**, *6*, 294–298. [CrossRef]

100. Karlage, R.E.; Wilson, C.L.; Zhang, N.; Kaste, S.; Green, D.M.; Armstrong, G.T.; Robison, L.L.; Chemaitilly, W.; Srivastava, D.K.; Hudson, M.M.; et al. Validity of Anthropometric Measurements for Characterizing Obesity among Adult Survivors of Childhood Cancer: A Report from the St. Jude Lifetime Cohort Study. *Cancer* **2015**, *121*, 2036–2043. [CrossRef]

101. Marriott, C.J.C.; Beaumont, L.F.; Farncombe, T.H.; Cranston, A.N.; Athale, U.H.; Yakemchuk, V.N.; Webber, C.E.; Barr, R.D. Body Composition in Long-Term Survivors of Acute Lymphoblastic Leukemia Diagnosed in Childhood and Adolescence: A Focus on Sarcopenic Obesity. *Cancer* **2018**, *124*, 1225–1231. [CrossRef]

102. Molinari, P.C.C.; Lederman, H.M.; Lee, M.L.D.M.; Caran, E.M.M. Assessment of The Late Effects on Bones and on Body Composition of Children and Adolescents Treated for Acute Lymphocytic Leukemia According To Brazilian Protocols. *Rev. Paul. Pediatr.* **2017**, *35*, 78–85. [CrossRef]

103. Wang, K.; Fleming, A.; Johnston, D.L.; Zelcer, S.M.; Rassekh, S.R.; Ladhani, S.; Socha, A.; Shinuda, J.; Jaber, S.; Burrow, S.; et al. Overweight, Obesity and Adiposity in Survivors of Childhood Brain Tumours: A Systematic Review and Meta-analysis. *Clin. Obes.* **2018**, *8*, 55–67. [CrossRef] [PubMed]

104. Warner, E.L.; Fluchel, M.; Wright, J.; Sweeney, C.; Boucher, K.M.; Fraser, A.; Smith, K.R.; Stroup, A.M.; Kinney, A.Y.; Kirchhoff, A.C. A Population-Based Study of Childhood Cancer Survivors' Body Mass Index. *J. Cancer Epidemiol.* **2014**, *2014*, 1–10. [CrossRef]

105. Prasad, M.; Arora, B.; Chinnaswamy, G.; Vora, T.; Narula, G.; Banavali, S.; Kurkure, P. Nutritional Status in Survivors of Childhood Cancer: Experience from Tata Memorial Hospital, Mumbai. *Indian J. Cancer* **2015**, *52*, 219.

106. McCarthy, H.D. Body Fat Measurements in Children as Predictors for the Metabolic Syndrome: Focus on Waist Circumference. *Proc. Nutr. Soc.* **2006**, *65*, 385–392.

107. Haddy, T.B.; Mosher, R.B.; Reaman, G.H. Osteoporosis in Survivors of Acute Lymphoblastic Leukemia. *Oncologist* **2001**, *6*, 278–285. [CrossRef]

108. Davies, J.H.; Evans, B.A.J.; Jenney, M.E.; Gregory, J.W. Skeletal Morbidity in Childhood Acute Lymphoblastic Leukaemia. *Clin. Endocrinol. (Oxf.)* **2005**, *63*, 1–9. [CrossRef]

109. Wasilewski-Masker, K.; Kaste, S.C.; Hudson, M.M.; Esiashvili, N.; Mattano, L.A.; Meacham, L.R. Bone Mineral Density Deficits in Survivors of Childhood Cancer: Long-Term Follow-up Guidelines and Review of the Literature. *Pediatrics* **2008**, *121*, 705–713. [CrossRef]

110. Hansen, J.A.; Stancel, H.H.; Klesges, L.M.; Tyc, V.L.; Hinds, P.S.; Wu, S.; Hudson, M.M.; Kahalley, L.S. Eating Behavior and BMI in Adolescent Survivors of Brain Tumor and Acute Lymphoblastic Leukemia. *J. Pediatr. Oncol. Nurs.* **2014**, *31*, 41–50. [CrossRef] [PubMed]

111. Wilson, C.L.; Liu, W.; Yang, J.J.; Kang, G.; Ojha, R.P.; Neale, G.A.; Srivastava, D.K.; Gurney, J.G.; Hudson, M.M.; Robison, L.L.; et al. Genetic and Clinical Factors Associated with Obesity among Adult Survivors of Childhood Cancer: A Report from the St. Jude Lifetime Cohort. *Cancer* **2015**, *121*, 2262–2270. [CrossRef] [PubMed]

112. Brouwer, C.A.J.; Gietema, J.A.; Vonk, J.M.; Tissing, W.J.E.; Boezen, H.M.; Zwart, N.; Postma, A. Body Mass Index and Annual Increase of Body Mass Index in Long-Term Childhood Cancer Survivors; Relationship to Treatment. *Support. Care Cancer* **2012**, *20*, 311–318. [CrossRef]

113. Meacham, L.R.; Gurney, J.G.; Mertens, A.C.; Ness, K.K.; Sklar, C.A.; Robison, L.L.; Oeffinger, K.C. Body Mass Index in Long-Term Adult Survivors of Childhood Cancer: A Report of the Childhood Cancer Survivor Study. *Cancer* **2005**, *103*, 1730–1739. [CrossRef]

114. Lustig, R.H. Hypothalamic Obesity after Craniopharyngioma: Mechanisms, Diagnosis, and Treatment. *Front. Endocrinol.* **2011**, *2*. [CrossRef]

115. Müller, H.L. Craniopharyngioma and Hypothalamic Injury: Latest Insights into Consequent Eating Disorders and Obesity. *Curr. Opin. Endocrinol. Diabetes Obes.* **2016**, *23*, 81–89. [CrossRef]

116. Armstrong, G.T.; Oeffinger, K.C.; Chen, Y.; Kawashima, T.; Yasui, Y.; Leisenring, W.; Stovall, M.; Chow, E.J.; Sklar, C.A.; Mulrooney, D.A.; et al. Modifiable Risk Factors and Major Cardiac Events among Adult Survivors of Childhood Cancer. *J. Clin. Oncol.* **2013**, *31*, 3673–3680. [CrossRef]

117. Elliot, D.L.; Lindemulder, S.J.; Goldberg, L.; Stadler, D.D.; Smith, J. Health Promotion for Adolescent Childhood Leukemia Survivors: Building on Prevention Science and Ehealth. *Pediatr. Blood Cancer* **2013**, *60*, 905–910. [CrossRef] [PubMed]

118. Rock, C.L.; Doyle, C.; Demark-Wahnefried, W.; Meyerhardt, J.; Courneya, K.S.; Schwartz, A.L.; Bandera, E.V.; Hamilton, K.K.; Grant, B.; McCullough, M.; et al. Nutrition and Physical Activity Guidelines for Cancer Survivors. *CA Cancer J. Clin.* **2012**, *62*, 243–274. [CrossRef]

119. Wiseman, M.; Cannon, G. *Food, Nutrition, Physical Activity and the Prevention of Cancer: A Global Perspective: Summary*; World Cancer Research Fund, American Institute for Cancer Research: Washington, DC, USA, 2007.

120. Children's Oncology Group. Long-Term Follow-Up Guidelines for Survivors of Childhood, Adolescent, and Young Adult Cancers. Available online: http://www.survivorshipguidelines.org/pdf/ltfuguidelines_40.pdf (accessed on 13 September 2020).

121. Brinkman, T.M.; Recklitis, C.J.; Michel, G.; Grootenhuis, M.A.; Klosky, J.L. Psychological Symptoms, Social Outcomes, Socioeconomic Attainment, and Health Behaviors Among Survivors of Childhood Cancer: Current State of the Literature. *J. Clin. Oncol.* **2018**, *36*, 2190–2197. [CrossRef]

122. Love, E.; Schneiderman, J.E.; Stephens, D.; Lee, S.; Barron, M.; Tsangaris, E.; Urbach, S.; Staneland, P.; Greenberg, M.; Nathan, P.C. A Cross-Sectional Study of Overweight in Pediatric Survivors of Acute Lymphoblastic Leukemia (ALL). *Pediatr. Blood Cancer* **2011**, *57*, 1204–1209. [CrossRef] [PubMed]

123. Zhang, F.F.; Saltzman, E.; Kelly, M.J.; Liu, S.; Must, A.; Parsons, S.K.; Roberts, S.B. Comparison of Childhood Cancer Survivors' Nutritional Intake with US Dietary Guidelines. *Pediatr. Blood Cancer* **2015**, *62*, 1461–1467. [CrossRef]

124. Landy, D.C.; Lipsitz, S.R.; Kurtz, J.M.; Hinkle, A.S.; Constine, L.S.; Adams, M.J.; Lipshultz, S.E.; Miller, T.L. Dietary Quality, Caloric Intake, and Adiposity of Childhood Cancer Survivors and Their Siblings: An Analysis from the Cardiac Risk Factors in Childhood Cancer Survivors Study. *Nutr. Cancer* **2013**, *65*, 547–555. [CrossRef]

125. Robien, K.; Ness, K.K.; Klesges, L.M.; Baker, K.S.; Gurney, J.G. Poor Adherence to Dietary Guidelines among Adult Survivors of Childhood Acute Lymphoblastic Leukemia. *J. Pediatr. Hematol. Oncol.* **2008**, *30*, 815–822. [CrossRef]

126. Smith, W.A.; Li, C.; Nottage, K.A.; Mulrooney, D.A.; Armstrong, G.T.; Lanctot, J.Q.; Chemaitilly, W.; Laver, J.H.; Srivastava, D.K.; Robison, L.L.; et al. Lifestyle and Metabolic Syndrome in Adult Survivors of Childhood Cancer: A Report from the St. Jude Lifetime Cohort Study. *Cancer* **2014**, *120*, 2742–2750. [CrossRef] [PubMed]

127. Tonorezos, E.S.; Robien, K.; Eshelman-Kent, D.; Moskowitz, C.S.; Church, T.S.; Ross, R.; Oeffinger, K.C. Contribution of Diet and Physical Activity to Metabolic Parameters among Survivors of Childhood Leukemia. *Cancer Causes Control CCC* **2013**, *24*, 313–321. [CrossRef] [PubMed]

128. Zhang, F.F.; Ojha, R.P.; Krull, K.R.; Gibson, T.M.; Lu, L.; Lanctot, J.; Chemaitilly, W.; Robison, L.L.; Hudson, M.M. Adult Survivors of Childhood Cancer Have Poor Adherence to Dietary Guidelines. *J. Nutr.* **2016**, *146*, 2497–2505. [CrossRef]

129. Freycon, F.; Trombert-Paviot, B.; Casagranda, L.; Bertrand, Y.; Plantaz, D.; Marec-Bérard, P. Trends in Treatment-Related Deaths (TRDs) in Childhood Cancer and Leukemia over Time: A Follow-up of Patients Included in the Childhood Cancer Registry of the Rhône-Alpes Region in France (ARCERRA). *Pediatr. Blood Cancer* **2008**, *50*, 1213–1220. [CrossRef]

130. Kaatsch, P. Epidemiology of Childhood Cancer. *Cancer Treat. Rev.* **2010**, *36*, 277–285. [CrossRef]

131. Bauer, J.; Jürgens, H.; Frühwald, M.C. Important Aspects of Nutrition in Children with Cancer1. *Adv. Nutr.* **2011**, *2*, 67–77. [CrossRef]

4

Evidence and Mechanisms of Fat Depletion in Cancer

Maryam Ebadi and Vera C. Mazurak *

Division of Human Nutrition, Department of Agricultural, Food and Nutritional Science, University of Alberta, 4-002 Li Ka Shing Centre for Health Research Innovation, Edmonton, AB T6G 2E1, Canada; ebadi@ualberta.ca
* Author to whom correspondence should be addressed; vmazurak@ualberta.ca

Abstract: The majority of cancer patients experience wasting characterized by muscle loss with or without fat loss. In human and animal models of cancer, body composition assessment and morphological analysis reveals adipose atrophy and presence of smaller adipocytes. Fat loss is associated with reduced quality of life in cancer patients and shorter survival independent of body mass index. Fat loss occurs in both visceral and subcutaneous depots; however, the pattern of loss has been incompletely characterized. Increased lipolysis and fat oxidation, decreased lipogenesis, impaired lipid depositionand adipogenesis, as well as browning of white adipose tissue may underlie adipose atrophy in cancer. Inflammatory cytokines such as interleukin-6 (IL-6), tumor necrosis factor alpha (TNF-α), and interleukin-1 beta (IL-1β) produced by the tumor or adipose tissue may also contribute to adipose depletion. Identifying the mechanisms and time course of fat mass changes in cancer may help identify individuals at risk of adipose depletion and define interventions to circumvent wasting. This review outlines current knowledge of fat mass in cancer and illustrates the need for further studies to assess alterations in visceral and subcutaneous adipose depots and possible mechanisms for loss of fat during cancer progression.

Keywords: adipose tissue; cancer; computed tomography; fat mobilization

1. Introduction

Adipose tissue (AT) is an active secretory organ that regulates energy balance, homeostasis, appetite, inflammation, insulin sensitivity, angiogenesis, and fat metabolism [1]. Adipose tissue metabolism and whole body fat mass are regulated through two major pathways: lipolysis (fat breakdown) and lipogenesis (fat synthesis) [2]. Adipose tissue dysfunction, fat mass changes and concurrent alterations in the production of adipokines, inflammatory cytokines, and lipid metabolites are common in metabolic disorders, such as insulin resistance, type 2 diabetes, cardiovascular disease, and obesity-related cancers such as colorectal and breast cancer [3,4].

The link between obesity and increased cancer incidence is well established [5,6], but the relationship between fat mass and cancer progression is much less clear. Studies indicate that the majority of cancer patients experience some degree of cancer-related wasting of both muscle and/or fat during the disease trajectory [7]. However, little is known about the importance of fat loss in cancer because the majority of studies of cancer-associated wasting typically focus on muscle. Potential links between fat loss and poor outcomes have been identified that indicate fat loss to be a poor prognostic factor in advanced cancer regardless of a patient' body weight [8,9]. This article reviews current knowledge of adipose tissue depletion in cancer, focusing on both assessment of fat tissue and morphological determination of adipose tissue in cancer populations. Possible mechanisms of fat loss are also discussed. Biological alterations in adipose tissue metabolism precede the physical manifestation of adipose tissue loss. Thus, understanding mechanisms and potential markers of fat loss in cancer are important for early detection which facilitates prevention of further loss to preserve fat and improve survival in cancer patients.

2. Adipose Atrophy in Cancer

Fat loss has been reported to be associated with shorter survival time [8,9]. Analysis of adipose tissue morphology and body composition has revealed body fat depletion in human and animal models of cancer cachexia. In the majority of human studies discussed in this review, cachexia is defined as ≥5% weight loss (WL) over 3 months or ≥10% within the previous 6 months. Weight loss does not necessarily reflect the severity of cachexia and fat loss but is the first outcome measurement typically used in studies of cancer. Validated data for classification of cachexia based on recent consensus are emerging [10].

The murine adenocarcinoma (MAC16) causes diminished adipocyte size with increased mitochondrial density, and elevated adipose tissue fibrosis in cachectic mice, compared to pair-fed and control animals [11]. The Walker 256 carcinoma, a well-established cancer cachexia model, affects adipose tissue in a time and depot-dependent manner [12–14]. Seven days after Walker 256 tumor injection, no significant changes were observed in adipocyte size. However, after 14 days, adipocyte size of retroperitoneal, and epididymal adipose tissue was decreased. On the other hand, mesenteric adipose tissue was not lost and size of mesenteric adipocytes increased after 14 days [13,14]. In support of these experimental studies, reduction in fat cell volume has been reported in weight-losing gastrointestinal (GI) cancer patients [15–17]. Cachectic patients exhibited smaller adipocytes compared to weight-stable controls [15–18] and non-cancer patients [16] but total body fat cell number was not altered [16,17]. Collectively, these studies suggest altered adipocyte size and reduced lipid storage capacity in the presence of a tumor.

3. Assessment of Fat Tissue over the Cancer Trajectory

The body mass index (BMI) has been used frequently as a clinically accessible measure of human body composition. However, the BMI does not differentiate between fat and fat-free mass or fat depots. Accumulation or loss of specific fat tissues are differentially associated with health outcomes. For example, there is a relationship between visceral adipose tissue (VAT) accumulation and insulin resistance [19]. Insulin resistant adipocytes that reside in VAT are more sensitive to catecholamine-induced lipolysis than subcutaneous adipose tissue (SAT) [1,20]. Lipolysis of fat from VAT enables direct delivery of free fatty acids to liver, which may lead to elevated hepatic triglyceride (TG) production, increased very low density lipoprotein secretion, and higher plasma TGs which exacerbates an already dysregulated metabolic state [20]. Therefore, an understanding of the intensity of loss and the type of fat being lost (VAT *vs.* SAT) is required. Potential differences in fat loss between depots has not been consistently demonstrated, partly due to the use of analytical techniques with limited applicability, as well as the variability among studies with regards to tumor type, stage and the time-point in the cancer trajectory that patients are studied. Discrepant methods of assessing fat and reporting values as cross sectional area (cm^2) or volume (cm^3), total fat mass (kg or %), change in area or the rate of changes also limit the ability to interpret and compare studies.

Body composition is assessed in cancer patients using a variety of methods including bioelectrical impedance analysis (BIA), dual-energy X-ray absorptiometry (DEXA), magnetic resonance imaging (MRI) and computed tomography (CT) scan analysis [21]. Body composition analysis using BIA has demonstrated lower body fat (% or kg) in cachectic patients compared to weight-stable cancer controls [15–17,22], healthy controls [23], or non-malignant controls [16,22]. When DEXA was applied to malnourished palliative cancer patients, no differences were observed in absolute fat mass (kg) during follow-up (4–62 months) [9]. However, the relative change (percentage of change from initial values) revealed a loss of fat concurrent with a marginal increase in lean mass during cancer progression [9]. As DEXA quantifies regional lean body mass, this study raised the possibility that patients may not have been gaining skeletal muscle per se but rather lean mass in internal organs such as the liver and spleen which has been reported as patients approached death in a subsequent study [24].

In an oncologic population, CT images are a routine part of treatment and are available from patient records as a chart review. CT image analysis has emerged as the gold standard for body composition assessment in cancer patients due to its ability to discriminate and quantify muscle, adipose tissue and organs. Shen *et al.* established that single slice tissue areas can be used to estimate whole body muscle and adipose tissue volumes [25]. Cachectic cancer patients exhibit lower adipose tissue mass compared to weight stable and/or controls [15–17,26]. Volumes of total adipose tissue, VAT and SAT were calculated in newly diagnosed GI cancer patients receiving no anticancer treatment [26]. Cachectic groups were separated into two groups, those with and without gastrointestinal obstruction that interfered with their food intake. Cachectic groups were compared to weight-stable cancer patients. Deterioration in nutritional status was confirmed by a higher Patient-Generated Subjective Global Assessment (PG-SGA) score in the cachectic patients with GI obstruction. Both BIA and CT analysis indicated that total fat mass (kg), and visceral and abdominal subcutaneous volumes were lower in cachectic patients compared to the weight-stable group. The cachectic patients with GI obstruction lost approximately two times more weight but VAT volume was greater compared to cachectic group without GI obstruction [26]. This study applied CT scans taken at one point in time; therefore, intensity of loss over time can not be determined. A lower amount of VAT, not the loss per se, was observed in cachectic group who did not have altered food intake.

Approaching death, the intensity of tissue loss increases and patients experience the greatest and most accelerated rate of loss [8,9,24,27]. Analysis of sequential CT images in 34 advanced colorectal cancer patients revealed that the greatest changes in body composition occur starting at 4.2 months from death [24]. One month from death, liver and spleen mass increase, whereas skeletal muscle and fat mass decrease [24]. A study by Murphy *et al.* quantified fat mass in 108 colorectal and lung cancer patients with at least two abdominal CT images in the last 500 days of life. Beginning seven months prior to death, both VAT and SAT mass decreased in cancer patients, reaching intensities of 10 kg of fat loss/100 days [8]. A recent study in pancreatic cancer patients suggested that the rate of visceral adipose tissue loss, rather than the absolute amount, may be an important indicator of survival [28]. Patients with at least two abdominal CT scans between diagnosis and death, receiving surgery (62%) or chemotherapy (88%) during cancer progression, were selected for this study. The rate of change (% change/100 days) for SAT was similar to VAT but a change in VAT was significantly correlated with survival in cancer patients. The presence of co-morbidities such as diabetes and anemia may have accelerated loss of VAT [28]. In another study, cachectic gastrointestinal cancer patients had significantly lower VAT and SAT three months prior to death compared to the benign controls. However, there was a tendency for cachectic patients to have smaller visceral and subcutaneous area compared to cancer patients without cachexia [27]. At present, no other studies exist regarding the pattern of fat loss in cancer and further studies are needed to establish the timeline and pattern of fat mass alterations in different adipose tissue depots during cancer progression. Further, the majority of studies assessing fat mass focus on gastrointestinal cancer patients so there is a gap in knowledge related to other malignant tumors.

While the majority of human studies focus on cachectic *vs.* non-cachectic patients, less is known about the effect of cancer treatments, which may also induce alterations in fat mass. For example, cancer surgery contributes to weight loss. Six months after surgery, weight is reduced from the baseline due to the catabolic response to the operation [29–31] and stabilizes after 12 months [31]. Adams reported that weight loss occurs rapidly in the three months following surgery [29]. Body composition assessment before, and 6 and 12 months after gastrectomy, measured from total body potassium and water, indicated 40% of fat mass was lost during the six months after surgery [30]. In a study by our group, two to six months after surgery, patients with colorectal liver metastasis were losing VAT at a greater rate than SAT, measured using consecutive CT scans (Figure 1). This supports the work of others in pancreatic cancer patients during early stages of disease progression. Intra-abdominal and subcutaneous adipose tissue mass were assessed before and after surgery using CT scans. Fat loss from intra-abdominal depot was greater than abdominal subcutaneous following surgery [32]. Therefore, surgical procedures may contribute to weight and fat loss due to the catabolic and inflammatory response to the surgery.

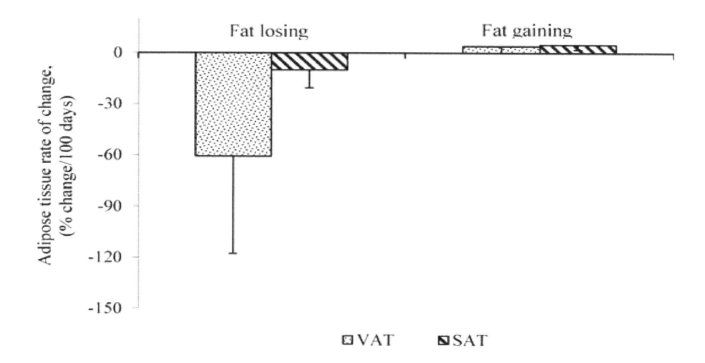

Figure 1. Mean rate of visceral adipose tissue (VAT) and subcutaneous adipose tissue (SAT) change in fat losing cancer patients assessed by consecutive computed tomography (CT) scans. Data are represented as Mean ± SD, $n = 5$ (Fat Losing) and $n = 2$ (Fat Stable), $p < 0.05$ VAT, visceral adipose tissue; SAT, subcutaneous adipose tissue.

Fat loss or gain after chemotherapy will depend on the tumor type, drug type, dose and overall response to chemotherapy. Following at least one cycle of chemotherapy treatment (cisplatin, 5-fluorouracil and/or epirubicin), patients with locally advanced oesophagogastric cancers lost an average of 1.3 ± 3.2 kg (6%) fat mass [33]. In advanced pancreatic cancer patients, a multivariate survival analysis revealed that VAT loss (determined from CT pre and post chemoradiation) but not muscle loss was significantly related to shorter survival [34].

Three months after chemotherapy initiation, testicular cancer patients who received 3 or 4 cycles of cisplatin-based chemotherapy had significantly higher VAT volume without changes in SAT [35]. However, nine months later, both VAT and SAT increased significantly, suggesting a capacity to rebuild lost adipose tissue [35]. A recent study using CT imaging to understand the loss and gain of muscle and adipose tissue during the year preceding death revealed that anabolic potential does exist, as some patients gained muscle and adipose tissue, but were only capable of doing this >3 months prior to death [36]. These results will initiate further research aiming to define the appropriate time to initiate nutritional intervention to preserve both muscle and fat tissue.

Fat loss may precede the loss of lean tissues (Table 1). The only patient group in which this question has been addressed is patients with newly diagnosed GI cancers. However, in all studies that have addressed this question to date, changes in adipose tissue were observed in absence of changes in lean tissues. The majority of these studies use BIA and DEXA for body composition assessments which are limited in ability to provide a direct estimate of muscle mass; further studies are needed to confirm that these findings are attributable to muscle loss or other lean body mass loss. Only one study used CT scans to assess body composition in GI cancer patients and that study showed no difference in abdominal muscle volume between cachectic and weight-stable cancer patients. However, that study assessed CT images at only one time point [26]. Adipose depletion may occur more rapidly than muscle during disease progress. Advanced pancreatic cancer patients lost both VAT and SAT over time, and the rate of change (%change/100 days) in total adipose tissue ($-40.4 \pm 25.4\%$/100 days) was much greater than muscle tissue ($-3.1 \pm 12.0\%$/100 days). No significant differences in adipose tissue mass were observed between patients who were or were not receiving chemotherapy [37]. These observations are supported by an experimental study in which lung carcinoma or melanoma cells were injected subcutaneously to induce cachexia in mice. Fat loss occurred prior to muscle loss, at early stages of tumor growth, at an intensity that was greater than muscle loss [38]. White adipose tissue browning, which contributes to fat loss in cancer, occurred before skeletal muscle wasting in mouse models of cancer cachexia [39].

Table 1. Articles reporting fat and lean tissue loss in newly diagnosed cancer patients.

Authors	Subjects [1]	Cancer Type	Body Composition Assessment	General Comments
Fouladiun et al., [9]	Malnourished patients (n = 132; 66 ± 3 years) advanced cancer with malnutrition (T4N1M1)	GI (n = 123) Breast (n = 1) Melanomas (n = 2) Other (n = 6), followed for 6–42 months	DEXA	Whole body fat loss was related to shorter survival Body fat loss more intense and pronounced compared to lean tissue
Agusstson et al., [15]	Weight stable cancer patients (n = 11), Weight-losing cachectic cancer patients with (n = 8) and without (n = 7) malnutrition	GI cancer with no treatment before surgery	BIA	No differences in lean body mass between groups Increased lipolysis in cancer cachectic patients
Dahlman et al., [17]	Cachectic patients (n = 13) Weight-stable cancer (n = 14)	GI cancer with no treatment before surgery	BIA	Decreased body fat mass but similar lean body mass between cachectic and control patients
Ryden et al., [16]	Cachectic patients (n = 13) Weight stable cancer patients (n = 10), Without cancer (n = 5)	GI cancer with no treatment before surgery	BIA	No difference in lean body mass between groups Elevated lipolysis with no changes in lipogenesis No local inflammation
Agustsson et al., [26]	Cancer cachectic without (n = 13) and with gastrointestinal obstruction (n = 10), Weight losing-cancer (n = 17)	GI cancer with no treatment before surgery	BIA, CT	No changes were observed in lean mass Visceral fat volume was lower in cachectic group compared to weight stable

[1] No patients received chemotherapy or radiotherapy.

4. Mechanisms for Adipose Depletion in Cancer

Elevated energy expenditure, decreased food intake and alterations in circulating levels of hormones including insulin, leptin, catecholamines, as well as elevated catabolism due to the tumor presence (high energy demands of tumor, inflammatory mediators produced by tumor) and tumor-host interactions are factors contributing to wasting in cancer [40]. These factors can cause abnormalities in lipid metabolism which may also lead to fat loss. Increased lipolytic activity, evidenced by elevated fasting plasma glycerol and free fatty acids is a driver of fat loss in advanced cancer patients [15,23,41] but the underlying causes of elevated lipolysis are not known. Other mechanisms including decreased lipogenesis [42,43], impairment in adipogenesis [11,14], elevated fat oxidation [17,23,44], and decreased lipid deposition [45–49] have also been attributed to fat loss in cancer (Figure 2).

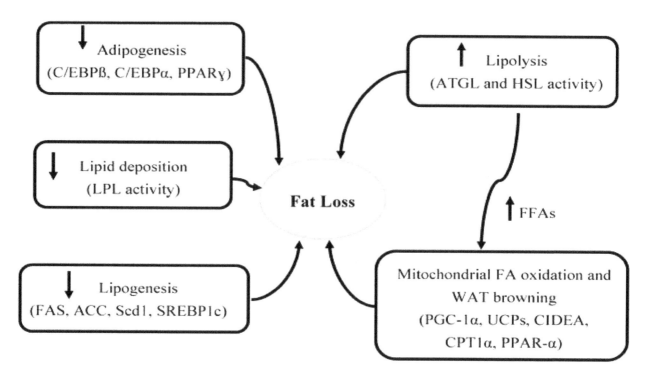

Figure 2. Summary of mechanisms and specific genes involved in adipose atrophy in cancer. WAT, white adipose tissue; FFAs, free fatty acids; ATGL, adipose triglyceride lipase, HSL, hormone sensitive lipase; PGC-1α, peroxisome proliferator-activated receptor-gamma coactivator 1 alpha; UCPs, un-coupling proteins; CIDEA, Cell death-inducing DFFA (DNA fragmentation factor-alpha)-like effector A; CPT1α, carnitine palmitoyltransferase 1 alpha; PPAR-γ, Peroxisome proliferator-activatedreceptor gamma; C/EBPα, CCAAT-enhancer-binding proteinα; LPL, lipoprotein lipase; FAS, fatty acid synthase; ACC, Acetyl-CoA carboxylase; Scd1, Stearoyl-CoA desaturase; SREBP1c, sterol regulatory element binding protein-1c.

Human and experimental models have been used to study the mechanisms of fat loss in cancer. Animal models are necessary to elevate our understanding of cancer associated weight-loss. However, each model may represent only some aspects of human cancer cachexia and choice of animal model is based on research objectives. For example, the MAC16 adenocarcinoma induces cachexia in the absence of anorexia and is suitable to study wasting related to the tumor produced factors rather than food intake. Yoshida ascites hepatoma AH130 (YAH-130), on the other hand, induces cachexia and anorexia accompanied by inflammation [50]. Therefore, the result of studies investigating the mechanisms underlying fat loss in cancer should be interpreted with caution as each specific tumor type, in various stages of growth, can affect various adipose tissue depots in a different manner.

4.1. Decreased Food Intake and Hypermetabolism

Anorexia alone does not explain reduced body weight or/and fat mass in cancer patients and cachexia-associated wasting can not be completely reversed by elevated nutritional intake [10]. Compared to pair-fed controls, the MAC-16 tumor leads to greater fat loss in mice indicating that tumors with high energy demands, rather than calorie restriction, may be responsible for adipose depletion [11]. Likewise, human studies have shown that in the absence of changes in food intake, hyper metabolism, characterized by elevated resting energy expenditure (REE), may be a contributing factor to the weight loss in cancer. Weight-losing and weight-stable cancer patients with various solid tumors had similar dietary intakes but weight losing patients had a higher REE determined by indirect calorimetry [51]. REE was also higher in weight-stable cancer patients compared to non-cancer controls which indicate that the tumor contributes to an elevated REE [52]. Johnson *et al.* reported no difference in measured REE between weight-losing and stable cancer patients but rather attributed higher REE in weight-losing cancer patients to elevated C-reactive protein (CRP) [53]. Although REE can contribute to weight loss in cancer, factors like tumor type, stage and duration of the disease also affect the REE in cancer [52,54].

In palliative cancer patients, during 4–62 months follow-up, body weight and fat mass (% change from baseline) decreased in the absence of changes in REE. Despite providing nutritional support to patients who had baseline calorie intake less than 90% of their energy requirement, body weight and fat mass did not increase [9]. Therefore, factors other than nutrient intake and hypermetabolism may contribute to fat loss in cancer.

4.2. Lipolysis and Elevated Fat Oxidation

It is well accepted that elevated lipolysis is the main cause of fat loss in cancer [15–17,22,23,55,56], however the specific mechanisms contributing to lipolysis have not been clearly defined. Hormone sensitive lipase (HSL) and adipose triglyceride lipase (ATGL) are major enzymes that contribute to TG breakdown in adipose tissue. Adipose triglyceride lipase catalyzes the first step in TG hydrolysis. During adipose tissue lipolysis, free fatty acids (FFA) and glycerol molecules are produced by the hydrolysis of triglyceride. HSL activity is regulated by hormones, i.e., catecholamines, insulin and glucagon, through a cAMP-mediated process [57,58]. Catecholamines stimulate lipolysis, whereas insulin has anti-lipolytic functions [59]. Binding of hormones to G-protein-coupled receptors results in up-regulation of adenylate cyclase which leads to an increase in intracellular cyclic adenosine monophosphate (cAMP) concentrations. cAMP stimulates a protein kinase which in turn phosphorylates and activates HSL [57,58]. Phosphorylated HSL translocates from the cytosol to the surface of lipid droplets to induce lipolysis.

Elevated expression of HSL mRNA [15,22,60] and protein [15,22] has been reported in cancer cachectic patients compared to weight-stable cancer. Higher mRNA expression of HSL in SAT was associated with higher serum FFAs in cancer patients, however, no significant differences were observed in mRNA expression of lipoprotein lipase (LPL), fatty acid synthase (FAS), insulin and tumor necrosis factor alpha (TNF-α) in adipose tissue of cancer patents compared to controls [60]. These results are supported by a study that reported HSL mRNA and protein over-expression, as well as increased hormone-stimulated lipolysis in cachectic cancer patients compared to malnourished weight-losing and weight stable cancer patients, explained the elevated adipose atrophy in cancer cachexia [15]. The ratio of plasma glycerol/body fat (index of in vivo lipolysis) was two times higher in cachectic patients. Ex vivo culture of adipocytes from the same patients revealed no difference in basal lipolysis (glycerol release to the media) between groups. However, incubation of adipocytes with catecholamines and natriuretic peptides elevated glycerol release to the media in the cachectic group suggesting that the adipocytes were more sensitive to the same amount of stimuli, and therefore more catabolic. There was no significant difference in plasma levels of catecholamines and natriuretic peptides between groups [15]. An explanation of the lack of difference in plasma hormone levels could be that lipolytic effects of hormones are elevated at the receptor level, evidenced by elevated β1-adrenoceptor (ADRB1) expression on adipocyte membranes in cachectic GI cancer patients [22]. Consequently, higher HSL expression and activity, which positively correlated with ADRB1 expression, were associated with higher plasma glycerol/fat mass and FFA/fat mass [22]. Therefore, lipolysis can be elevated in cancer cachectic patients due to increased expression of receptors on adipocytes membrane and their response to lipolytic effects of hormones, rather than elevated levels of mediators.

In study by Agustsson et al. [15], elevated HSL mRNA and protein expression contributed to the increased lipolysis. No significant difference in mRNA expression of ATGL was observed between cachectic cancer patients and controls; however, protein expression was not measured in this study [15]. Das and Hoefler [61] reported that ATGL mRNA expression may not translate to enzyme activity as its function is regulated via post-translational modifications. In another study, Das et al. reported higher ATGL and HSL activity in VAT of cachectic patients compared to non-cancer and cancer patients without cachexia, which has been previously reported [38]. Animal studies suggest that ATGL plays a more important role in adipose tissue lipolysis than HSL [38,62]. In mice bearing cachexia-inducing lung carcinoma or melanoma cells, lower body weight, decreased fat and muscle mass and elevated lipolysis were observed in tumor group compared to the controls. In HSL deficient mice, the tumor could reduce body weight and fat mass due to elevated ATGL activity. However, in ATGL deficient mice, the tumor did not induce elevated lipolysis and there was no significant difference in weight and fat mass between control and tumor group. Fat preservation in ATGL deficient mice, prevented muscle loss in tumor bearing animals [38]. Consistent with these findings, a recent study in mice bearing cachectic Colon-26 carcinoma revealed lower fat mass and increased lipolysis in cachectic mice compared to control mice. Increased lipolysis was induced by ATGL rather than the PKA/HSL pathway during late stages of cancer cachexia. ATGL protein levels increased in cachectic mice, however, no changes were observed in ATGL mRNA expression [62]. Therefore, not only mRNA expression but also protein expression and/or activity of these enzymes need to be determined in adipose tissue to investigate mechanisms that underlie elevated lipolysis.

The majority of studies indicated elevated lipolysis as a reason for fat loss in cancer; and consequently, increasing fatty acid oxidation could be a tentative approach to utilize surplus fatty acids (FAs). By increasing fatty acid oxidation within adipose tissue, liberated FAs are oxidized and can not be re-esterified into TG. Zuijdgeest-van Leeuwen *et al.* [23] reported higher lipolysis and reduced food intake in weight-losing cancer patients compared to healthy weight-stable adults. Whole body lipolysis and fatty acid oxidation were higher in cancer patients compared to healthy subjects, even after adjusting for food intake. However, this heterogeneous population of cancer patients had varying degrees of weight loss (5.3%–25%/6 months) and were at different stages in the disease trajectory (1–180 months since diagnosis) [23]. Up-regulation of genes involved in mitochondrial fat oxidation such as peroxisome proliferator-activated receptor-gamma coactivator 1 alpha (PGC-1α), and uncoupling protein 2 (UCP-2) have been demonstrated in animal models of cancer cachexia [11]. Enhanced fat oxidation reflected by a decreased respiratory quotient (RQ) [17,44], higher expression of genes related to energy and FA metabolism pathways such as Krebs TCA cycle, oxidative phosphorylation, and FA degradation have been reported in patients with cachexia [17]. No differences were observed in expression of genes involved in fatty acid oxidation including PPARα, PGC-1α, carnitine palmitoyltransferase 1 alpha (CPT1α) in mice bearing Colon-26 carcinoma compared to controls. However, mRNA expression of peroxisomal bifunctional enzyme (Pbe), specific for peroxisomal fatty acid oxidation, was higher in cachectic mice [62]. Another study found that mRNA levels of Cell death-inducing DFFA (DNA fragmentation factor-alpha)-like effector A (Cidea), which mediates oxidation of excess FAs rather than glucose, is increased in SAT of cachectic patients. In addition, cachectic patients had lower plasma TGs, increased FAs and glycerol, and lower RQ indicating elevated FA oxidation [44]. In pancreatic cancer patients, Cidea expression was higher in intra-abdominal adipose tissue compared to subcutaneous in early stages of tumor progression. CT image analysis of these same patients revealed that patients were losing intra-abdominal fat more than subcutaneous fat [32].

Excess fatty acids from enhanced lipolysis are oxidized by mitochondria to produce energy. However, the appearance of brown adipocytes within the white adipose tissue can dissipate energy of substrate oxidation as heat through uncoupling fatty acid oxidation from ATP production by uncoupling protein-1 (UCP1) [63]. Recently, studies found that white adipose tissue browning can contribute to adipose atrophy in cancer by enhancing white fat thermogenesis [39,64]. Small adipocytes with large nuclei were observed during early stages of cachexia in SAT of mouse models of lung and pancreatic cancer. Multi-locular cells interspersed in the white adipose tissue, resembling brown adipocytes, positively stained for UCP-1 [39]. White adipose tissue browning was associated with increased expression of brown fat markers including UCP-1, PGC-1α, PPARγ and Cidea in cachectic mice compared to the controls [39,64]. β-adrenergic signaling, inflammatory cytokines like interleukin-6 (IL-6) [39] and tumor-derived parathyroid hormone-related protein (PTHrP) [64] can mediate white adipose browning by inducing expression of thermogenic genes. Blocking of these mediators might help to prevent adipose atrophy in cancer cachexia [39,64]. Collectively, lipolysis, increase fatty acid oxidation and elevated white adipose tissue thermogenesis play an important role in AT depletion in cancer.

4.3. Lipogenesis and Lipid Deposition

Despite the importance of lipolysis in fat loss in cancer, fat depletion can also occur when lipogenesis is limited in white adipose tissue. In murine cachectic models (Yoshida AH-130 ascites hepatoma), decreased AT lipogenesis was accompanied by an increase in liver lipogenesis and hypertriglyceridemia [42]. Decreased lipogenesis was accompanied by lower activities of FAS, citrate cleavage enzyme, and malic enzyme in rats bearing a mammary adenocarcinoma during late phases of tumor progression [43]. Deterioration in lipid synthesis capacity of epidydimal adipose tissue was observed in MAC16 bearing rats, evidenced by decreased mRNA levels of important lipogenic enzymes such as acetyl-CoA carboxylase, FAS, stearoyl-CoA desaturase-1 and glycerol-3-phosphate acyltransferase [11].

Increased lipolysis and decreased lipogenesis has been reported in male Japanese white rabbits bearing the VX2 tumor cells compared to food-restricted animals. Body weight reduction and fat loss occurred before any decrease in food intake [65]. Adipocyte apoptosis (20–30 days after tumor implantation) was also observed in tumor groups, however no changes in total body fat cell numbers has been reported in previous human studies [15–17]. Discrepancies may be caused by the fact that patients in previous studies were at early stages of disease and also the fat cell numbers were extrapolated based on the total body fat and mean fat cell volume. In contrast to those human studies, animals were followed during cancer progression and also biological differences and limitations of extrapolating results between different species may contribute to the discrepancies.

LPL mediate FAs uptake in adipose tissue by hydrolysis of very-low-density lipoproteins and chylomicrons. Numerous animal studies suggest reduced LPL activity in cancer [42,43,45,46]. Reduction in AT LPL activity in tumor bearing mice to the levels of starved animals was associated with impaired lipid deposition, fat loss, reduced breakdown of plasma lipoproteins and increased circulating lipid concentrations [47]. Decreased adipose tissue LPL activity was associated with hypertriglyceridemia during early stages of tumor growth in Lewis rats bearing a mammary adenocarcinoma [43]. Decreased fat content and LPL activity in WAT was accompanied by increasing circulating triglycerides, and body weight loss induced by the Yoshida AH-130 ascites hepatoma in rats [42,45,46]. In mice bearing MAC16, plasma TGs decreased during cancer progression, regardless of the amount of weight loss. At early stages, plasma FFA decreased and LPL activity increased; however, at advanced stages of tumor, LPL activity decreased [49].

While the majority of studies have utilized animal models to investigate lipogenesis and LPL activity during cancer progression, the human studies have reported decreased mRNA expression and activity of LPL and FAS in VAT in proximity to a tumor compared to distal adipose tissue in colorectal cancer patients [48]. Decreased FAS activity in adipose tissue and elevated activity in tumor cells might be important for tumor cell growth [48]. No changes were observed in lipogenesis in adipocytes isolated from cancer patients' SAT, compared to controls [16]. Lower plasma TG and higher glycerol and FFAs have been observed in cachectic patients [16,17,27] but the activity or expression of LPL was not determined in these studies. Further studies are required to determine the lipogenesis capacity and fatty acid uptake by adipose tissue in various groups of cancer patients at different stages during disease trajectory.

4.4. Adipogenesis

Fat loss may arise from impairment in the adipose tissue development and ability for fat synthesis and storage capacity. Adipogenesis is a highly regulated process which encompasses preadipocyte proliferation and differentiation into mature adipocytes. Adipogenesis is then followed by lipogenesis to store lipid in fat cells. TNF-α, a proinflammatory cytokine produced by both tumor and adipose tissue regulates adipocyte differentiation [66]. Therefore, higher production of TNF-α in cancer-associated cachexia may lead to the altered differentiation status of adipocytes. A reduction in mRNA levels of adipogenic transcription factors including CCAAT-enhancer-binding proteins (c/EBPβ), PPARγ, c/EBPα, sterol regulatory element binding protein-1c (SREBP-1c) in epididymal adipose tissue of mice bearing MAC16 tumor was associated with diminished adipocytes size [11]. Expression of adipogenic factors including C/EBPα, SREBP1C and PPARγ decreased in rats bearing Walker 256 during early stages of cachexia. Morphological changes evident by smaller adipocytes occurred during late stages of cachexia which supports a reduction in expression of adipogenic genes [14]. Lower expression of adipogenic genes such as C/EBPα, Reverba, Per2 and PPARγ has been reported in cachectic mice bearing the Colon-26 carcinoma [62]. More research in both animal and human models is required to demonstrate the possible alterations in adipogenesis during cancer progression.

5. Local Adipose Tissue Inflammation

Proinflammatory cytokines, *i.e.*, IL-1β, TNF-α, IL-6 produced by tumor or host tissue due to tumor presence leads to both systemic and local inflammation in cancer [67,68]. Visceral adipose tissue is a more active producer of inflammatory cytokines IL-6, TNF-α [69,70]. However, data on local adipose tissue inflammation in cancer are inconsistent, being reported as either increased [14,62,71] or unchanged [11,16,17,31,32]. Walker 256 carcinoma caused elevated expression of macrophage markers (f4/80, CD68) especially during late stages of tumor progression [14]. Mesenteric and epididymal adipose tissue were the most and least commonly affected fat depots by macrophages, respectively [14]. In mice bearing Colon-26 carcinoma, depleted fat mass was associated with enhanced inflammatory IL-6/STAT3 cytokine signaling pathway [62]. IL-6 induces signal transducer and activator of transcription-3 (STAT3) activation through phosphorylation. Elevated levels of phosphorylated STAT3 in cachectic mice compared to the control group were observed [62]. Higher mRNA expression of TNF-α in SAT, not VAT, of cachectic GI cancer patients compared to weight-stable cancer patients was reported in newly diagnosed cancer patients. [71]. Contrary to those studies, no change in mRNA expression of inflammatory markers including IL-6 and TNF-α were observed in SAT from cancer patients [16,17] or in an animal model [11]. This paralleled the observation that macrophages or lymphocytes did not infiltrate SAT, as there were no changes in mRNA levels of CD68 (macrophages infiltration marker), CD3 (T-lymphocytes marker) [16] in humans, and MAC1 and F4/80 (macrophage markers) expression in animals [11]. Monocyte chemoattractant protein-1 (MCP-1) and TNF-α mRNA levels in both intra-abdominal and subcutaneous depots did not differ between pancreatic cancer patient and non-cancer controls. However, mRNA expression of MCP-1 and TNF-α in intra-abdominal adipose tissue negatively correlated with post-operative change in intra-abdominal mass assessed by CT scans [32]. This paradox may be due to differences in tumor stages between studies, involvement of other cytokines such as transforming growth factor-b (TGF-b), IL-1 or interferon gamma in cancer associated cachexia or the balance between anti- and pro-inflammatory cytokines of might be important for cachexia-associated inflammation [61,72]. Another explanation is that a cytokine like TNF-α is involved in early stages of cachexia but is transient in nature. Therefore, due to its short half-life and different assay sensitivities, results should be interpreted with caution (reviewed by Das and Hoefler) [61]. Alternate markers such as TNF-R1 and TNF-R2 (Soluble TNF-α membrane receptors) may be more accurate markers than TNF-α due to their longer half-life and stability [73]. Overall, a major gap remains related to comparison of local inflammatory markers in both visceral and subcutaneous depots. Inflammatory cytokines can mediate fat loss in cancer (reviewed by Bing [74]), therefore, assessing whether depot-specific differences in inflammatory cytokines transcription may contribute to inflammatory factors production and subsequent alterations in fat mass would be of great value.

6. Conclusions

Alterations in adipose tissue fat metabolism including changes in expression of genes involved in fat synthesis, storage, mobilization or oxidation, browning of white adipose tissue, adipocytes development, and elevated inflammatory signaling may have a role in fat loss in cancer patients. Fat accumulation at the time of diagnosis may contribute to cancer progression but the accelerated rate of adipose tissue loss would be expected to be associated with shorter survival time during cancer progression. Alterations in fat mass and composition between visceral and subcutaneous depots are equivocal in cancer trajectory and little is known regarding these alterations. The prognostic significance of these depots needs to be investigated in large populations throughout the cancer progression. Due to various roles of adipose tissue in controlling human metabolism, further identification of mechanisms and mediators of fat loss in cancer would help in the identifying fat-losing cancer patients that would benefit from early therapeutic interventions which could improve survival and prevent muscle atrophy in these patients. Finally, results need to be interpreted carefully as factors including tumor type, cancer stage, response to treatment and metabolic capacity of patients may influence findings.

Author Contributions: Maryam Ebadi and Vera C. Mazurak contributed to the conception and intellectual content of the paper.

References

1. Ibrahim, M.M. Subcutaneous and visceral adipose tissue: Structural and functional differences. *Obes. Rev.* **2010**, *11*, 11–18.

2. Ntambi, J.M.; Young-Cheul, K. Adipocyte differentiation and gene expression. *J. Nutr.* **2000**, *130*, 3122–3126.

3. Park, J.; Euhus, D.M.; Scherer, P.E. Paracrine and endocrine effects of adipose tissue on cancer development and progression. *Endocr. Rev.* **2011**, *32*, 550–570. [PubMed]

4. Guilherme, A.; Virbasius, J.V.; Puri, V.; Czech, M.P. Adipocyte dysfunctions linking obesity to insulin resistance and type 2 diabetes. *Nat. Rev. Mol. Cell Biol.* **2008**, *9*, 367–377. [CrossRef] [PubMed]

5. Calle, E.E.; Kaaks, R. Overweight, obesity and cancer: Epidemiological evidence and proposed mechanisms. *Nat. Rev. Cancer* **2004**, *4*, 579–591. [CrossRef] [PubMed]

6. Prieto-Hontoria, P.L.; Perez-Matute, P.; Fernandez-Galilea, M.; Bustos, M.; Martinez, J.A.; Moreno-Aliaga, M.J. Role of obesity-associated dysfunctional adipose tissue in cancer: A molecular nutrition approach. *Biochim. Biophys. Acta* **2011**, *1807*, 664–678. [CrossRef] [PubMed]

7. Fearon, K.C. Cancer cachexia: Developing multimodal therapy for a multidimensional problem. *Eur. J. Cancer* **2008**, *44*, 1124–1132. [CrossRef] [PubMed]

8. Murphy, R.A.; Wilke, M.S.; Perrine, M.; Pawlowicz, M.; Mourtzakis, M.; Lieffers, J.R.; Maneshgar, M.; Bruera, E.; Clandinin, M.T.; Baracos, V.E.; *et al.* Loss of adipose tissue and plasma phospholipids: Relationship to survival in advanced cancer patients. *Clin. Nutr.* **2010**, *29*, 482–487. [CrossRef] [PubMed]

9. Fouladiun, M.; Korner, U.; Bosaeus, I.; Daneryd, P.; Hyltander, A.; Lundholm, K.G. Body composition and time course changes in regional distribution of fat and lean tissue in unselected cancer patients on palliative care—Correlations with food intake, metabolism, exercise capacity, and hormones. *Cancer* **2005**, *103*, 2189–2198. [CrossRef] [PubMed]

10. Fearon, K.; Strasser, F.; Anker, S.D.; Bosaeus, I.; Bruera, E.; Fainsinger, R.L.; Jatoi, A.; Loprinzi, C.; MacDonald, N.; Mantovani, G.; *et al.* Definition and classification of cancer cachexia: An international consensus. *Lancet Oncol.* **2011**, *12*, 489–495. [CrossRef] [PubMed]

11. Bing, C.; Russell, S.; Becket, E.; Pope, M.; Tisdale, M.J.; Trayhurn, P.; Jenkins, J.R. Adipose atrophy in cancer cachexia: Morphologic and molecular analysis of adipose tissue in tumour-bearing mice. *Br. J. Cancer* **2006**, *95*, 1028–1037. [CrossRef]

12. Machado, A.P.; Costa Rosa, L.F.; Seelaender, M.C. Adipose tissue in walker 256 tumour-induced cachexia: Possible association between decreased leptin concentration and mononuclear cell infiltration. *Cell Tissue Res.* **2004**, *318*, 503–514. [CrossRef] [PubMed]

13. Bertevello, P.S.; Seelaender, M.C. Heterogeneous response of adipose tissue to cancer cachexia. *Braz. J. Med. Biol. Res.* **2001**, *34*, 1161–1167. [CrossRef] [PubMed]

14. Batista, M.L., Jr.; Neves, R.X.; Peres, S.B.; Yamashita, A.S.; Shida, C.S.; Farmer, S.R.; Seelaender, M. Heterogeneous time-dependent response of adipose tissue during the development of cancer cachexia. *J. Endocrinol.* **2012**, *215*, 363–373. [CrossRef] [PubMed]

15. Agustsson, T.; Ryden, M.; Hoffstedt, J.; van Harmelen, V.; Dicker, A.; Laurencikiene, J.; Isaksson, B.; Permert, J.; Arner, P. Mechanism of increased lipolysis in cancer cachexia. *Cancer Res.* **2007**, *67*, 5531–5537. [CrossRef] [PubMed]

16. Ryden, M.; Agustsson, T.; Laurencikiene, J.; Britton, T.; Sjolin, E.; Isaksson, B.; Permert, J.; Arner, P. Lipolysis—Not inflammation, cell death, or lipogenesis—Is involved in adipose tissue loss in cancer cachexia. *Cancer* **2008**, *113*, 1695–1704. [CrossRef] [PubMed]

17. Dahlman, I.; Mejhert, N.; Linder, K.; Agustsson, T.; Mutch, D.M.; Kulyte, A.; Isaksson, B.; Permert, J.; Petrovic, N.; Nedergaard, J.; *et al.* Adipose tissue pathways involved in weight loss of cancer cachexia. *Br. J. Cancer* **2010**, *102*, 1541–1548. [CrossRef] [PubMed]

18. Mracek, T.; Stephens, N.A.; Gao, D.; Bao, Y.; Ross, J.A.; Ryden, M.; Arner, P.; Trayhurn, P.; Fearon, K.C.; Bing, C.; *et al.* Enhanced ZAG production by subcutaneous adipose tissue is linked to weight loss in gastrointestinal cancer patients. *Br. J. Cancer* **2011**, *104*, 441–447. [CrossRef] [PubMed]

19. Otake, S.; Takeda, H.; Suzuki, Y.; Fukui, T.; Watanabe, S.; Ishihama, K.; Saito, T.; Togashi, H.; Nakamura, T.; Matsuzawa, Y.; *et al.* Association of visceral fat accumulation and plasma adiponectin with colorectal adenoma: Evidence for participation of insulin resistance. *Clin. Cancer Res.* **2005**, *11*, 3642–3646. [CrossRef] [PubMed]

20. Hellmer, J.; Marcus, C.; Sonnenfeld, T.; Arner, P. Mechanisms for differences in lipolysis between human subcutaneous and omental fat cells. *J. Clin. Endocrinol. Metab.* **1992**, *75*, 15–20. [PubMed]

21. Fabbro, E.D.; Bruera, E.; Demark-Wahnefried, W.; Bowling, T.; Hopkinson, J.B.; Baracos, V.E. *Nutrition and the Cancer Patient*; Oxford University Press: New York, NY, USA, 2010; pp. 24–28.

22. Cao, D.X.; Wu, G.H.; Yang, Z.A.; Zhang, B.; Jiang, Y.; Han, Y.S.; He, G.D.; Zhuang, Q.L.; Wang, Y.F.; Huang, Z.L.; *et al.* Role of beta1-adrenoceptor in increased lipolysis in cancer cachexia. *Cancer Sci.* **2010**, *101*, 1639–1645. [CrossRef] [PubMed]

23. Zuijdgeest-van Leeuwen, S.D.; van den Berg, J.W.; Wattimena, J.L.; van der Gaast, A.; Swart, G.R.; Wilson, J.H.; Dagnelie, P.C. Lipolysis and lipid oxidation in weight-losing cancer patients and healthy subjects. *Metabolism* **2000**, *49*, 931–936. [CrossRef] [PubMed]

24. Lieffers, J.R.; Mourtzakis, M.; Hall, K.D.; McCargar, L.J.; Prado, C.M.; Baracos, V.E. A viscerally driven cachexia syndrome in patients with advanced colorectal cancer: Contributions of organ and tumor mass to whole-body energy demands. *Am. J. Clin. Nutr.* **2009**, *89*, 1173–1179. [CrossRef] [PubMed]

25. Shen, W.; Punyanitya, M.; Wang, Z.; Gallagher, D.; St-Onge, M.P.; Albu, J.; Heymsfield, S.B.; Heshka, S. Total body skeletal muscle and adipose tissue volumes: Estimation from a single abdominal cross-sectional image. *J. Appl. Physiol.* **2004**, *97*, 2333–2338. [CrossRef] [PubMed]

26. Agustsson, T.; Wikrantz, P.; Ryden, M.; Brismar, T.; Isaksson, B. Adipose tissue volume is decreased in recently diagnosed cancer patients with cachexia. *Nutrition* **2012**, *28*, 851–855. [CrossRef] [PubMed]

27. Ogiwara, H.; Takahashi, S.; Kato, Y.; Uyama, I.; Takahara, T.; Kikuchi, K.; Iida, S. Diminished visceral adipose tissue in cancer cachexia. *J. Surg. Oncol.* **1994**, *57*, 129–133. [CrossRef] [PubMed]

28. Di Sebastiano, K.M.; Yang, L.; Zbuk, K.; Wong, R.K.; Chow, T.; Koff, D.; Moran, G.R.; Mourtzakis, M. Accelerated muscle and adipose tissue loss may predict survival in pancreatic cancer patients: The relationship with diabetes and anaemia. *Br. J. Nutr.* **2013**, *109*, 302–312. [CrossRef] [PubMed]

29. Adams, J.F. The clinical and metabolic consequences of total gastrectomy. I. Morbidity, weight, and nutrition. *Scand. J. Gastroenterol.* **1967**, *2*, 137–149. [CrossRef] [PubMed]

30. Liedman, B.; Andersson, H.; Bosaeus, I.; Hugosson, I.; Lundell, L. Changes in body composition after gastrectomy: Results of a controlled, prospective clinical trial. *World J. Surg.* **1997**, *21*, 416–421. [CrossRef] [PubMed]

31. Bachmann, J.; Heiligensetzer, M.; Krakowski-Roosen, H.; Buchler, M.W.; Friess, H.; Martignoni, M.E. Cachexia worsens prognosis in patients with resectable pancreatic cancer. *J. Gastrointest. Surg.* **2008**, *12*, 1193–1201. [CrossRef] [PubMed]

32. Haugen, F.; Labori, K.J.; Noreng, H.J.; Buanes, T.; Iversen, P.O.; Drevon, C.A. Altered expression of genes in adipose tissues associated with reduced fat mass in patients with pancreatic cancer. *Arch. Physiol. Biochem.* **2011**, *117*, 78–87. [CrossRef] [PubMed]

33. Awad, S.; Tan, B.H.; Cui, H.; Bhalla, A.; Fearon, K.C.; Parsons, S.L.; Catton, J.A.; Lobo, D.N. Marked changes in body composition following neoadjuvant chemotherapy for oesophagogastric cancer. *Clin. Nutr.* **2012**, *31*, 74–77. [CrossRef] [PubMed]

34. Dalal, S.; Hui, D.; Bidaut, L.; Lem, K.; del Fabbro, E.; Crane, C.; Reyes-Gibby, C.C.; Bedi, D.; Bruera, E. Relationships among body mass index, longitudinal body composition alterations, and survival in patients with locally advanced pancreatic cancer receiving chemoradiation: A pilot study. *J. Pain Symptom Manag.* **2012**, *44*, 181–191. [CrossRef]

35. Willemse, P.P.; van der Meer, R.W.; Burggraaf, J.; van Elderen, S.G.; de Kam, M.L.; de Roos, A.; Lamb, H.J.; Osanto, S. Abdominal visceral and subcutaneous fat increase, insulin resistance and hyperlipidemia in testicular cancer patients treated with cisplatin-based chemotherapy. *Acta Oncol.* **2014**, *53*, 351–360. [CrossRef]

36. Prado, C.M.; Sawyer, M.B.; Ghosh, S.; Lieffers, J.R.; Esfandiari, N.; Antoun, S.; Baracos, V.E. Central tenet of cancer cachexia therapy: Do patients with advanced cancer have exploitable anabolic potential? *Am. J. Clin. Nutr.* **2013**, *98*, 1012–1019. [CrossRef]

37. Tan, B.H.; Birdsell, L.A.; Martin, L.; Baracos, V.E.; Fearon, K.C. Sarcopenia in an overweight or obese patient is an adverse prognostic factor in pancreatic cancer. *Clin. Cancer Res.* **2009**, *15*, 6973–6979. [CrossRef] [PubMed]

38. Das, S.K.; Eder, S.; Schauer, S.; Diwoky, C.; Temmel, H.; Guertl, B.; Gorkiewicz, G.; Tamilarasan, K.P.; Kumari, P.; Trauner, M.; *et al.* Adipose triglyceride lipase contributes to cancer-associated cachexia. *Science* **2011**, *333*, 233–238. [CrossRef] [PubMed]

39. Petruzzelli, M.; Schweiger, M.; Schreiber, R.; Campos-Olivas, R.; Tsoli, M.; Allen, J.; Swarbrick, M.; Rose-John, S.; Rincon, M.; Robertson, G.; *et al.* A switch from white to brown fat increases energy expenditure in cancer-associated cachexia. *Cell Metab.* **2014**, *20*, 433–447. [CrossRef] [PubMed]

40. Tisdale, M.J. Cachexia in cancer patients. *Nat. Rev. Cancer* **2002**, *2*, 862–871. [CrossRef] [PubMed]

41. Ryden, M.; Arner, P. Fat loss in cachexia—Is there a role for adipocyte lipolysis? *Clin. Nutr.* **2007**, *26*, 1–6. [CrossRef] [PubMed]

42. Lopez-Soriano, J.; Argiles, J.M.; Lopez-Soriano, F.J. Lipid metabolism in rats bearing the Yoshida AH-130 ascites hepatoma. *Mol. Cell. Biochem.* **1996**, *165*, 17–23. [CrossRef] [PubMed]

43. Lanza-Jacoby, S.; Lansey, S.C.; Miller, E.E.; Cleary, M.P. Sequential changes in the activities of lipoprotein lipase and lipogenic enzymes during tumor growth in rats. *Cancer Res.* **1984**, *44*, 5062–5067. [PubMed]

44. Laurencikiene, J.; Stenson, B.M.; Arvidsson Nordstrom, E.; Agustsson, T.; Langin, D.; Isaksson, B.; Permert, J.; Ryden, M.; Arner, P. Evidence for an important role of CIDEA in human cancer cachexia. *Cancer Res.* **2008**, *68*, 9247–9254. [CrossRef] [PubMed]

45. Lopez-Soriano, J.; Argiles, J.M.; Lopez-Soriano, F.J. Sequential changes in lipoprotein lipase activity and lipaemia induced by the Yoshida AH-130 ascites hepatoma in rats. *Cancer Lett.* **1997**, *116*, 159–165. [CrossRef] [PubMed]

46. Lopez-Soriano, J.; Argiles, J.M.; Lopez-Soriano, F.J. Marked hyperlipidaemia in rats bearing the Yoshida AH-130 ascites hepatoma. *Biochem. Soc. Trans.* **1995**, *23*, 492.

47. Thompson, M.P.; Koons, J.E.; Tan, E.T.; Grigor, M.R. Modified lipoprotein lipase activities, rates of lipogenesis, and lipolysis as factors leading to lipid depletion in C57BL mice bearing the preputial gland tumor, ESR-586. *Cancer Res.* **1981**, *41*, 3228–3232. [PubMed]

48. Notarnicola, M.; Miccolis, A.; Tutino, V.; Lorusso, D.; Caruso, M.G. Low levels of lipogenic enzymes in peritumoral adipose tissue of colorectal cancer patients. *Lipids* **2012**, *47*, 59–63. [CrossRef] [PubMed]

49. Briddon, S.; Beck, S.A.; Tisdale, M.J. Changes in activity of lipoprotein lipase, plasma free fatty acids and triglycerides with weight loss in a cachexia model. *Cancer Lett.* **1991**, *57*, 49–53. [CrossRef] [PubMed]

50. Bennani-Baiti, N.; Walsh, D. Animal models of the cancer anorexia-cachexia syndrome. *Support. Care Cancer* **2011**, *19*, 1451–1463. [CrossRef] [PubMed]

51. Bosaeus, I.; Daneryd, P.; Lundholm, K. Dietary intake, resting energy expenditure, weight loss and survival in cancer patients. *J. Nutr.* **2002**, *132*, 3465–3466.

52. Cao, D.X.; Wu, G.H.; Zhang, B.; Quan, Y.J.; Wei, J.; Jin, H.; Jiang, Y.; Yang, Z.A. Resting energy expenditure and body composition in patients with newly detected cancer. *Clin. Nutr.* **2010**, *29*, 72–77. [CrossRef] [PubMed]

53. Johnson, G.; Salle, A.; Lorimier, G.; Laccourreye, L.; Enon, B.; Blin, V.; Jousset, Y.; Arnaud, J.P.; Malthiery, Y.; Simard, G.; *et al.* Cancer cachexia: Measured and predicted resting energy expenditures for nutritional needs evaluation. *Nutrition* **2008**, *24*, 443–450. [CrossRef] [PubMed]

54. Fredrix, E.W.; Soeters, P.B.; Wouters, E.F.; Deerenberg, I.M.; von Meyenfeldt, M.F.; Saris, W.H. Effect of different tumor types on resting energy expenditure. *Cancer Res.* **1991**, *51*, 6138–6141. [PubMed]

55. Klein, S.; Wolfe, R.R. Whole-body lipolysis and triglyceride-fatty acid cycling in cachectic patients with esophageal cancer. *J. Clin. Investig.* **1990**, *86*, 1403–1408. [CrossRef]

56. Jeevanandam, M.; Horowitz, G.D.; Lowry, S.F.; Brennan, M.F. Cancer cachexia and the rate of whole body lipolysis in man. *Metabolism* **1986**, *35*, 304–310. [CrossRef] [PubMed]

57. Jaworski, K.; Sarkadi-Nagy, E.; Duncan, R.E.; Ahmadian, M.; Sul, H.S. Regulation of triglyceride metabolism. IV. Hormonal regulation of lipolysis in adipose tissue. *Am. J. Physiol. Gastrointest. Liver Physiol.* **2007**, *293*, 1–4. [CrossRef]

58. Jocken, J.W.; Blaak, E.E. Catecholamine-induced lipolysis in adipose tissue and skeletal muscle in obesity. *Physiol. Behav.* **2008**, *94*, 219–230. [CrossRef] [PubMed]

59. Holm, C. Molecular mechanisms regulating hormone-sensitive lipase and lipolysis. *Biochem. Soc. Trans.* **2003**, *31*, 1120–1124. [CrossRef] [PubMed]

60. Thompson, M.P.; Cooper, S.T.; Parry, B.R.; Tuckey, J.A. Increased expression of the mRNA for hormone-sensitive lipase in adipose tissue of cancer patients. *Biochim. Biophys. Acta* **1993**, *1180*, 236–242. [CrossRef] [PubMed]

61. Das, S.K.; Hoefler, G. The role of triglyceride lipases in cancer associated cachexia. *Trends Mol. Med.* **2013**, *19*, 292–301. [CrossRef] [PubMed]

62. Tsoli, M.; Schweiger, M.; Vanniasinghe, A.S.; Painter, A.; Zechner, R.; Clarke, S.; Robertson, G. Depletion of white adipose tissue in cancer cachexia syndrome is associated with inflammatory signaling and disrupted circadian regulation. *PLoS One* **2014**, *9*. [CrossRef] [PubMed]

63. Harms, M.; Seale, P. Brown and beige fat: Development, function and therapeutic potential. *Nat. Med.* **2013**, *19*, 1252–1263. [CrossRef] [PubMed]

64. Kir, S.; White, J.P.; Kleiner, S.; Kazak, L.; Cohen, P.; Baracos, V.E.; Spiegelman, B.M. Tumour-derived PTH-related protein triggers adipose tissue browning and cancer cachexia. *Nature* **2014**, *513*, 100–104. [CrossRef] [PubMed]

65. Ishiko, O.; Nishimura, S.; Yasui, T.; Sumi, T.; Hirai, K.; Honda, K.; Ogita, S. Metabolic and morphologic characteristics of adipose tissue associated with the growth of malignant tumors. *Jpn. J. Cancer Res.* **1999**, *90*, 655–659. [CrossRef] [PubMed]

66. Cawthorn, W.P.; Heyd, F.; Hegyi, K.; Sethi, J.K. Tumour necrosis factor-alpha inhibits adipogenesis *via* a beta-catenin/TCF4 (TCF7L2)-dependent pathway. *Cell Death Differ.* **2007**, *14*, 1361–1373. [CrossRef] [PubMed]

67. Bing, C.; Trayhurn, P. New insights into adipose tissue atrophy in cancer cachexia. *Proc. Nutr. Soc.* **2009**, *68*, 385–392. [CrossRef] [PubMed]

68. Lin, W.W.; Karin, M. A cytokine-mediated link between innate immunity, inflammation, and cancer. *J. Clin. Investig.* **2007**, *117*, 1175–1183. [CrossRef] [PubMed]

69. Harman-Boehm, I.; Bluher, M.; Redel, H.; Sion-Vardy, N.; Ovadia, S.; Avinoach, E.; Shai, I.; Kloting, N.; Stumvoll, M.; Bashan, N.; *et al.* Macrophage infiltration into omental *versus* subcutaneous fat across different populations: Effect of regional adiposity and the comorbidities of obesity. *J. Clin. Endocrinol. Metab.* **2007**, *92*, 2240–2247. [CrossRef] [PubMed]

70. Fain, J.N.; Madan, A.K.; Hiler, M.L.; Cheema, P.; Bahouth, S.W. Comparison of the release of adipokines by adipose tissue, adipose tissue matrix, and adipocytes from visceral and subcutaneous abdominal adipose tissues of obese humans. *Endocrinology* **2004**, *145*, 2273–2282. [CrossRef] [PubMed]

71. Batista, M.L., Jr.; Olivan, M.; Alcantara, P.S.; Sandoval, R.; Peres, S.B.; Neves, R.X.; Silverio, R.; Maximiano, L.F.; Otoch, J.P.; Seelaender, M.; *et al.* Adipose tissue-derived factors as potential biomarkers in cachectic cancer patients. *Cytokine* **2013**, *61*, 532–539. [CrossRef] [PubMed]

72. Argiles, J.M.; Alvarez, B.; Lopez-Soriano, F.J. The metabolic basis of cancer cachexia. *Med. Res. Rev.* **1997**, *17*, 477–498. [CrossRef] [PubMed]

73. Hosono, K.; Yamada, E.; Endo, H.; Takahashi, H.; Inamori, M.; Hippo, Y.; Nakagama, H.; Nakajima, A. Increased tumor necrosis factor receptor 1 expression in human colorectal adenomas. *World J. Gastroenterol.* **2012**, *18*, 5360–5368. [CrossRef] [PubMed]

74. Bing, C. Lipid mobilization in cachexia: Mechanisms and mediators. *Curr. Opin. Support. Palliat. Care* **2011**, *5*, 356–360. [CrossRef] [PubMed]

5

Inflammaging and Cancer: A Challenge for the Mediterranean Diet

Rita Ostan [1], Catia Lanzarini [1,2], Elisa Pini [1], Maria Scurti [1], Dario Vianello [1], Claudia Bertarelli [1], Cristina Fabbri [1], Massimo Izzi [2], Giustina Palmas [2], Fiammetta Biondi [2], Morena Martucci [1], Elena Bellavista [1,2], Stefano Salvioli [1,2], Miriam Capri [1,2], Claudio Franceschi [1,3,4] and Aurelia Santoro [1,*]

[1] Department of Experimental, Diagnostic and Specialty Medicine (DIMES), University of Bologna, Via San Giacomo 12, 40126 Bologna, Italy; rita.ostan3@unibo.it (R.O.); catia.lanzarini2@unibo.it (C.L.); elisa.pini5@unibo.it (E.P.); maria.scurti@unibo.it (M.S.); dario.vianello@unibo.it (D.V.); claudia.bertarelli@unibo.it (C.B.); cristina.fabbri12@unibo.it (C.F.); morena.martucci3@unibo.it (M.M.); elena.bellavista2@unibo.it (E.B.); stefano.salvioli@unibo.it (S.S.); miriam.capri@unibo.it (M.C.); claudio.franceschi@unibo.it (C.F.)

[2] Interdepartmental Centre "L. Galvani" (CIG) University of Bologna, Via San Giacomo 12, 40126 Bologna, Italy; massimo.izzi@unibo.it (M.I.); mariagiustina.palmas@unibo.it (G.P.); fiammetta.biondi2@unibo.it (F.B.)

[3] IRCCS, Institute of Neurological Sciences, Via Altura 3, 40139 Bologna, Italy

[4] National Research Council of Italy, CNR, Institute for Organic Synthesis and Photoreactivity (ISOF), Via P. Gobetti 101, 40129 Bologna, Italy

* Author to whom correspondence should be addressed; aurelia.santoro@unibo.it

Abstract: Aging is considered the major risk factor for cancer, one of the most important mortality causes in the western world. Inflammaging, a state of chronic, low-level systemic inflammation, is a pervasive feature of human aging. Chronic inflammation increases cancer risk and affects all cancer stages, triggering the initial genetic mutation or epigenetic mechanism, promoting cancer initiation, progression and metastatic diffusion. Thus, inflammaging is a strong candidate to connect age and cancer. A corollary of this hypothesis is that interventions aiming to decrease inflammaging should protect against cancer, as well as most/all age-related diseases. Epidemiological data are concordant in suggesting that the Mediterranean Diet (MD) decreases the risk of a variety of cancers but the underpinning mechanism(s) is (are) still unclear. Here we review data indicating that the MD (as a whole diet or single bioactive nutrients typical of the MD) modulates multiple interconnected processes involved in carcinogenesis and inflammatory response such as free radical production, NF-κB activation and expression of inflammatory mediators, and the eicosanoids pathway. Particular attention is devoted to the capability of MD to affect the balance between pro- and anti-inflammaging as well as to emerging topics such as maintenance of gut microbiota (GM) homeostasis and epigenetic modulation of oncogenesis through specific microRNAs.

Keywords: aging; inflammation; inflammaging; cancer; mediterranean diet; nutrients; microRNAs; NU-AGE project

1. Inflammaging as a Major Component of Aging, Age-Related Diseases and Cancer

Human aging is a complex, extremely heterogeneous and dynamic trait determined by a number of environmental, genetic, epigenetic, and stochastic factors [1]. A pervasive feature of human aging and probably one of its major causes, is represented by the chronic, low-level state of systemic and sterile (in the absence of overt infection) inflammation called "inflammaging" [2,3]. Indeed, inflammation has been recently included among the seven pillars of aging [4]. It can be beneficial as an acute, transient immune response to harmful conditions, facilitating the repair, turnover and adaptation of many tissues. However, during aging, inflammatory response tends to become chronic and of low grade, leading to tissue degeneration.

Indeed, inflammaging is characterized by a general increase in plasma levels and cell capability to produce pro-inflammatory cytokines such as Interleukin-6 (IL-6), Interleukin-1 (IL-1) and Tumour Necrosis Factor-α (TNF-α) and by a subsequent increase of the main inflammatory markers, such as C-reactive protein (CRP) and serum amyloid A (A-SAA) [2,5]. This generalized pro-inflammatory status, interacting with the genetic background and environmental factors, potentially triggers the onset of the most important age-related diseases, such as cardiovascular diseases, atherosclerosis, metabolic syndrome, type 2 diabetes, obesity, neurodegeneration, arthrosis and arthritis, osteoporosis and osteoarthritis, sarcopenia, major depression, frailty and cancer [6,7].

The hypothesis of a possible correlation between cancer and inflammation was firstly formulated by the Greek physician Galenus [8,9]. In 1863 Rudolph Virchow, a pioneer of cellular pathology, noted inflammatory cells within tumor mass and that tumors arise at sites of chronic inflammation [10,11]. A functional framework developed by Hanahan and Weinberg (2000) characterizes cancer by six biological hallmarks, able to regulate the conversion of normal cells in cancer cells: self-sufficiency in growth signals, insensitivity to growth inhibitory signals, limitless replicative potential, the ability to evade programmed cell-death (apoptosis), the ability to sustain angiogenesis, the ability to invade tissues and metastasize [12]. Studies have also supported the important role of inflammatory cells and cytokines in the tumor microenvironment [13–15]. In 2011, Weinberg and Hanahan proposed four additional new cancer hallmarks: ability to evade the immune system, presence of inflammation, tendency towards genomic instability and dysregulated metabolism [16]. The correlation between chronic inflammation and cancer has been supported by epidemiological and experimental studies on humans and animal models [13,15,17] along with the observation that preventive treatments with anti-inflammatory drugs such as aspirin or cyclooxygenase-2 (COX-2) inhibitors reduce the risk of developing colorectal and breast cancer and even mortality [15,18,19]. Chronic inflammation affects all cancer stages, increasing the onset risk, supporting the initial genetic mutation or epigenetic mechanism leading to cancer initiation [20–22], promoting tumor progression, and supporting metastatic diffusion [9,22–25].

We recently hypothesised that it is important to distinguish between systemic inflammaging and local inflammaging. While the pathological and pathogenetic role of circulating pro-inflammatory compounds and cytokines is unclear and possibly negligible (a marker of inflammation rather than an active player), there are a number of observations and papers suggesting that the local production of inflammatory cytokines can have strong deleterious effects, as we recently suggested in the case of breast cancer niche as a paradigmatic example [26,27]. Therefore, it is tempting to speculate that the important aspect to be considered in inflammaging and cancer is not the mere increase in inflammatory mediators but rather the source, and therefore the local targets, of these mediators. The tangled interplay among local immune responses and systemic inflammation and their influence on clinical outcomes in cancer has been recently reviewed [28].

Different types of tissues (muscle, adipose tissue), organs (brain and liver), systems (immune system) and ecosystems (gut microbiota, GM) may contribute to the systemic inflammatory state, through altered production of pro-inflammatory and/or anti-inflammatory mediators [5,7,26,29,30].

Inflammaging can be influenced by many other factors, such as microRNAs (miRs) and agalactosylated N-glycans, together with the products and metabolites of the intestinal microbiota.

Additionally, some mitochondrial components, including mtDNA and other "cellular debris" released outside of the cells, as a consequence of natural cell turnover/damage, could trigger and sustain a sort of "physiological inflammatory tone" that increases with age [31]. This conceptualization can be extended to nutrients, whereby an excess of nutrients could be therefore capable of triggering an inflammatory response [32–34] that has been dubbed "metaflammation" [35], contributing to the above-mentioned physiological inflammatory tone.

Inflammatory Sources for Cancer Development

Apart from inflammaging, viruses, bacteria and parasite infections as well as the exposure to chemical or physical agents can support chronic inflammation and have been linked to several cancer types [36–38]. Similarly, unresolved inflammation unrelated to infections can also contribute to carcinogenesis as observed in Barrett's metaplasia, chronic pancreatitis or esophagitis [21,38–43] or in autoimmune diseases [21].

Obesity plays a central role in carcinogenesis since adipose tissue has been recognized as an endocrine source of mediators (hormones, acute-phase proteins, cytokines, adipokines and growth factors, [44]) able to sustain a chronic low-grade inflammation. During the last fifteen years, obesity has been associated with several types of tumors such as breast, endometrium, prostate, kidney, esophagus, stomach, colon, pancreas, gallbladder, and liver [45–49] and also with an increased cancer aggressiveness, risk of relapse and mortality [49].

A large amount of data indicates that inflammation is closely connected to oxidative stress. Reactive oxygen species (ROS) are continuously produced by our cells as a by-product of oxidative metabolism and are essential for several physiological functions and signalling pathways. However, an excessive accumulation of ROS may cause cellular oxidative damage to nucleic acids and proteins in cells of several systems including the endocrine and the immune systems [26,50]. We have recently hypothesised that most of the deleterious effects of excessive oxidative stress in tissues and organs can be mediated by the induction of unwanted inflammatory reactions [50].

Indeed, an important characteristic of tumor promoters is their ability to recruit inflammatory cells and to stimulate them to generate ROS [51]. Mast cells and leukocytes recruited to the site of damage lead to a "respiratory burst" due to an increased uptake of oxygen and, thus, an increased release and accumulation of ROS at the site of damage [20]. On the other hand, inflammatory cells also produce soluble mediators, such as metabolites of arachidonic acid, CRP, cytokines (IL-1, IL-6), and chemokines, which act by further recruiting inflammatory cells to the site of damage and producing more reactive species. This sustained inflammatory/oxidative environment leads to a vicious cycle, which can affect healthy neighboring epithelial and stromal cells, by inducing DNA damage and activating epigenetic mechanisms, and over a long period of time may lead to carcinogenesis.

During tumor progression, immune and inflammatory cells produce cytokines and chemokines, which facilitate cancer cell survival and proliferation, and promote the angiogenic switch enhancing tumor growth [52]. Cytokines and chemokines also induce further recruitment and differentiation of immune cells in the tumor microenvironment [53]. The key mediators can activate signal transduction cascades and induce changes in transcription factors, such as nuclear factor-κB (NF-κB), signal transducer and activator of transcription 3 (STAT3), PPAR-γ, β-catenin, p53, hypoxia-inducible factor-1α (HIF-1α), activator protein-1 (AP-1), nuclear factor of activated T cells (NFAT), and NF-E2 related factor-2 (Nrf2), which mediates immediate cellular stress responses [54]. All these molecules are regulated by the transcription factor NF-κB [55], which could be considered as a "hub" in tumorigenesis linking cellular senescence, inflammaging and cancer [23]. As summarized in Figure 1, almost all gene products involved in inflammation are indeed regulated by the activation of NF-κB (e.g., TNF-α, IL-1, IL-6, chemokines, COX-2, 5LOX, CRP) [56] and NF-κB is activated in response to several well known cancer risk factors such as smoke, stress, dietary agents, obesity, infectious agents and irradiation. Moreover, NF-κB has been associated with transformation of cells [57] and is constitutively active in most tumor cells. Cellular senescence, a tumour suppressive stress response, is associated with a secretory phenotype that might be an important additional contributor to chronic inflammation [58]. Senescent cells are in fact characterized by the capability to produce high amounts of pro-inflammatory proteins [59,60]. The senescent phenotype is also accompanied by an upregulation of the DNA damage-response system and recently it has been proposed that the accrual of DNA damage with age can contribute significantly to inflammaging via the production of IL-6 [27]. In the cancer field this phenomenon, related to the propagation to bystander cells of DNA damage, DNA damage response and inflammation, has been conceptualized as "para-flammation" [61].

All these exogenous and endogenous danger signals (viruses, bacteria, including the GM and its products, damaged and senescent cells, cell debris, altered/modified proteins, N-glycans, mtDNA, ROS, *etc.*) are overall conceptualized by our group as "garbage", able to trigger inflammaging and inflammation. Indeed, all these "dysfunctional" molecules can be sensed by receptors of the innate immune response and thus are potential stimulants of pro-inflammatory responses. This "garbage" is an inevitable byproduct of the normal metabolism, but its accumulation becomes evident with advancing age and/or in pathological conditions [3], due to the lifelong exposure to exogenous/endogenous insults on one side, and to the decreased capacity of the ubiquitin-proteasome system [62,63] and autophagy [64] to cope with these products on the other side.

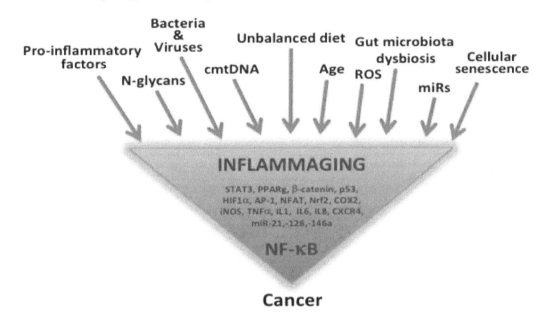

Figure 1. Among the main causes of inflammaging, we found the accumulation of pro-inflammatory factors, viruses and bacteria, age, reactive oxygen species (ROS) and cellular senescence. Inflammaging can also be influenced by many other factors, including non-immunological ones, and those not directly related to inflammation, such as microRNAs (miRs), circulating mitochondrial DNA (cmtDNA) and agalactosylated N-glycans, together with the products and related metabolites of the intestinal microbiota. Several pathways and molecules are triggered by these factors, which then are able to activate the nuclear transcription factor NF-κB which could be considered as a hub in carcinogenesis, linking inflammaging, cellular senescence and cancer.

2. The Mediterranean Diet

2.1. The Mediterranean Diet: Definitions and Characteristics

In literature, there are various definitions of the Mediterranean Diet (MD) but they generally share the main components: a high consumption of vegetables, fruits, whole grains, legumes, olive oil and fish (especially marine species), a low intake of saturated fats such as butter and other animal fats, red meat, poultry, dairy products and a regular but moderate consume of ethanol mainly consisting of red wine during meals. Some of these features overlap with other healthy dietary patterns, whereas other aspects are unique to the MD.

The MD is the typical dietary pattern of the populations bordering the Mediterranean area. The traditional MD has been accepted and acknowledged by the scientific community following the publication by Ancel Keys and colleagues showing results from the Seven Countries Study. The purpose of this longitudinal epidemiological study, started in the late 1950s, was to examine the relationships between lifestyle and dietary factors and cardiovascular diseases in populations from different regions of the world (the USA, Northern Europe, Southern Europe and Japan). Resulting data indicated that the mortality rate for coronary heart disease was higher in the USA and Northern Europe in comparison to Southern Europe. In particular, subjects from Greece and Italy showed the lowest mortality for cardiovascular diseases [65]. In 2003, the PREDIMED study found that the MD supplemented with extra virgin olive oil or tree nuts was able to prevent cardiovascular diseases in comparison to a low-fat diet [66].

Between 2005 and 2010, the Moli-sani study showed that higher adherence to the MD was associated with a reduction of leukocytes and platelets suggesting that the set of foods composing the MD could have an anti-inflammatory action and a protective effect on many diseases (primarily atherosclerosis) with an inflammatory pathogenesis [67]. Overall, these and other studies indicated the existence of inverse associations between MD and total mortality [68], the incidence of coronary heart disease [69,70], thrombotic stroke [71], and with the development of various forms of cancer [72,73].

The international scientific community has accepted the role of the MD in increasing life expectancy and improving general health contributing to the spread of the MD pattern as a central pillar of programs and public health policy in many countries, from the USA to Europe. The MD is not only a diet but represents a lifestyle. The "Mediterranean Diet Foundation" developed a chart of the food pyramid, which includes information closely related to the Mediterranean lifestyle, cultural and social order as well as the importance of exercise and conviviality. Figure 2 highlights the importance of the Mediterranean lifestyle, including factors not associated with the use of particular foods.

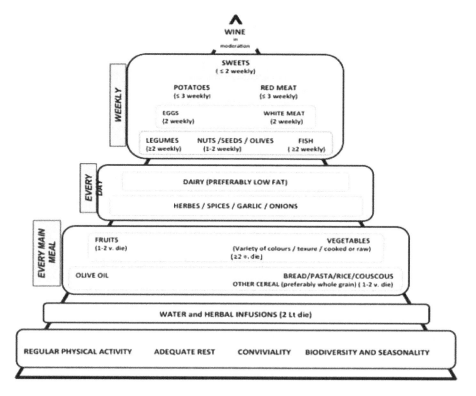

Figure 2. Pyramid of Mediterranean lifestyle (inspired by the "Mediterranean Diet Foundation" Barcelona Spain). The size of different sectors of the pyramid is directly proportional to the frequency of use of that particular food or food group. At the base of the pyramid there are healthy habits and groups of foods to be eaten daily and in large quantities (*i.e.*, fruit, vegetables, *etc.*). The upper levels show the foods to be eaten moderately (*i.e.*, sweets, red meat, *etc.*).

The carbohydrate composition of the MD deserves special attention. Consumption of unrefined whole grain carbohydrates as a preferred choice has a double action: it limits the elevation of postprandial blood glucose and ensures a good supply of fiber. In fact, whole grain cereals have a lower glycemic index (GI) than refined products made with white flour, white rice and sugar. The consumption of low-GI foods avoids sudden increases in blood glucose, limits the secretion of insulin, and, therefore, inflammation [74]. Moreover, low-GI products have an anti-atherogenic action, decreasing the production of atherogenic lipoproteins, oxidized LDL and inflammatory markers [75]. The consumption of whole grains, legumes and other plant foods recommended by the MD brings a high amount of fiber (β-glucans, arabinoxylans, galactomannans, pectins) that increases satiety and helps to control weight. Numerous scientific results showed that dietary fiber promotes gut health and prevents cardiovascular disease, cancer, obesity and diabetes [76]. In the gut, prebiotic fiber (inulin, lactulose and galactooligosaccharides) can be selectively fermented by Bifidobacteria and/or Lactobacilli. The growth of these microorganisms maintains homeostasis and functionality of the intestinal microbiota and reduces the risk of dysbiosis [77]. Moreover, fiber is an effective "carrier" of bioactive antioxidants (vitamins C and E, carotenoids, and polyphenols).

The MD is characterized by a high content of "good fats", monounsaturated (MUFA) and polyunsaturated (PUFA) fatty acids, present in marine fish, vegetable oils (especially olive oil), in nuts and seeds, and by a low intake of saturated fatty acids and hydrogenated oils (trans fats). In particular, the MD provides an optimal dietary fat profile characterized by a low intake of saturated and ω-6 fatty acids and a moderate intake of ω-3 fatty acids [78]. The ratio between ω-6 and ω-3 PUFAs plays an important role in the modulation of inflammation and blood coagulation [79] and is one of the most powerful anti-inflammatory features of this diet.

In terms of micronutrients, the MD is rich in B vitamins (B1, B2, niacin, B6, folate or B12), antioxidant vitamins (vitamins E and C) and minerals, especially iron, selenium, phosphorus and potassium.

Plant foods constitute the core of MD and are characterized by a high content of "non-nutritive" components (phytochemicals), including polyphenols, phytosterols and carotenoids. Phytochemicals are bioactive substances known to combat cellular inflammation due to their powerful antioxidant action. Data from PREDIMED and other studies suggested that the efficiency of the dietary antioxidants in modulating the plasma antioxidant capacity depends on the health status of individuals. In fact, the best results are obtained in people with some risk factors (for example, smokers) or cardiovascular disease or in subjects with a low initial plasma antioxidant capacity. The healthy subjects with low levels of oxidative stress showed a reduced responsiveness to antioxidants. In addition, some studies indicate a negative effect of antioxidant supplements in overall mortality and mortality caused by cardiovascular disease, diabetes and some types of cancer. This is certainly due to the complexity of the interactions between endogenous and exogenous antioxidants and to the existence of homestatic mechanisms of control intended to prevent an overload of reducing agents maintaining the physiological state of homeostasis [80,81]. Therefore, although an adequate intake of antioxidants is needed to counteract oxidative stress, these compounds should be introduced through plant foods such as fruits, vegetables, whole grains, nuts and seeds naturally present in a healthy and complete nutritional model such as the MD.

Diet scores are increasingly being employed to define MD adherence in epidemiological studies [82]. Trichopoulou and colleagues proposed in 1995, and subsequently updated, the Mediterranean Diet Score (MDS) [83]. This simple score was constructed by assigning a value of 0 or 1 for each of the nine components. Therefore, the total MDS ranges from 0 (minimal adherence to the traditional Mediterranean diet) to 9 (maximum adherence) [70]. The NIH-AARP Diet, the Health Study, the European Prospective Investigation into Cancer and Nutrition (EPIC) and other studies used the MDS and other scores later derived from it to confirm the correlation between adherence to MD and mortality reduction, demonstrating the MD protective role in regard to the prevention of cancer, cardiovascular and other chronic diseases [72,73,84,85].

2.2. The Preventive Role of the Mediterranean Diet on Cancer

2.2.1. Epidemiological Studies

Nutrition represents an easily modifiable factor able to contrast inflammation and oxidative stress. Growing evidence indicates the beneficial and preventive role of the Mediterranean Diet (MD) in the onset of cancer and other diseases associated with increased level of inflammation, oxidative damage and angiogenesis. A recent metanalysis of all the observational studies regarding the adherence to MD in relation to cancer risk [86] showed that MD is associated with a significant reduction of overall risk of cancer incidence and mortality by 10%. In particular, increased adherence to the MD reduces the likelihood of having colorectal cancer CRC, even among obese and diabetic patients suggesting potential benefits of this dietary model on CRC risk factors [87–89]. Contrasting data are reported on other forms of neoplasms. While the metanalysis by Schwingshackl and Hoffmann indicates a reduction of the risk of prostate cancer by 4%, a recent paper reported that a higher Mediterranean Diet Score (MDS, see Section 2.1 for details) was not associated with risk of advanced prostate cancer or disease progression in a cohort of 47867 men prospectively followed for 24 years. However, in the same subjects, the adherence to the MD was associated with lower overall mortality after diagnosis of nonmetastatic prostate cancer [90]. Some studies investigating the role of the MD on oral and pharyngeal cancer reported an inverse association between the risk of this neoplasm and adherence to the MD, as measured by various indexes, and indicated a stronger effect in younger subjects [91–93]. A meta-analysis by Schwingshackl and Hoffmann did not seem to confirm an effect of the MD on the risk of breast cancer, even if a subgroup of case-control study showed that the risk of this cancer could be reduced by 18% in women adhering to the MD. In particular, a recent study on 500 Greek middle-aged women showed that one unit increase in MDS was associated with 9% lower risk of breast cancer. It is worth noting that the protective effect of the MD against breast cancer seemed to depend on individual's characteristics and potential risk factors, *i.e.* obesity, physical activity, smoking, age at the menarche, menopausal status. In the above described cohort, the beneficial effect of MD on breast cancer risk is observed only in normal weight, non smoking women and in women who did not present an early menarche (<12 year old) [94]. The studies describing the MD preventive action against various types of cancer suggested that this healthful dietary pattern acts through several mechanisms, decreasing the dysregulated free radical production and inflammation [80,95,96].

2.2.2. Chemoprotective Effects of Polyphenols on Inflammation and Cancer

The abundant consumption of fruit, vegetables, grains, legumes, olive oil and the moderate intake of red wine introduces, in the organism, high levels of different polyphenols and plant bioactive compounds that initially were known as antioxidants but later were studied for their anti-inflammatory, anti-tumor, anti-atherogenic abilities that could not be explained solely on the basis of their antioxidant properties. In fact, a series of investigations into the mechanism of action of these molecules have shed light on the fact that polyphenols do not merely exert their effects only as free radical scavengers, but may also modulate cellular signaling processes involved in inflammatory response or may themselves serve as signaling agents [97]. In particular, dietary polyphenols from olive oil (oleuropein, hydroxyltyrosol) and from red wine (resveratrol) were shown to modulate the eicosanoids pathway through the inhibition of cellular enzymes such as phospholipase A2 (PLA2), cyclooxygenase (COX-1 and COX-2) and lipoxigenase (LOX). This action reduces the cellular production of arachidonic acid and inflammatory prostaglandins and leukotrienes [98]. Other studies showed that also quercitin, the most abundant and widespread natural flavonoid present in a variety of fruit and vegetables, inhibited COX and LOX in different cellular animal models exerting an anti-inflammatory action [99–101]; quercitin is also able to rejuvenate senescent fibroblasts by activating proteasome function [102]. Olive oil and red wine polyphenols reduce inflammatory angiogenesis, a key pathogenic process in cancer and atherosclerosis, in human cultured endothelial cell through the inibithion of COX-2 protein expression, prostaglandin production and MMP-9 release. This effect is accompanied by a substantial reduction of ROS levels and NF-κB activation [103]. A variety of polyphenols (quercitin, apigenin, luteolin, kaempferol, myricetin) are able to modulate the inflammatory process through the inhibition of nitric oxide (NO) production by supressing nitric oxide synthase (NOS) enzyme expression and/or activity [104–106]. A plethora of studies on human and animal cellular models have shown that different flavonoids such as quercitin and phenolic compounds from extra virgin olive oil interfere with the expression, production and/or function of cytokines/chemokines such as TNF-α, IL-1β, IL-6, IL-8, MCP-1, IFN-γ and IL-10, contributing to the control of the balance between pro- and anti-inflammatory mediators and exerting a potent anti-inflammatory activity. These compounds, as natural antioxidants are able to efficiently modulate the redox status of cells and strictly regulate the inducible gene expression of inflammatory mediators [107–112]. Moreover, polyphenols are involved in multiple steps of the NF-κB activation process, which represent an important and very promising pathway for the treatment and prevention of inflammatory diseases and cancer [113]. A recent review described the action played by dietary polyphenols in the inhibition of cancer cell growth due to their ability to modulate the activity of multiple targets involved in carcinogenesis through simultaneous direct interaction or modulation of gene expression. In particular, polyphenols are able to reduce and prevent the cross-talk between ErbB receptors, NF-κB and the Hedgehog (HH)/glioma-associated oncogene (GLI) pathways representing three of the main signal transduction pathways for neoplastic transformation [114].

Phenolic compounds are able to modulate the pathways of mitogen-activated protein kinases (MAPKs). These specific transcription factors play a central role in cell growth, proliferation, death and differentiation by modulating gene transcription in response to changes in the cellular environment. MAPKs regulate the transcription and traslocation of inflammatory mediators and represent potential targets for new anti-inflammatory molecules. Kaempferol, chrysin, apigenin and luteolin inhibit the activity of the three mitogen activated protein kinases, ERK, JNK and p38, blocking TNF-α stimulated ICAM-1 expression in respiratory epithelial cells [115]. Even quercitin inhibits a wide range of pro-inflammatory genes through the regulation of the MAPK pathway. In particular, this compound inhibits ERK, JNK and their phosphorylated forms, suppressing the transcription and the production of TNF-α in human monocytes [116].

In this context, quercitin and other dietary polyphenols typical in the MD, are able to reduce inflammation through a series of different but interconnected mechanisms, and may represent very attractive anti-inflammatory agents and safe non-pharmacological tools for the prevention and treatment of cancer (Figure 3). Moreover, polyphenols exerted their anti-cancer and chemopreventive action through the regulation of mTOR (mammalian target of rapamycin) and the sirtuins pathways by mechanisms that mimic caloric restriction [117]. In particular, quercitin is able to inhibit mTOR activity by multiple pathways. The signalling pathway of mTOR stimulates cell growth and proliferation inducing protein synthesis and inhibiting autophagy in case of food wealth. When essential cellular functions are endangered by insufficient nutrient supply, as in the case of caloric restriction, mTOR activity is blocked and cytosolic compounds are recruited for degradation and recycled by autophagy. On the contrary, the mTOR complex is often hyperactivated in cancer [118] and therefore is considered to be an interesting and attractive therapeutic target for anti-cancer therapy. Sirtuins role in cancer development is very complex and contradictory since different members of the sirtuin family are implicated in various cancer types. Several studies corroborate the possibility of the inhibitory effect of sirtuins on inflammation [119,120] by influencing mainly the NF-κB pathway [121,122] or TNF-α and IL-6 expression (SIRT6) [123,124]. A series of polyphenols have been shown to induce SIRTt1, defined as a guardian against oxidative stress and DNA damage [117], acting as tumor suppressor and attenuating cellular proliferation, but also speeding up tumorigenesis activating oncoproteins. Such dual functions of SIRT1 may be determined, at least in part, by its subcellular localization [125,126]. Data from mice indicated that a diet rich in olive oil polyphenols reduced oxidative stress, inducing NRF2 and the expression of its target genes coding for antioxidant enzymes, and increasing SIRT1 gene expression [127]. Systematic molecular analysis of olive oil phenolic extracts identified secoiridoids as a family of compounds with a strong anti-cancer activity related to the activation of anti-aging/cellular stress-like gene signatures, including endoplasmic reticulum (ER) stress and the unfolded protein response as well as SIRT1 and NRF2 signaling [128]. Several studies demonstrated that resveratrol is able to induce Sirt1 and clinical investigations indicated a role of this compound in the modulation of enzyme systems involved in carcinogen activation and detoxification, suggesting a possible mechanism by which resveratrol inhibits carcinogenesis. Unfortunately, phase II studies have failed to confirm the safety and efficacy of resveratrol in patients with relapsed/refractory multiple myeloma [129].

While many epidemiological studies have associated the consumption of polyphenols with a decreased risk of developing several diseases such as cancer, intervention studies have not always confirmed these effects. This discrepancy may in part depend on potential differences in doses, interactions with the food matrix, and differences in polyphenol bioavailability that limit their overall biological effectiveness. In addition to endogenous factors such as microbiota and digestive enzymes, the food matrix considerably affects bioaccessibility, uptake, and further metabolism of polyphenols. In particular, dietary fiber (such as hemicellulose), divalent minerals, and viscous and protein-rich meals are likely to cause detrimental effects on polyphenol bioaccessibility. In addition, certain food preparation techniques may alter nutrient composition and structure reducing polyphenol bioavailability [130].

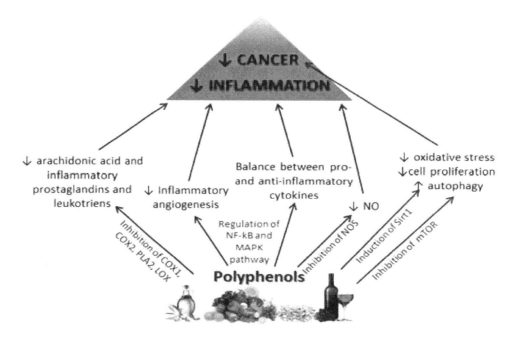

Figure 3. Polyphenols control and reduce inflammation through a series of pathways preventing cancer and other age-related diseases with an inflammatory pathogenesis. Moreover, resveratrol, quercitin and other polyphenols exerted their anti-cancer and chemopreventive action through mechanism that mimic caloric restriction (sirtuin and mTOR pathways).

2.2.3. Other Mediterranean Diet Components and Their Effects on Inflammation and Cancer

Several epidemiological studies have linked the increased consumption of lycopene, the red and lipophilic carotenoid representing the most relevant functional component of tomatoes, with decreased prostate cancer risk. *In vitro*, several experiments showed that lycopene enhances the antioxidant response of prostate cells, inhibits proliferation, induces apoptosis and decreases the metastatic capacity of prostate cancer cells. However, the *in vivo* effectiveness of lycopene as a chemoprotective has still to be proven [131]. Several clinical trials have shown that carotenoids, vitamin A, and vitamin E based antioxidant supplements do not possess preventive effects on cancer and may be harmful and increase mortality especially in well-nourished populations. Therefore, the optimal source of antioxidants seems to come from diet, not from antioxidant supplements in pills or tablets [132].

The high presence of fiber typical of the MD is probably at the basis of the reduced incidence of colorectal cancer. Dietary fibers possess a proven anti-inflammatory action decreasing systemic inflammation-associated biomarkers such as CRP, IL-6, and TNF-α [133–135], as well as inhibiting COX-2 and iNOS activities and gene expression [136].

Fermentable dietary fibers shift the gut microbial populations by providing substrates for bacterial fermentation. In particular, fructooligosaccharides and galactooligosaccharides increase the fecal populations of *Bifidobacteria* and *Lactobacillus* [137] and these changes in gut flora population can result in a modulation of inflammatory processes [138]. Moreover, the consumption of fiber-rich foods avoids glycemic "spikes" and rapid insulin release that may adversely regulate multiple mechanisms, including (acutely and/or chronically) oxidative stress, inflammation, low-density lipoprotein oxidation, protein glycation, and blood coagulation [74]. Finally, dietary fibers favour an enlargement of the bulk of stool fasting intestinal transit and reducing the contact of potentially carcinogenic and toxic coumpounds with gastrointestinal epithelium [139].

Data from PREDIMED and other studies indicated an association between walnut consumption and reduced risk of cancer and mortality particularly in the context of the MD. Numerous components of walnuts, including α-linolenic acid (ALA), ellagitannins, γ-tocopherol, melatonin, β-sisterol and fiber may counter inflammation-related cancer mechanisms [140]. In particular, one-year of the MD supplemented with either extra virgin olive oil or mixed nuts (walnuts, almonds, and hazelnuts) *versus* a low fat diet decreased intercellular adhesion molecule-1 (ICAM-1), IL-6, TNFR60, and TNFR80 levels in adults [141].

The frequent consumption of marine fish typical in the MD provides a high quantity of ω-3 polyunsatured fatty acids. A high ω-3 to ω-6 fatty acids ratio has been associated with a reduced risk of cancer, especially breast cancer, and with improved prognosis [78,142]. ω-3 Fatty acids exert anti-angiogenic effects and have anti-inflammatory and immunosuppressive properties reducing inflammation through different mechanisms. In particular, EPA (eicosapentaenoic) and DHA (docosahexanoic) ω-3 fatty acids partially replace arachidonic acid as eicosanoid substrate in all cell membranes but especially in erythrocytes, neutrophils, monocytes and liver cells, thus suppressing the production of ω-6 pro-inflammatory eicosanoids. In addition, EPA and DHA suppress the NF-κB pathway and modulate plasma membrane micro-organization (lipid rafts), in particular relatively to the function of Toll-like receptors (TLRs), and T-lymphocyte signaling molecule recruitment to the immunological synapse [143].

The traditional MD is characterized by a low consumption of red and processed meat, which is often associated with an increased risk of colorectal cancer. Processed meat intake is linked to cancer risk through different mechanisms including the production of carcinogenic heterocyclic amines, polycyclic aromatic hydrocarbons and N-nitroso compounds as well as the high content of saturated fatty acids that enhances the prostaglandin system feeding the arachidonic acid and PGE$_2$ pro-inflammatory pathways [144].

In contrast to the MD, the Western diet, characterized by a low intake of nutrient-rich food (fruit, vegetables, whole grain cereals, legumes and fish) and by an over consumption of salt, refined sugars, saturated fatty acids and a low ω-6:ω-3 fatty acids ratio, damages the immune system leading to an increased level of inflammation and increased onset of cancer [145].

2.3. The Mediterranean Diet Epigenetic Regulation: the Role of microRNAs

MiRs are small non-coding RNAs involved in the post-transcriptional regulation of gene expression and are recently recognized as diagnostic and prognostic biomarkers for many age-related diseases and aging [59,146].

MiRs play a critical role in basic biological processes such as cellular differentiation, apoptosis, cell proliferation, metabolism, inflammation, stem cells development, immune modulation and carcinogenesis [147,148]. It has also been shown that miR expression is tissue specific, altered with age, and can define the physiological context of the cell, including disease [149]. Alterations in the expression of specific miRs have also been reported to play a role in oxidative stress-induced inflammation [20,51–54,150]. Recently, our team identified three miRs we named "inflamma-miRs": miR-21, -126 and -146a, which target mRNAs belonging to the NF-κB pathway [151].

Several patterns of expression of miRs were exclusive of certain tumors and reflect the differentiation state of tumor development [152]. Especially in the last 10 years, many studies have shown that dysregulation of miR expression underlies many human cancers, both as oncogenes (oncomirs) or tumor suppressors [153–155]. Therefore, the possibility of using miRs to block accumulation of senescent cells to inhibit the establishment of a microenvironment favoring cancer development and progression could be a potential new approach to cancer prevention.

In this regard, it is extremely important to know which type of miRs can be modulated by nutrients typical of MD, and to evaluate the possible role of nutrient-induced miRs as chemoprevention therapy.

MiRs are also present in all the biological fluids of our body. The possibility to monitor the changes of metabolic miR profiling in the blood stream after prolonged diet intervention in humans could be a relevant achievement. Currently, this topic is in its infancy; in cancer, the study of the association between miRs expression and diet has been carried out mainly using tumor cell lines or animal models. The absorption and metabolism of nutrients at the molecular level have been studied with high-throughput "omics" technologies. The results obtained led to the recognition of certain nutrients able to regulate gene expression, at the base of nutrigenomics [156]. It is expected that miRs expression may also change in response to certain dietary bioactive agents, such as PUFAs, vitamins and phytochemicals and some important data are reviewed as follows:

2.3.1. Fatty Acids

The development of tumors such as colon cancer [157–160], breast cancer [161], and glioblastoma [162] is inversely related to the intake of ω-3 PUFA. In contrast, diets rich in ω-6 PUFA (linoleic acid, arachidonic acid and LA, AA) favor both the initiation and promotion of colon cancer [163,164]. In mice, Davidson and colleagues studied the effect of a diet based on corn oil-cellulose compared with a diet based on fish oil (EPA and DHA) and pectin in the presence of carcinogens: their results demonstrated an increased expression of miR-16, miR-19b, miR-21, miR-26b, miR-27b, miR -93, 200c, and miR-203 and the decreased expression of some of their direct targets, such as, PTK2B, TCF4, PDE4B, HDAC4, and IGF1 [158], thus suggesting some different molecular mechanisms involving the fish oil diet. Vinciguerra et al. observed that unsaturated fatty acids inhibit PTEN expression in human hepatocytes by up-regulating miR-21 synthesis via mTOR/NF-κB-dependent signaling, exemplifying a regulatory mechanism by which fatty acids affect PTEN expression and trigger liver disorders [165].

Butyrate has chemoprotective properties acting as an inhibitor of histone deacetylase, decreasing proliferation and increasing apoptosis in tumor cells of the colon-rectum [166–169]. Human colon cancer cells (HCT116) treated with butyrate reduce the expression of different miRs belonging to the miR-17-92-18b, miR-106a and miR-106b-25 clusters [170] mediated by p21, which is a direct target of miR-106b. Experiments in rats showed that butyrate, generated by fermentable fiber and fish oil (EPA and DHA) have a synergistic protective action towards colon tumorigenesis. The increased expression of miR-19b, -26b, -27b, -200c, -203 and the concomitant decrease of their targets expression mediate the tumor suppression mechanisms [171].

2.3.2. Vitamins

All-trans-retinoic acid, the most biologically active metabolite of vitamin A, acts as a tumor suppressor factor in lung, liver, bladder, prostate, breast, and pancreatic cancer models [172]. In breast cancer cells (MCF-7), exposure to retinoic acid inhibited cell proliferation by inducing miR-21 [173].

Recent studies show that vitamin D may exert its protective effects by modulating the expression of miRs and their targets. Vitamin D3 down-regulated miR-181a and miR-181b in human myeloid leukemia cells, resulting in an up-regulation of p27Kip1 and p21Cip1 and cell cycle arrest [174].

2.3.3. Phytochemicals

As described in previous paragraphs, many studies showed that the consumption of foods rich in polyphenols was associated with the prevention of chronic diseases [175–178]. In particular, quercetin, hesperidin, narangin, anthocyanins, catechins, proanthocyanin, caffeic acid, ferulic acid, and curcumin, act through a common mechanism envisaging the modulation of five miRs, *i.e.*, miR-30c, miR-291b-5p, miR-296-5p, miR -373, and miR-467b [179].

The treatment of human pancreatic cancer cells with curcumin led to a significant up-regulation of eleven miRs and down-regulation of eighteen miRs [180]. Among all, miR-22 was the most significantly up-regulated and was associated with the suppression of Sp1 and estrogen receptor 1, while miR-199a* was the most significantly down-regulated miR. Curcumin and its synthetic analogue, curcumin diflourinated (CDF), alone or in combination, down-regulate miR-200 and miR-21 expression, inducing the up-regulation of its target PTEN in pancreatic cancer cells [181].

Hereafter, changes in blood levels of miRs after the consumption of specific nutrients could be used as biomarkers to monitor the metabolic effects of dietary intervention over time and thus identify dietary interventions that may protect our body from the development of cancer.

3. Gut Microbiota, Inflammation and Cancer

Inflammaging and immunosenescence are the main culprits of the changes in microbiota composition in older people [182,183]. It is well known that the human digestive tract is colonized by over 100 trillions of bacteria, which constitute the so-called "gut microbiota" (GM) [184]. These microorganisms, responsible for the degradation of certain complex substances ingested by diet, allowing their digestion and the absorption of certain micronutrients, contribute substantially to our metabolism, and are also essential for the normal development of the immune system. Longitudinal studies have shown that the intestinal microbiota is extremely malleable and could be altered in response to changes in the environment, geography, genetics, metabolism, age, antibiotic treatments, stress, and diet. This plasticity allows the human body to optimize performance while preserving metabolic and immune homestasis as well as health [185].

The impact of the habitual diet on the GM of the elderly [186,187] has been recently highlighted in a study demonstrating the correlation of diet with the inflammatory status, residence and a different rate of health decline upon aging [188]. The balance of carbohydrates, proteins and fats has a profound influence on the maintenance of GM homeostasis [189–191]. The adoption of a specific diet, of animal origin, rather than a predominantly vegetable one, determines a different composition of the GM at the expense of interindividual differences in microbial gene expression [192]. Moreover, a diet rich in animal fats induces the development of inflammation and intestinal diseases by modification of the GM.

Our group has shown that centenarians have a different composition of the GM in respect to young subjects and that this is associated with an increase of the "inflammatory state" represented by high levels of pro-inflammatory cytokines (IL-6 and IL-8) [193].

The dysbiosis condition of GM in the elderly can trigger the development of carcinogenic processes in the intestinal mucosa. The number of cases of colorectal cancer (CRC), in fact, increases in the elderly population. The greatest number of CRC occurs in the elderly, with nearly 70% of cases diagnosed in those older than age 65 and 40% diagnosed in those over 75 years of age [194].

It has been demonstrated that mice with a compromised GM homeostasis are prone to developing an inflammatory state in the intestinal mucosa, which, in turn, predisposes them to cancer development [195].

The next generation sequencing techniques allowed, with extreme accuracy, the identification of the composition of GM associated with CRC. The feces of CRC patients compared with those of healthy subjects are particularly rich in pro-inflammatory opportunistic pathogens and microorganisms responsible for metabolic disorders. The "good" GM, with protective function on the mucous membrane, is rather very poor. It is therefore possible to assume that there are "families" of microorganisms able to perform a pro-carcinogenic function (*Fusobacterium*, *Prevotella*, *Coprobacillus*), as well as other families able to perform a protective function of the intestinal mucosa such as *Bifidobacterium* and *Faecalibacterium* [196].

The mechanisms by which microorganisms induce the development of the CRC are varied and include the development of a chronic inflammatory process, the production of toxic metabolites, the development of genotoxins that acts directly on the cell cycle, on the development of DNA and the activation of food heterocyclic amine which are pro-carcinogenic compounds [197].

Among the various metabolites produced by the intestinal microbiota, pro-carcinogenic molecules and molecules with important protective functions have been identified. Secondary bile acids, ammonia, certain amines, phenols and hydrogen sulfide are toxic metabolites, while butyrate plays an anti-proliferative action, energizes the intestinal cells and has shown an apoptotic action against CRC cells *in vitro* [198].

Thus, due to the strong influence of nutrition on GM composition and metabolism [187], the adoption of an anti-inflammatory dietary pattern such as the Mediterranean Diet will contribute to the maintenance of a "good" GM with healthy outcomes.

4. A Systems Biology Approach to Diet, Inflammation and Cancer

Systems biology aims to understand how a biological system as a whole responds to internal and external stimuli. Metabolomics [199], instead, aims to measure the global dynamic metabolic response of a living system to biological stimuli or genetic manipulation as a whole, and represents the cutting-edge methodology to fully understand the system-wide effects that diet has on any living organism. The latter approach neatly superimposes to the first: the final result is in both cases a "top-down" view of all the biochemistry processes involved in a complex organism, even if at distinct levels.

Important efforts were made to allow researchers to readily process metabolomics data. The Human Metabolome Project [200] seeks to reproduce what the Human Genome Project did in the genome field, hosting a rapidly growing database of thousands of human metabolites, along with their spectroscopic data. Similarly, the LIPID Metabolites and Pathway Strategy [201] is progressively characterizing human lipids. Metabolomics represents a first-class tool to understand diseases where other approaches are falling short [202]. Metabolome-wide association (MWA) studies, deeply intertwining genome-derived concepts to the "metabolome" world, will in the near future represent a standard approach [203–206]. A recent study by Watson *et al.* [207] successfully identified metabolites that affect *Caenorhabditis elegans* gene expression and physiology, exploiting an interspecies systems biology approach. Influence of a herring-based diet on sterol metabolism and protein turnover in mice was recently identified, with clear implications also on disease development [208].

The common thread connecting cancer, inflammation and diet is now the focus of metabolomics studies, where the goal is to identify individual metabolites representing end-points of perturbed molecular pathways. These altered molecular pathways may then be further investigated in depth, exploiting other "-omics" techniques [209–211]. In a work by Sreekumar *et al.* (2009), the authors were able to successfully identify 87 metabolites distinguishing prostate cancer from benign prostate tissue [212]. More recently, de Boer *et al.* designed a protocol to easily screen the population to detect CRC [213] (or its precursor, advanced adenoma) relying only on volatile organic compound (VOC) analysis. This finding, if confirmed, will pave the way to new, effective and cost-saving methods to perform preventative, large-scale screening, of the population.

To strengthen the proofs in favour of this inter-systems link, focused cohort-based studies are needed. The European Prospective Investigation into Cancer and Nutrition (EPIC) did exactly that: starting from a cohort of 2380 subjects they analysed a panel of 127 serum metabolites [214], looking for correlations among metabolite networks and different conditions, *i.e.*, physical activity energy expenditure, obesity, and waist circumference, shedding light on the possible adoption of some of the metabolites under analysis as markers to evaluate subjects health. Additionally, an independent cohort study investigating the effect of a diet based on healthy Nordic foods [208], found a lower incidence of colorectal cancer in women following such a diet. The same study also suggests that the Nordic population could better improve their health following diets centered on Nordic food, breaking the dogma that a "Mediterranean Diet" represents the best possible nutritional intervention in all cases, independently from anthropological considerations.

In our bird's eye voyage through the three different worlds of diet, inflammation and cancer, we showed how these worlds are indeed deeply intertwined. The modulatory effect that unsaturated fatty acids has on the immune systems, the inflammatory response of which can then fuel the micro-environment propelling tumour progression, is just one of the examples of these extensive and branched connections. Any effort to understand the functioning of one of these phenomena must take into consideration all of them, or faces a highly probable failure. In some of the just cited articles, authors fruitfully applied systems biology approaches to unravel the mechanistic reasons underlining the effects they observed. Most of these efforts led to results indicating important advances in the field. In the future, widespread adoption of these analysis techniques will permit breakthrough discoveries that may eventually have a deep impact on public health.

5. The Mediterranean Diet and Healthy Aging: the European Project NU-AGE Targeted on Inflammaging to Prevent Age-Related Diseases as a Whole

EU member states are experiencing an extraordinary increase in the life expectancy, which is predicted to reach 84.6 years for women and 82.5 years for men in 2060 [215]. As a direct consequence of the improvement of socio-economic-environmental conditions, the increasing longevity of European citizens will also imply a wide range of societal responsibilities, such as the increased incidence of age-related diseases and the resulting impact on health care cost. Consequently, there is an urgent need to provide policies for preventing aging and related disorders, such as cancer and neurodegenerative disorders among others, allowing the maintenance of reasonably good health as long as possible.

One of the most fascinating anti-aging strategies seems to be the possibility of reducing inflammaging without compromising the physiological role of inflammation, which is essential for survival [5]. At present, nutrition represents the most powerful and flexible tool that we have to reach a chronic and systemic modulation of the aging process in order to improve the health status of the elderly population.

Several studies analized the effect of an individual food or nutrient on a particular form of cancer. However, the overall dietary pattern is more than the sum of the single foods or nutrients eaten and the effect of a dietary intervention on any health outcome is strongly influenced by genetic and environmental factors. Studies regarding the role of the MD on cancer prevention are often conducted analyzing the association between MD adherence and the onset of a specific neoplasia. Studies considering in a comprehensive and integrated way the effect of a balanced whole MD, followed for a consistent period of time, on the chronic and systemic inflammation typical of aging are still scant in the scientific literature.

To rectify this gap in knowledge, the European Project NU-AGE (ClinicalTrials.gov Identifier, NCT01754012) [216,217] will study in a comprehensive and integrated way, the effect of a whole MD newly designed according to the nutritional needs of people over 65 years of age called "NU-AGE diet" [218] on the health status of elderly people in the EU.

The specific rationale of NU-AGE is to enroll in the study free-living, apparently healthy, elderly people including pre-frail subjects (a large segment of the elderly population having the potential to benefit from diet change). All the volunteers will be characterized before and after dietary intervention by measuring a number of robust parameters capable of providing reliable data about different domains/subsystems (health and nutritional status, physical and cognitive functions, immunological, biochemical and metabolic parameters). A sub-group of subjects will be further characterized by advanced techniques (genetics, epigenetics) and highthroughput "omics" (transcriptomics, metagenomics, pyrosequencing, HITChip array) in order to identify cellular and molecular targets and mechanisms responsible for the effects of the whole diet intervention.

The massive amount of data collected from the NU-AGE nutritional intervention will be stored in an ad-hoc built database that, based on an integrated statistical analysis and a system biology approach, will allow the identification of nutritional risk factors in the elderly associated with inflammaging, and to identify the pathways and networks responsive to the NU-AGE diet [219].

This approach will allow an evaluation of the whole-organism response considering several tissues and organs/systems as a functional network instead of assessing the single tissue and organ responses separately, as in previously funded projects, which thereby missed the fundamental cross-talk between tissues and organs/systems. For a detailed description of the entire project it is suggested to read the recently published NU-AGE project dedicated special issue [220].

6. Conclusions

Chronic inflammation plays a pivotal role in each stage of carcinogenesis from the initial genetic or epigenetic changes to tumour progression and metastatic diffusion [23,25]. Thus, the chronic, low-level inflammatory state typical in the elderly, that we have named "inflammaging", likely represents one of the links between aging and cancer.

Inflammaging is both local and systemic, and a variety of organs and systems provide inflammatory stimuli that accumulate lifelong [3]. The key mediators of the inflammatory response activate, in turn, the NF-κB pathway that can be considered the link among cellular senescence, inflammaging and cancer.

A suitable intervention to combat inflammation is a modification of dietary habits. Actually, several studies reported that a healthy lifestyle and a balanced diet might provide benefits to health not only by preventing the risk of diseases but also through facilitating recovery and improving survival. The MD represents one of the best examples of a healthy diet, considered a heritage of humanity by UNESCO, and is considered pivotal in many public health programs in Europe. The acceptance of a Mediterranean lifestyle indeed has a beneficial and preventive role in the onset of cancer and other diseases associated with increased level of inflammation, oxidative damage and angiogenesis.

However, even if the outcomes of the MD on health are well known, knowledge of the reasons of these outcomes is still rather poor. While recent nutrition research focused on the effects of specific dietary constituents, it is still unclear which are the molecular and cellular pathways triggered by the MD as a whole. To this aim, the NU-AGE project is studying in depth the effects of a one-year whole MD in a representative sample of four geographic and cultural areas of Europe (Northern, Eastern, Central and Southern) by measuring an unprecedented number of parameters, including those obtained from "omic" high-throughput analyses, and considering them in a systems biology perspective in order to get a comprehensive view of this dietary intervention on inflammation in old age. This strategy could also hopefully provide insight on diet as cancer prevention; NU-AGE and its study design were noted, in a special issue of the journal *Nature*, devoted to aging studies, as "the kind of large, longitudinal study that scientists the world over are clamouring for" [221].

Acknowledgments: This study was supported by the European Union's Seventh Framework Program under the grant agreement No. 266486 ("NU-AGE: New dietary strategies addressing the specific needs of the elderly population for healthy aging in Europe") and No. 259679 (IDEAL) to CF, by Progetto Made in Italy Alimentazione Over 50 (MIAO50) to CF and by the Roberto and Cornelia Pallotti Legacy for cancer research to SS and MC.

Author Contributions: R.O., C.L.: contributed to the review of the literature on nutrition, the Mediterranean Diet and cancer and wrote the paper; E.P., M.S., M.I., G.P.: wrote the paragraph on inflammation and cancer; D.V.:

wrote on systems biology; C.B., C.Fa., F.B., M.M.: reviewed the literature with particular attention to inflammation and cancer; EB: reviewed the literature on aging and inflammaging; S.S. and M.C.: critically revised the whole manuscript; C.Fr. and A.S.: designed the structure of the paper and wrote on aging and inflammaging.

References

1. López-Otín, C.; Blasco, M.A.; Partridge, L.; Serrano, M.; Kroemer, G. The hallmarks of aging. *Cell* **2013**, *153*, 1194–1217. [CrossRef] [PubMed]

2. Franceschi, C.; Bonafè, M.; Valensin, S.; Olivieri, F.; de Luca, M.; Ottaviani, E.; de Benedictis, G. Inflamm-aging. An evolutionary perspective on immunosenescence. *Ann. N.Y. Acad. Sci.* **2000**, *908*, 244–254. [CrossRef] [PubMed]

3. Franceschi, C.; Campisi, J. Chronic inflammation (inflammaging) and its potential contribution to age-associated diseases. *J. Gerontol. A Biol. Sci. Med. Sci.* **2014**, *69*, 4–9. [CrossRef]

4. Kennedy, B.K.; Berger, S.L.; Brunet, A.; Campisi, J.; Cuervo, A.M.; Epel, E.S.; Franceschi, C.; Lithgow, G.J.; Morimoto, R.I.; Pessin, J.E.; *et al.* Geroscience: Linking aging to chronic disease. *Cell* **2014**, *159*, 709–713. [CrossRef]

5. Franceschi, C. Inflammaging as a major characteristic of old people: Can it be prevented or cured? *Nutr. Rev.* **2007**, *65*, 173–176. [CrossRef] [PubMed]

6. Franceschi, C.; Capri, M.; Monti, D.; Giunta, S.; Olivieri, F.; Sevini, F.; Panourgia, M.P.; Invidia, L.; Celani, L.; Scurti, M.; *et al.* Inflammaging and anti-inflammaging: A systemic perspective on aging and longevity emerged from studies in humans. *Mech. Ageing. Dev.* **2007**, *128*, 92–105. [CrossRef] [PubMed]

7. Cevenini, E.; Monti, D.; Franceschi, C. Inflammaging. *Curr. Opin. Clin. Nutr. Metab. Care* **2013**, *16*, 14–20. [CrossRef] [PubMed]

8. Reedy, J. Galen on cancer and related diseases. *Clio Med.* **1975**, *10*, 227–238. [PubMed]

9. Trinchieri, G. Cancer and inflammation: An old intuition with rapidly evolving new concepts. *Annu. Rev. Immunol.* **2012**, *30*, 677–706. [CrossRef] [PubMed]

10. Virchow, R. *Cellular Pathology as Based upon Physiological and Pathological Histology*; J.B. Lippincott: Philadelphia, PA, USA, 1863.

11. Balkwill, F.; Mantovani, A. Inflammation and cancer: Back to Virchow? *Lancet* **2001**, *357*, 539–545. [CrossRef] [PubMed]

12. Hanahan, D.; Weinberg, R.A. The Hallmarks of Cancer. *Cell* **2000**, *100*, 57–70. [CrossRef] [PubMed]

13. Coussens, L.M.; Werb, Z. Inflammation and cancer. *Nature* **2002**, *420*, 860–867. [CrossRef]

14. Luo, J.L.; Tan, W.; Ricono, J.M.; Korchynskyi, O.; Zhang, M.; Gonias, S.L.; Cheresh, D.A.; Karin, M. Nuclear cytokine-activated IKKalpha controls prostate cancer metastasis by repressing Maspin. *Nature* **2007**, *446*, 690–694. [CrossRef] [PubMed]

15. Mantovani, A.; Allavena, P.; Sica, A.; Balkwill, F. Cancer-related inflammation. *Nature* **2008**, *454*, 436–444. [CrossRef] [PubMed]

16. Hanahan, D.; Weinberg, R.A. Hallmarks of cancer: The next generation. *Cell* **2011**, *144*, 646–674. [CrossRef] [PubMed]

17. Karin, M. Nuclear factor-κB in cancer development and progression. *Nature* **2006**, *441*, 431–436. [CrossRef] [PubMed]

18. Chia, W.K.; Ali, R.; Toh, H.C. Aspirin as adjuvant therapy for colorectal cancer—Reinterpreting paradigms. *Nat. Rev. Clin. Oncol.* **2012**, *9*, 561–570. [CrossRef] [PubMed]

19. Giraldo, N.A.; Becht, E.; Remark, R.; Damotte, D.; Sautès-Fridman, C.; Fridman, W.H. The immune contexture of primary and metastatic human tumours. *Curr. Opin. Immunol.* **2014**, *27*, 8–15. [CrossRef]

20. Hussain, S.P.; Hofseth, L.J.; Harris, C.C. Radical causes of cancer. *Nat. Rev. Cancer* **2003**, *3*, 276–285. [CrossRef] [PubMed]

21. Colotta, F.; Allavena, P.; Sica, A.; Garlanda, C.; Mantovani, A. Cancer-related inflammation, the seventh hallmark of cancer: Links to genetic instability. *Carcinogenesis* **2009**, *30*, 1073–1081. [CrossRef] [PubMed]

22. Grivennikov, S.I.; Greten, F.R.; Karin, M. Immunity, inflammation, and cancer. *Cell* **2010**, *140*, 883–899. [CrossRef] [PubMed]

23. Aggarwal, B.B.; Gehlot, P. Inflammation and cancer: How friendly is the relationship for cancer patients? *Curr. Opin. Pharmacol.* **2009**, *9*, 351–369. [CrossRef] [PubMed]

24. Multhoff, G.; Molls, M.; Radons, J. Chronic inflammation in cancer development. *Front. Immunol.* **2012**, *2*, 98. [CrossRef] [PubMed]

25. De Lerma Barbaro, A.; Perletti, G.; Bonapace, I.M.; Monti, E. Inflammatory cues acting on the adult intestinal stem cells and the early onset of cancer (review). *Int. J. Oncol.* **2014**, *45*, 959–968. [PubMed]

26. Salvioli, S.; Monti, D.; Lanzarini, C.; Conte, M.; Pirazzini, C.; Bacalini, M.G.; Garagnani, P.; Giuliani, C.; Fontanesi, E.; Ostan, R.; *et al.* Immune system, cell senescence, aging and longevity—inflamm-aging reappraised. *Curr. Pharm. Des.* **2013**, *19*, 1675–1679. [PubMed]

27. Bonafè, M.; Storci, G.; Franceschi, C. Inflamm-aging of the stem cell niche: Breast cancer as a paradigmatic example: Breakdown of the multi-shell cytokine network fuels cancer in aged people. *Bioessays* **2012**, *34*, 40–49. [CrossRef] [PubMed]

28. Diakos, C.I.; Charles, K.A.; McMillan, D.C.; Clarke, S.J. Cancer-related inflammation and treatment effectiveness. *Lancet Oncol.* **2014**, *15*, 493–503. [CrossRef]

29. Cevenini, E.; Caruso, C.; Candore, G.; Capri, M.; Nuzzo, D.; Duro, G.; Rizzo, C.; Colonna-Romano, G.; Lio, D.; di Carlo, D.; *et al.* Age-related inflammation: The contribution of different organs, tissues and systems. How to face it for therapeutic approaches. *Curr. Pharm. Des.* **2010**, *16*, 609–618. [CrossRef] [PubMed]

30. Ostan, R.; Bucci, L.; Capri, M.; Salvioli, S.; Scurti, M.; Pini, E.; Monti, D.; Franceschi, C. Immunosenescence and immunogenetics of human longevity. *Neuroimmunomodulation* **2008**, *15*, 224–240. [CrossRef] [PubMed]

31. Grignolio, A.; Franceschi, C. *History of Research into Aging/Senescence*; John Wiley & Sons: Chichester, UK, 2012.

32. Wellen, K.E.; Fucho, R.; Gregor, M.F.; Furuhashi, M.; Morgan, C.; Lindstad, T.; Vaillancourt, E.; Gorgun, C.Z.; Saatcioglu, F.; Hotamisligil, G.S. Coordinated regulation of nutrient and inflammatory responses by STAMP2 is essential for metabolic homeostasis. *Cell* **2007**, *129*, 537–548. [CrossRef] [PubMed]

33. Erridge, C.; Attina, T.; Spickett, C.M.; Webb, D.J. A high-fat meal induces low-grade endotoxemia: Evidence of a novel mechanism of postprandial inflammation. *Am. J. Clin. Nutr.* **2007**, *86*, 1286–1292. [PubMed]

34. Cani, P.D.; Amar, J.; Iglesias, M.A.; Poggi, M.; Knauf, C.; Bastelica, D.; Neyrinck, A.M.; Fava, F.; Tuohy, K.M.; Chabo, C.; *et al.* Metabolic endotoxemia initiates obesity and insulin resistance. *Diabetes* **2007**, *56*, 1761–1772. [CrossRef] [PubMed]

35. Gregor, M.F.; Hotamisligil, G.S. Inflammatory mechanisms in obesity. *Annu. Rev. Immunol.* **2011**, *29*, 415–445. [CrossRef] [PubMed]

36. De Martel, C.; Franceschi, S. Infections and cancer: Established associations and new hypotheses. *Crit. Rev. Oncol. Hematol.* **2009**, *70*, 183–194. [CrossRef] [PubMed]

37. De Visser, K.E.; Eichten, A.; Coussens, L.M. Paradoxical roles of the immune system during cancer development. *Nat. Rev. Cancer* **2006**, *6*, 24–37. [CrossRef] [PubMed]

38. Lu, H.; Ouyang, W.; Huang, C. Inflammation, a key event in cancer development. *Mol. Cancer Res.* **2006**, *4*, 221–233. [CrossRef] [PubMed]

39. Macarthur, M.; Hold, G.L.; El-Omar, E.M. Inflammation and Cancer II. Role of chronic inflammation and cytokine polymorphisms in the pathogenesis of gastrointestinal malignancy. *Am. J. Physiol. Gastrointest. Liver Physiol.* **2004**, *286*, G515–G520. [CrossRef] [PubMed]

40. Whitcomb, D.C. Inflammation and Cancer V. chronic pancreatitis and pancreatic cancer. *Am. J. Physiol. Gastrointest. Liver Physiol.* **2004**, *287*, 315–319. [CrossRef]

41. Baan, R.; Grosse, Y.; Straif, K.; Secretan, B.; El Ghissassi, F.; Bouvard, V. A review of human carcinogens Part F. Chemical agents and related occupations. *Lancet Oncol.* **2009**, *10*, 1143–1144. [CrossRef] [PubMed]

42. Houghton, A.M. Mechanistic links between COPD and lung cancer. *Nat. Rev. Cancer* **2013**, *13*, 233–245. [CrossRef] [PubMed]

43. Askling, J.; Grunewald, J.; Eklund, A.; Hillerdal, G.; Ekbom, A. Increased risk for cancer following sarcoidosis. *Am. J. Respir. Crit. Care Med.* **1999**, *160*, 1668–1672. [CrossRef] [PubMed]

44. Calder, P.C.; Ahluwalia, N.; Brouns, F.; Buetler, T.; Clement, K.; Cunningham, K.; Esposito, K.; Jönsson, L.S.; Kolb, H.; Lansink, M.; *et al.* Dietary factors and low-grade inflammation in relation to overweight and obesity. *Br. J. Nutr.* **2011**, *106*, S5–S78. [CrossRef] [PubMed]

45. Wolk, A.; Gridley, G.; Svensson, M.; Nyrén, O.; McLaughlin, J.K.; Fraumeni, J.F.; Adam, H.O. A prospective study of obesity and cancer risk (Sweden). *Cancer Causes Control* **2001**, *12*, 13–21. [CrossRef] [PubMed]

46. Calle, E.E.; Rodriguez, C.; Walker-Thurmond, K.; Thun, M.J. Overweight, obesity, and mortality from cancer in a prospectively studied cohort of U.S. adults. *N. Engl. J. Med.* **2003**, *348*, 1625–1638. [CrossRef] [PubMed]

47. Renehan, A.G.; Tyson, M.; Egger, M.; Heller, R.F.; Zwahlen, M. Body-mass index and incidence of cancer: A systematic review and meta-analysis of prospective observational studies. *Lancet* **2008**, *371*, 569–578. [CrossRef] [PubMed]

48. Basen-Engquist, K.; Chang, M. Obesity and cancer risk: Recent review and evidence. *Curr. Oncol. Rep.* **2011**, *13*, 71–76. [CrossRef] [PubMed]

49. Karagozian, R.; Derdák, Z.; Baffy, G. Obesity-associated mechanisms of hepatocarcinogenesis. *Metabolism* **2014**, *63*, 607–617. [CrossRef] [PubMed]

50. Vitale, G.; Salvioli, S.; Franceschi, C. Oxidative stress and the ageing endocrine system. *Nat. Rev. Endocrinol.* **2013**, *9*, 228–240. [CrossRef] [PubMed]

51. Reuter, S.; Gupta, S.C.; Chaturvedi, M.M.; Aggarwal, B.B. Oxidative stress, inflammation, and cancer: How are they linked? *Free Radic. Biol. Med.* **2010**, *49*, 1603–1616. [CrossRef] [PubMed]

52. Mantovani, A. Cancer: inflammation by remote control. *Nature* **2005**, *435*, 752–753.

53. Lin, W.W.; Karin, M.A. A cytokine-mediated link between innate immunity, inflammation, and cancer. *J. Clin. Investig.* **2007**, *117*, 1175–1183. [CrossRef] [PubMed]

54. Hoesel, B.; Schmid, J.A. The complexity of NF-κB signaling in inflammation and cancer. *Mol. Cancer* **2013**, *2*, 12–86.

55. Tieri, P.; Termanini, A.; Bellavista, E.; Salvioli, S.; Capri, M.; Franceschi, C. Charting the NF-κB pathway interactome map. *PLoS ONE* **2012**, *7*, e32678. [CrossRef] [PubMed]

56. Aggarwal, B.B.; Sung, B. NF-κB in cancer: A matter of life and death. *Cancer Discov.* **2011**, *1*, 469–471. [CrossRef] [PubMed]

57. Fan, Y.; Mao, R.; Yang, J. NF-κB and STAT3 signaling pathways collaboratively link inflammation to cancer. *Protein Cell* **2013**, *4*, 176–185. [CrossRef] [PubMed]

58. Freund, A.; Orjalo, A.V.; Desprez, P.Y.; Campisi, J. Inflammatory networks during cellular senescence: causes and consequences. *Trends Mol. Med.* **2010**, *16*, 238–246. [CrossRef] [PubMed]

59. Olivieri, F.; Lazzarini, R.; Recchioni, R.; Marcheselli, F.; Rippo, M.R.; di Nuzzo, S.; Albertini, M.C.; Graciotti, L.; Babini, L.; Mariotti, S.; *et al.* MiR-146a as marker of senescence-associated pro-inflammatory status in cells involved in vascular remodelling. *Age (Dordr)* **2012**, *35*, 1157–1172. [CrossRef]

60. Rodier, F.; Campisi, J. Four faces of cellular senescence. *J. Cell Biol.* **2011**, *192*, 547–556. [CrossRef] [PubMed]

61. Martin, O.A.; Redon, C.E.; Dickey, J.S.; Nakamura, A.J.; Bonner, W.M. Para-inflammation mediates systemic DNA damage in response to tumor growth. *Commun. Integr. Biol.* **2011**, *4*, 78–81. [CrossRef] [PubMed]

62. Bellavista, E.; Andreoli, F.; Parenti, M.D.; Martucci, M.; Santoro, A.; Salvioli, S.; Capri, M.; Baruzzi, A.; Del Rio, A.; Franceschi, C.; *et al.* Immunoproteasome in cancer and neuropathologies: a new therapeutic target? *Curr. Pharm. Des.* **2013**, *19*, 702–718. [CrossRef] [PubMed]

63. Bellavista, E.; Martucci, M.; Vasuri, F.; Santoro, A.; Mishto, M.; Kloss, A.; Capizzi, E.; Degiovanni, A.; Lanzarini, C.; Remondini, D.; *et al.* Lifelong maintenance of composition, function and cellular/subcellulardistribution of proteasomes in human liver. *Mech. Ageing Dev.* **2014**, *141–142*, 26–34. [CrossRef] [PubMed]

64. Morimoto, R.I.; Cuervo, A.M. Proteostasis and the aging proteome in health and disease. *J. Gerontol. A Biol. Sci. Med. Sci.* **2014**, *69*, 33–38. [CrossRef]

65. Keys, A.; Arvanis, C.; Blackburn, H. *Seven Countries: A Multivariate Analysis of Death and Coronary Heart Disease*; Harvard University Press: Cambridge, MA, USA, 1980.

66. Estruch, R.; Ros, E.; Salas-Salvadó, J.; Covas, M.I.; Corella, D.; Arós, F.; Gómez-Gracia, E.; Ruiz-Gutiérrez, V.; Fiol, M.; Lapetra, J.; *et al.* PREDIMED Study Investigators. Primary prevention of cardiovascular disease with a Mediterranean diet. *N. Engl. J. Med.* **2013**, *368*, 1279–1290. [CrossRef] [PubMed]

67. Bonaccio, M.; di Castelnuovo, A.; de Curtis, A.; Costanzo, S.; Persichillo, M.; Donati, M.B.; Cerletti, C.; Iacoviello, L.; de Gaetano, G. Moli-sani Project Investigators. Adherence to the Mediterranean diet is associated with lower platelet and leukocyte counts: Results from the Moli-sani study. *Blood* **2014**, *123*, 3037–3044. [CrossRef] [PubMed]

68. Trichopoulou, A.; Orfanos, P.; Norat, T.; Bueno-de-Mesquita, B.; Ocké, M.C.; Peeters, P.H.; van der Schouw, Y.T.; Boeing, H.; Hoffmann, K.; Boffetta, P.; *et al.* Modified Mediterranean diet and survival: EPIC-elderly prospective cohort study. *BMJ* **2005**, *330*, 991. [CrossRef] [PubMed]

69. Mente, A.; de Koning, L.; Shannon, H.S.; Anand, S.S. A systematic review of the evidence supporting a causal link between dietary factors and coronary heart disease. *Arch. Intern. Med.* **2009**, *169*, 659–669. [CrossRef] [PubMed]

70. Trichopoulou, A.; Costacou, T.; Bamia, C.; Trichopoulos, D. Adherence to a Mediterranean diet and survival in a Greek population. *N. Engl. J. Med.* **2003**, *348*, 2599–2608. [CrossRef] [PubMed]

71. Misirli, G.; Benetou, V.; Lagiou, P.; Bamia, C.; Trichopoulos, D.; Trichopoulou, A. Relation of the traditional Mediterranean diet to cerebrovascular disease in a Mediterranean population. *Am. J. Epidemiol.* **2012**, *176*, 1185–1192. [CrossRef] [PubMed]

72. Benetou, V.; Trichopoulou, A.; Orfanos, P.; Naska, A.; Lagiou, P.; Boffetta, P.; Trichopoulos, D.; Greek, E. Conformity to traditional Mediterranean diet and cancer incidence: The Greek EPIC cohort. *Br. J. Cancer* **2008**, *99*, 191–195. [CrossRef] [PubMed]

73. Couto, E.; Boffetta, P.; Lagiou, P.; Ferrari, P.; Buckland, G.; Overvad, K.; Dahm, C.C.; Tjonneland, A.; Olsen, A.; Clavel-Chapelon, F.; *et al.* Mediterranean dietary pattern and cancer risk in the EPIC cohort. *Br. J. Cancer* **2011**, *104*, 1493–1499. [CrossRef] [PubMed]

74. Brand-Miller, J.; Dickinson, S.; Barclay, A.; Celermajer, D. The glycemic index and cardiovascular disease risk. *Curr. Atheroscler. Rep.* **2007**, *9*, 479–485. [CrossRef] [PubMed]

75. Mirrahimi, A.; Chiavaroli, L.; Srichaikul, K.; Augustin, L.S.; Sievenpiper, J.L.; Kendall, C.W.; Jenkins, D.J. The role of glycemic index and glycemic load in cardiovascular disease and its risk factors: A review of the recent literature. *Curr. Atheroscler. Rep.* **2014**, *16*, 381. [CrossRef] [PubMed]

76. Sofi, F.; Macchi, C.; Abbate, R.; Gensini, G.F.; Casini, A. Mediterranean diet and health. *Biofactors* **2013**, *39*, 335–342. [CrossRef] [PubMed]

77. De Vrese, M.; Schrezenmeir, J. Probiotics, prebiotics, and synbiotics. *Adv. Biochem. Eng. Biotechnol.* **2008**, *111*, 1–66.

78. De Lorgeril, M.; Salen, P. New insights into the health effects of dietary saturated and omega-6 and omega-3 polyunsaturated fatty acids. *BMC Med.* **2012**, *10*, 50. [CrossRef] [PubMed]

79. Kalogeropoulos, N.; Chiou, A.; Ioannou, M.S.; Karathanos, V.T. Nutritional evaluation and health promoting activities of nuts and seeds cultivated in Greece. *Int. J. Food Sci. Nutr.* **2013**, *64*, 757–767. [CrossRef] [PubMed]

80. Zamora-Ros, R.; Serafini, M.; Estruch, R.; Lamuela-Raventós, R.M.; Martínez-González, M.A.; Salas-Salvadó, J.; Fiol, M.; Lapetra, J.; Arós, F.; Covas, M.I.; *et al.* PREDIMED Study Investigators. Mediterranean diet and non enzymatic antioxidant capacity in the PREDIMED study: Evidence for a mechanism of antioxidant tuning. *Nutr. Metab. Cardiovasc. Dis.* **2013**, *23*, 1167–1174. [CrossRef] [PubMed]

81. Kolomvotsou, A.I.; Rallidis, L.S.; Mountzouris, K.C.; Lekakis, J.; Koutelidakis, A.; Efstathiou, S.; Nana-Anastasiou, M.; Zampelas, A. Adherence to Mediterranean diet and close dietetic supervision increase total dietary antioxidant intake and plasma antioxidant capacity in subjects with abdominal obesity. *Eur. J. Nutr.* **2013**, *52*, 37–48. [CrossRef] [PubMed]

82. Trichopoulou, A.; Martínez-González, M.A.; Tong, T.Y.; Forouhi, N.G.; Khandelwal, S.; Prabhakaran, D.; Mozaffarian, D.; de Lorgeril, M. Definitions and potential health benefits of the Mediterranean diet: views from experts around the world. *BMC Med.* **2014**, *12*, 112. [CrossRef] [PubMed]

83. Trichopoulou, A.; Kouris-Blazos, A.; Wahlqvist, M.L.; Gnardellis, C.; Lagiou, P.; Polychronopoulos, E.; Vassilakou, T.; Lipworth, L.; Trichopoulos, D. Diet and overall survival in elderly people. *BMJ* **1995**, *311*, 1457–1460. [CrossRef] [PubMed]

84. Bosire, C.; Stampfer, M.J.; Subar, A.F.; Park, Y.; Kirkpatrick, S.I.; Chiuve, S.E.; Hollenbeck, A.R.; Reedy, J. Index-based dietary patterns and the risk of prostate cancer in the NIH-AARP diet and health study. *Am. J. Epidemiol.* **2013**, *177*, 504–513. [CrossRef] [PubMed]

85. Mitrou, P.N.; Kipnis, V.; Thiébaut, A.C.; Reedy, J.; Subar, A.F.; Wirfält, E.; Flood, A.; Mouw, T.; Hollenbeck, A.R.; Leitzmann, M.F.; *et al.* Mediterranean dietary pattern and prediction of all-cause mortality in a US population: results from the NIH-AARP Diet and Health Study. *Arch. Intern. Med.* **2007**, *167*, 2461–2468. [CrossRef] [PubMed]

86. Schwingshackl, L.; Hoffmann, G. Adherence to Mediterranean diet and risk of cancer: A systematic review and meta-analysis of observational studies. *Int. J. Cancer* **2014**, *135*, 1884–1897. [CrossRef] [PubMed]

87. Grosso, G.; Biondi, A.; Galvano, F.; Mistretta, A.; Marventano, S.; Buscemi, S.; Drago, F.; Basile, F. Factors associated with colorectal cancer in the context of the Mediterranean diet: A case-control study. *Nutr. Cancer* **2014**, *66*, 558–565. [CrossRef] [PubMed]

88. Agnoli, C.; Grioni, S.; Sieri, S.; Palli, D.; Masala, G.; Sacerdote, C.; Vineis, P.; Tumino, R.; Giurdanella, M.C.; Pala, V.; *et al.* Italian Mediterranean Index and risk of colorectal cancer in the Italian section of the EPIC cohort. *Int. J. Cancer* **2013**, *132*, 1404–1411. [CrossRef] [PubMed]

89. Reedy, J.; Mitrou, P.N.; Krebs-Smith, S.M.; Wirfält, E.; Flood, A.; Kipnis, V.; Leitzmann, M.; Mouw, T.; Hollenbeck, A.; Schatzkin, A.; *et al.* Index-based dietary patterns and risk of colorectal cancer: the NIH-AARP Diet and Health Study. *Am. J. Epidemiol.* **2008**, *168*, 38–48. [CrossRef] [PubMed]

90. Kenfield, S.A.; DuPre, N.; Richman, E.L.; Stampfer, M.J.; Chan, J.M.; Giovannucci, E.L. Mediterranean diet and prostate cancer risk and mortality in the health professionals follow-up study. *Eur. Urol.* **2014**, *65*, 887–894. [CrossRef] [PubMed]

91. Filomeno, M.; Bosetti, C.; Garavello, W.; Levi, F.; Galeone, C.; Negri, E.; la Vecchia, C. The role of a Mediterranean diet on the risk of oral and pharyngeal cancer. *Br. J. Cancer* **2014**, *111*, 981–986. [CrossRef] [PubMed]

92. Bosetti, C.; Gallus, S.; Trichopoulou, A.; Talamini, R.; Franceschi, S.; Negri, E.; la Vecchia, C. Influence of the Mediterranean diet on the risk of cancers of the upper aerodigestive tract. *Cancer Epidemiol. Biomarkers Prev.* **2003**, *12*, 1091–1094. [PubMed]

93. Samoli, E.; Lagiou, A.; Nikolopoulos, E.; Lagogiannis, G.; Barbouni, A.; Lefantzis, D.; Trichopoulos, D.; Brennan, P.; Lagiou, P. Mediterranean diet and upper aerodigestive tract cancer: the Greek segment of the Alcohol-Related Cancers and Genetic Susceptibility in Europe study. *Br. J. Nutr.* **2010**, *104*, 1369–1374. [CrossRef] [PubMed]

94. Mourouti, N.; Papavagelis, C.; Plytzanopoulou, P.; Kontogianni, M.; Vassilakou, T.; Malamos, N.; Linos, A.; Panagiotakos, D. Dietary patterns and breast cancer: A case-control study in women. *Eur. J. Nutr.* **2014**, in press.

95. De la Torre-Carbot, K.; Chávez-Servín, J.L.; Jaúregui, O.; Castellote, A.I.; Lamuela-Raventós, R.M.; Nurmi, T.; Poulsen, H.E.; Gaddi, A.V.; Kaikkonen, J.; Zunft, H.F.; *et al.* Elevated circulating LDL phenol levels in men who consumed virgin rather than refined olive oil are associated with less oxidation of plasma LDL. *J. Nutr.* **2010**, *140*, 501–508. [CrossRef] [PubMed]

96. Camargo, A.; Delgado-Lista, J.; Garcia-Rios, A.; Cruz-Teno, C.; Yubero-Serrano, E.M.; Perez-Martinez, P.; Gutierrez-Mariscal, F.M.; Lora-Aguilar, P.; Rodriguez-Cantalejo, F.; Fuentes-Jimenez, F.; *et al.* Expression of proinflammatory, proatherogenic genes is reduced by the Mediterranean diet in elderly people. *Br. J. Nutr.* **2012**, *108*, 500–508. [CrossRef] [PubMed]

97. Aggarwal, B.B.; Shisodia, S. Suppression of the nuclear factor-kappaB activation pathway by spice-derived phytochemicals: reasoning for seasoning. *Ann. N.Y. Acad. Sci.* **2004**, *1030*, 434–441. [CrossRef] [PubMed]

98. Santangelo, C.; Varì, R.; Scazzocchio, B.; Di Benedetto, R.; Filesi, C.; Masella, R. Polyphenols, intracellular signalling and inflammation. *Ann. Ist. Super Sanita* **2007**, *43*, 394–405. [PubMed]

99. Laughton, M.J.; Evans, P.J.; Moroney, M.A.; Hoult, J.R.; Halliwell, B. Inhibition of mammalian 5-lipoxygenase and cyclo-oxygenase by flavonoids and phenolic dietary additives. Relationship to antioxidant activity and to iron ion-reducing ability. *Biochem. Pharmacol.* **1991**, *42*, 1673–1681. [CrossRef] [PubMed]

100. Ferrándiz, M.L.; Alcaraz, M.J. Anti-inflammatory activity and inhibition of arachidonic acid metabolism by flavonoids. *Agents Actions* **1991**, *32*, 283–288. [CrossRef] [PubMed]

101. Kim, H.P.; Mani, I.; Iversen, L.; Ziboh, V.A. Effects of naturally-occurring flavonoids and biflavonoids on epidermal cyclooxygenase and lipoxygenase from guinea-pigs. *Prostaglandins Leukot. Essent. Fatty Acids* **1998**, *58*, 17–24. [CrossRef] [PubMed]

102. Chondrogianni, N.; Kapeta, S.; Chinou, I.; Vassilatou, K.; Papassideri, I.; Gonos, E.S. Anti-ageing and rejuvenating effects of quercetin. *Exp. Gerontol.* **2010**, *45*, 763–771. [CrossRef] [PubMed]

103. Scoditti, E.; Calabriso, N.; Massaro, M.; Pellegrino, M.; Storelli, C.; Martines, G.; de Caterina, R.; Carluccio, M.A. Mediterranean diet polyphenols reduce inflammatory angiogenesis through MMP-9 and COX-2 inhibition in human vascular endothelial cells: A potentially protective mechanism in atherosclerotic vascular disease and cancer. *Arch. Biochem. Biophys.* **2012**, *527*, 81–89. [CrossRef] [PubMed]

104. Liang, Y.C.; Huang, Y.T.; Tsai, S.H.; Lin-Shiau, S.Y.; Chen, C.F.; Lin, J.K. Suppression of inducible cyclooxygenase and inducible nitric oxide synthase by apigenin and related flavonoids in mouse macrophages. *Carcinogenesis* **1999**, *20*, 1945–1952. [CrossRef] [PubMed]

105. Kim, H.K.; Cheon, B.S.; Kim, Y.H.; Kim, S.Y.; Kim, H.P. Effects of naturally occurring flavonoids on nitric oxide production in the macrophage cell line RAW 264.7 and their structure-activity relationships. *Biochem. Pharmacol.* **1999**, *58*, 759–765. [CrossRef] [PubMed]
106. Chen, Y.C.; Shen, S.C.; Lee, W.R.; Hou, W.C.; Yang, L.L.; Lee, T.J. Inhibition of nitric oxide synthase inhibitors and lipopolysaccharide induced inducible NOS and cyclooxygenase-2 gene expressions by rutin, quercetin, and quercetin pentaacetate in RAW 264.7 macrophages. *J. Cell Biochem.* **2001**, *82*, 537–548. [CrossRef] [PubMed]
107. Miles, E.A.; Zoubouli, P.; Calder, P.C. Differential anti-inflammatory effects of phenolic compounds from extra virgin olive oil identified in human whole blood cultures. *Nutrition* **2005**, *21*, 389–394. [CrossRef] [PubMed]
108. Calixto, J.B.; Campos, M.M.; Otuki, M.F.; Santos, A.R. Anti-inflammatory compounds of plant origin. Part II. modulation of pro-inflammatory cytokines, chemokines and adhesion molecules. *Plant. Med.* **2004**, *70*, 93–103. [CrossRef]
109. Comalada, M.; Ballester, I.; Bailón, E.; Sierra, S.; Xaus, J.; Gálvez, J.; de Medina, F.S.; Zarzuelo, A. Inhibition of pro-inflammatory markers in primary bone marrow-derived mouse macrophages by naturally occurring flavonoids: Analysis of the structure-activity relationship. *Biochem. Pharmacol.* **2006**, *72*, 1010–1021. [CrossRef] [PubMed]
110. Blonska, M.; Czuba, Z.P.; Krol, W. Effect of flavone derivatives on interleukin-1beta (IL-1beta) mRNA expression and IL-1beta protein synthesis in stimulated RAW 264.7 macrophages. *Scand. J. Immunol.* **2003**, *57*, 162–166. [CrossRef] [PubMed]
111. Sharma, V.; Mishra, M.; Ghosh, S.; Tewari, R.; Basu, A.; Seth, P.; Sen, E. Modulation of interleukin-1beta mediated inflammatory response in human astrocytes by flavonoids: Implications in neuroprotection. *Brain Res. Bull.* **2007**, *73*, 55–63. [CrossRef] [PubMed]
112. Min, Y.D.; Choi, C.H.; Bark, H.; Son, H.Y.; Park, H.H.; Lee, S.; Park, J.W.; Park, E.K.; Shin, H.I.; Kim, S.H. Quercetin inhibits expression of inflammatory cytokines through attenuation of NF-kappaB and p38 MAPK in HMC-1 human mast cell line. *Inflamm. Res.* **2007**, *5*, 210–215. [CrossRef]
113. Rahman, I.; Biswas, S.K.; Kirkham, P.A. Regulation of inflammation and redox signaling by dietary polyphenols. *Biochem. Pharmacol.* **2006**, *72*, 1439–1452. [CrossRef] [PubMed]
114. Benvenuto, M.; Fantini, M.; Masuelli, L.; de Smaele, E.; Zazzeroni, F.; Tresoldi, I.; Calabrese, G.; Galvano, F.; Modesti, A.; Bei, R. Inhibition of ErbB receptors, Hedgehog and NF-kappaB signaling by polyphenols in cancer. *Front. Biosci. (Landmark Ed.)* **2013**, *18*, 1290–1310. [CrossRef]
115. Chen, C.C.; Chow, M.P.; Huang, W.C.; Lin, Y.C.; Chang, Y.J. Flavonoids inhibit tumor necrosis factor-alpha-induced up-regulation of intercellular adhesion molecule-1 (ICAM-1) in respiratory epithelial cells through activator protein-1 and nuclear factor-kappaB: Structure-activity relationships. *Mol. Pharmacol.* **2004**, *66*, 683–693. [CrossRef] [PubMed]
116. Huang, S.M.; Wu, C.H.; Yen, G.C. Effects of flavonoids on the expression of the pro-inflammatory response in human monocytes induced by ligation of the receptor for AGEs. *Mol. Nutr. Food. Res.* **2006**, *50*, 1129–1139. [CrossRef] [PubMed]
117. Pallauf, K.; Giller, K.; Huebbe, P.; Rimbach, G. Nutrition and healthy ageing: Calorie restriction or polyphenol-rich "MediterrAsian" diet? *Oxid. Med. Cell. Longev.* **2013**, *2013*, 707421. [PubMed]
118. Bruning, A. Inhibition of mTOR signaling by quercetin in cancer treatment and prevention. *Anticancer Agents Med. Chem.* **2013**, *13*, 1025–1031. [CrossRef] [PubMed]
119. Galli, M.; van Gool, F.; Leo, O. Sirtuins and inflammation: friends or foes? *Biochem. Pharmacol.* **2011**, *81*, 569–576. [CrossRef] [PubMed]
120. Horio, Y.; Hayashi, T.; Kuno, A.; Kunimoto, R. Cellular and molecular effects of sirtuins in health and disease. *Clin. Sci. (Lond)* **2011**, *121*, 191–203. [CrossRef]
121. Yeung, F.; Hoberg, J.E.; Ramsey, C.S.; Keller, M.D.; Jones, D.R.; Frye, R.A.; Mayo, M.W. Modulation of NF-kappaB-dependent transcription and cell survival by the SIRT1 deacetylase. *EMBO J.* **2004**, *23*, 2369–2380. [CrossRef] [PubMed]
122. Kawahara, T.L.; Michishita, E.; Adler, A.S.; Damian, M.; Berber, E.; Lin, M.; McCord, R.A.; Ongaigui, K.C.; Boxer, L.D.; Chang, H.Y.; *et al.* SIRT6 links histone H3 lysine 9 deacetylation to NF-kappaB-dependent gene expression and organismal life span. *Cell* **2009**, *136*, 62–74. [CrossRef] [PubMed]

123. Alhazzazi, T.Y.; Kamarajan, P.; Verdin, E.; Kapila, Y.L. Sirtuin-3 (SIRT3) and the Hallmarks of Cancer. *Genes Cancer* **2013**, *4*, 164–171. [CrossRef] [PubMed]
124. Van Gool, F.; Galli, M.; Gueydan, C.; Kruys, V.; Prevot, P.P.; Bedalov, A.; Mostoslavsky, R.; Alt, F.W.; de Smedt, T.; Leo, O. Intracellular NAD levels regulate tumor necrosis factor protein synthesis in a sirtuin-dependent manner. *Nat. Med.* **2009**, *15*, 206–210. [CrossRef] [PubMed]
125. Parbin, S.; Kar, S.; Shilpi, A.; Sengupta, D.; Deb, M.; Rath, S.K.; Patra, S.K. Histone deacetylases: A saga of perturbed acetylation homeostasis in cancer. *J. Histochem. Cytochem.* **2014**, *62*, 11–33. [CrossRef] [PubMed]
126. Song, N.Y.; Surh, Y.J. Janus-faced role of SIRT1 in tumorigenesis. *Ann. N. Y. Acad. Sci.* **2012**, *1271*, 10–19. [CrossRef] [PubMed]
127. Bayram, B.; Ozcelik, B.; Grimm, S.; Roeder, T.; Schrader, C.; Ernst, I.M.; Wagner, A.E.; Grune, T.; Frank, J.; Rimbach, G. A diet rich in olive oil phenolics in the heart of SAMP8 mice by induction of Nrf2-dependent gene expression. *Rejuvenation Res.* **2012**, *15*, 71–81. [CrossRef] [PubMed]
128. Menendez, J.A.; Joven, J.; Aragonès, G.; Barrajón-Catalán, E.; Beltrán-Debón, R.; Borrás-Linares, I.; Camps, J.; Corominas-Faja, B.; Cufí, S.; Fernández-Arroyo, S.; et al. Xenohormetic and anti-aging activity of secoiridoid polyphenols present in extra virgin olive oil: A new family of gerosuppressant agents. *Cell Cycle* **2013**, *12*, 555–578. [CrossRef] [PubMed]
129. Popat, R.; Plesner, T.; Davies, F.; Cook, G.; Cook, M.; Elliott, P.; Jacobson, E.; Gumbleton, T.; Oakervee, H.; Cavenagh, J. A phase 2 study of SRT501 (resveratrol) with bortezomib for patients with relapsed and or refractory multiple myeloma. *Br. J. Haematol.* **2013**, *160*, 714–717. [CrossRef] [PubMed]
130. Bohn, T. Dietary factors affecting polyphenol bioavailability. *Nutr. Rev.* **2014**, *72*, 429–452. [CrossRef] [PubMed]
131. Holzapfel, N.P.; Holzapfel, B.M.; Champ, S.; Feldthusen, J.; Clements, J.; Hutmacher, D.W. The potential role of lycopene for the prevention and therapy of prostate cancer: from molecular mechanisms to clinical evidence. *Int. J. Mol. Sci.* **2013**, *14*, 14620–14646. [CrossRef] [PubMed]
132. Bjelakovic, G.; Nikolova, D.; Gluud, C. Antioxidant supplements and mortality. *Curr. Opin. Clin. Nutr. Metab. Care* **2014**, *17*, 40–44. [PubMed]
133. Ma, Y.; Hébert, J.R.; Li, W.; Bertone-Johnson, E.R.; Olendzki, B.; Pagoto, S.L.; Tinker, L.; Rosal, M.C.; Ockene, I.S.; Ockene, J.K.; et al. Association between dietary fiber and markers of systemic inflammation in the Women's Health Initiative Observational Study. *Nutrition* **2008**, *24*, 941–949. [CrossRef] [PubMed]
134. Ma, Y.; Griffith, J.A.; Chasan-Taber, L.; Olendzki, B.C.; Jackson, E.; Stanek, E.J., 3rd; Li, W.; Pagoto, S.L.; Hafner, A.R.; Ockene, I.S. Association between dietary fiber and serum C-reactive protein. *Am. J. Clin. Nutr.* **2006**, *83*, 760–766. [PubMed]
135. Chuang, S.C.; Vermeulen, R.; Sharabiani, M.T.; Sacerdote, C.; Fatemeh, S.H.; Berrino, F.; Krogh, V.; Palli, D.; Panico, S.; Tumino, R.; et al. The intake of grain fibers modulates cytokine levels in blood. *Biomarkers* **2011**, *16*, 504–510. [CrossRef] [PubMed]
136. Reddy, B.S.; Hirose, Y.; Cohen, L.A.; Simi, B.; Cooma, I.; Rao, C.V. Preventive potential of wheat bran fractions against experimental colon carcinogenesis: implications for human colon cancer prevention. *Cancer Res.* **2000**, *60*, 4792–4797. [PubMed]
137. Guigoz, Y.; Rochat, F.; Perruisseau-Carrier, G.; Rochat, I.; Schiffrin, E.J. Effects of oligosaccharide on the faecal flora and nonspecific immune system in elderly people. *Nutr. Res.* **2002**, *22*, 13–25. [CrossRef]
138. Kaczmarczyk, M.M.; Miller, M.J.; Freund, G.G. The health benefits of dietary fiber: Beyond the usual suspects of type 2 diabetes mellitus, cardiovascular disease and colon cancer. *Metabolism* **2012**, *61*, 1058–1066. [CrossRef] [PubMed]
139. Durko, L.; Malecka-Panas, E. Lifestyle Modifications and Colorectal Cancer. *Curr. Colorectal. Cancer Rep.* **2014**, *10*, 45–54. [CrossRef] [PubMed]
140. Toner, C.D. Communicating clinical research to reduce cancer risk through diet: Walnuts as a case example. *Nutr. Res. Pract.* **2014**, *8*, 347–351. [CrossRef] [PubMed]
141. Urpi-Sarda, M.; Casas, R.; Chiva-Blanch, G.; Romero-Mamani, E.S.; Valderas-Martínez, P.; Salas-Salvadó, J.; Covas, M.I.; Toledo, E.; Andres-Lacueva, C.; Llorach, R.; et al. The Mediterranean diet pattern and its main components are associated with lower plasma concentrations of tumor necrosis factor receptor 60 in patients at high risk for cardiovascular disease. *J. Nutr.* **2012**, *142*, 1019–1025. [CrossRef] [PubMed]

142. Patterson, R.E.; Flatt, S.W.; Newman, V.A.; Natarajan, L.; Rock, C.L.; Thomson, C.A.; Caan, B.J.; Parker, B.A.; Pierce, J.P. Marine fatty acid intake is associated with breast cancer prognosis. *J. Nutr.* **2011**, *141*, 201–206. [CrossRef] [PubMed]

143. Chapkin, R.S.; Kim, W.; Lupton, J.R.; McMurray, D.N. Dietary docosahexaenoic and eicosapentaenoic acid: emerging mediators of inflammation. *Prostaglandins Leukot. Essent. Fatty Acids* **2009**, *81*, 187–191. [CrossRef] [PubMed]

144. Santarelli, R.L.; Pierre, F.; Corpet, D.E. Processed meat and colorectal cancer: A review of epidemiologic and experimental evidence. *Nutr. Cancer* **2008**, *60*, 131–144. [CrossRef] [PubMed]

145. Myles, I.A. Fast food fever: reviewing the impacts of the Western diet on immunity. *Nutr. J.* **2014**, *13*, 61. [CrossRef] [PubMed]

146. Olivieri, F.; Spazzafumo, L.; Santini, G.; Lazzarini, R.; Albertini, M.C.; Rippo, M.R.; Galeazzi, R.; Abbatecola, A.M.; Marcheselli, F.; Monti, D.; *et al.* Age-related differences in the expression of circulating microRNAs: miR-21 as a new circulating marker of inflammaging. *Mech. Ageing Dev.* **2012**, *133*, 675–685. [CrossRef] [PubMed]

147. Esquela-Kerscher, A.; Slack, F.J. Oncomirs—microRNAs with a role in cancer. *Nat. Rev. Cancer* **2006**, *6*, 259–269. [CrossRef] [PubMed]

148. Winter, J.; Jung, S.; Keller, S.; Gregory, R.I.; Diederichs, S. Many roads to maturity: microRNA biogenesis pathways and their regulation. *Nat. Cell Biol.* **2009**, *11*, 228–234. [CrossRef] [PubMed]

149. Tzur, G.; Israel, A.; Levy, A.; Benjamin, H.; Meiri, E.; Shufaro, Y.; Meir, K.; Khvalevsky, E.; Spector, Y.; Rojansky, N.; *et al.* Comprehensive gene and microRNA expression profiling reveals a role for microRNAs in human liver development. *PLoS ONE* **2009**, *4*, e7511. [CrossRef] [PubMed]

150. Hussain, S.P.; Harris, C.C. Inflammation and cancer: an ancient link with novel potentials. *Int. J. Cancer* **2007**, *121*, 2373–2380. [CrossRef] [PubMed]

151. Olivieri, F.; Rippo, M.R.; Monsurrò, V.; Salvioli, S.; Capri, M.; Procopio, A.D.; Franceschi, C. MicroRNAs linking inflamm-aging, cellular senescence and cancer. *Ageing Res. Rev.* **2013**, *12*, 1056–1068. [CrossRef] [PubMed]

152. Lu, J.; Getz, G.; Miska, E.A.; Alvarez-Saavedra, E.; Lamb, J.; Peck, D.; Sweet-Cordero, A.; Ebert, B.L.; Mak, R.H.; Ferrando, A.A.; *et al.* MicroRNA expression profiles classify human cancers. *Nature* **2005**, *435*, 834–838. [CrossRef] [PubMed]

153. Piepoli, A.; Tavano, F.; Copetti, M.; Mazza, T.; Palumbo, O.; Panza, A.; di Mola, F.F.; Pazienza, V.; Mazzoccoli, G.; Biscaglia, G.; *et al.* miRNA expression profiles identify drivers in colorectal and pancreatic cancers. *PLoS ONE* **2012**, *7*, e33663. [CrossRef] [PubMed]

154. Lu, Y.; Govindan, R.; Wang, L.; Liu, P.Y.; Goodgame, B.; Wen, W.; Sezhiyan, A.; Pfeifer, J.; Li, Y.F.; Hua, X.; *et al.* MicroRNA profiling and prediction of recurrence/relapse-free survival in stage I lung cancer. *Carcinogenesis* **2012**, *33*, 1046–1054. [CrossRef] [PubMed]

155. Zhang, Y.; Li, M.; Wang, H.; Fisher, W.E.; Lin, P.H.; Yao, Q.; Chen, C. Profiling of 95 microRNAs in pancreatic cancer cell lines and surgical specimens by real-time PCR analysis. *World. J. Surg.* **2009**, *33*, 698–709. [CrossRef] [PubMed]

156. Fenech, M.; El-Sohemy, A.; Cahill, L.; Ferguson, L.R.; French, T.A.; Tai, E.S.; Milner, J.; Koh, W.P.; Xie, L.; Zucker, M.; *et al.* Nutrigenetics and nutrigenomics: Viewpoints on the current status and applications in nutrition research and practice. *J. Nutrigenet. Nutrigenomics* **2011**, *4*, 69–89. [CrossRef] [PubMed]

157. Chang, W.L.; Chapkin, R.S.; Lupton, J.R. Fish oil blocks azoxymethane-induced rat colon tumorigenesis by increasing cell differentiation and apoptosis rather than decreasing cell proliferation. *J. Nutr.* **1998**, *128*, 491–497. [PubMed]

158. Davidson, L.A.; Wang, N.; Ivanov, I.; Goldsby, J.; Lupton, J.R.; Chapkin, R.S. Identification of actively translated mRNA transcripts in a rat model of early-stage colon carcinogenesis. *Cancer Prev. Res.* **2009**, *2*, 984–994. [CrossRef]

159. Kachroo, P.; Ivanov, I.; Davidson, L.A.; Chowdhary, B.P.; Lupton, J.R.; Chapkin, R.S. Classification of diet-modulated gene signatures at the colon cancer initiation and progression stages. *Dig. Dis. Sci.* **2011**, *5*, 2595–2604. [CrossRef]

160. Turk, H.F.; Barhoumi, R.; Chapkin, R.S. Alteration of EGFR spatiotemporal dynamics suppresses signal transduction. *PLoS ONE* **2012**, *7*, e39682. [CrossRef] [PubMed]

161. Dimri, M.; Bommi, P.V.; Sahasrabuddhe, A.A.; Khandekar, J.D.; Dimri, G.P. Dietary omega-3 polyunsaturated fatty acids suppress expression of EZH2 in breast cancer cells. *Carcinogenesis* **2010**, *31*, 489–495. [CrossRef] [PubMed]

162. Leaver, H.A.; Wharton, S.B.; Bell, H.S.; Leaver-Yap, I.M.; Whittle, I.R. Highly unsaturated fatty acid induced tumour regression in glioma pharmacodynamics and bioavailability of gamma linolenic acid in an implantation glioma model: effects on tumour biomass, apoptosis and neuronal tissue histology. *Prostaglandins Leukot. Essent. Fatty Acids* **2002**, *67*, 283–292. [CrossRef] [PubMed]

163. Reddy, B.S.; Burill, C.; Rigotty, J. Effect of diets high in omega-3 and omega-6 fatty acids on initiation and postinitiation stages of colon carcinogenesis. *Cancer Res* **1991**, *51*, 487–491. [PubMed]

164. Whelan, J.; McEntee, M.F. Dietary (n-6) PUFA and intestinal tumorigenesis. *J Nutr.* **2004**, *134*, 3421–3426.

165. Vinciguerra, M.; Sgroi, A.; Veyrat-Durebex, C.; Rubbia-Brandt, L.; Buhler, L.H.; Foti, M. Unsaturated fatty acids inhibit the expression of tumor suppressor phosphatase and tensin homolog (PTEN) via microRNA-21 up-regulation in hepatocytes. *Hepatology* **2009**, *49*, 1176–1184. [CrossRef] [PubMed]

166. Hodin, R.A.; Meng, S.; Archer, S.; Tang, R. Cellular growth state differentially regulates enterocyte gene expression in butyrate-treated HT-29 cells. *Cell Growth Differ.* **1996**, *7*, 647–653. [PubMed]

167. Hinnebusch, B.F.; Meng, S.; Wu, J.T.; Archer, S.Y.; Hodin, R.A. The effects of short-chain fatty acids on human colon cancer cell phenotype are associated with histone hyperacetylation. *J. Nutr.* **2002**, *132*, 1012–1017. [PubMed]

168. Chirakkal, H.; Leech, S.H.; Brookes, K.E.; Prais, A.L.; Waby, J.S.; Corfe, B.M. Upregulation of BAK by butyrate in the colon is associated with increased Sp3 binding. *Oncogene* **2006**, *25*, 7192–7200. [CrossRef] [PubMed]

169. Comalada, M.; Bailón, E.; de Haro, O.; Lara-Villoslada, F.; Xaus, J.; Zarzuelo, A.; Gálvez, J. The effects of short-chain fatty acids on colon epithelial proliferation and survival depend on the cellular phenotype. *J. Cancer Res. Clin. Oncol.* **2006**, *132*, 487–497. [CrossRef] [PubMed]

170. Hu, S.; Dong, T.S.; Dalal, S.R.; Wu, F.; Bissonnette, M.; Kwon, J.H.; Chang, E.B. The microbe-derived short chain fatty acid butyrate targets miRNA-dependent p21 gene expression in human colon cancer. *PLoS ONE* **2011**, *6*, e16221. [CrossRef] [PubMed]

171. Shah, M.S.; Schwartz, S.L.; Zhao, C.; Davidson, L.A.; Zhou, B.; Lupton, J.R.; Ivanov, I.; Chapkin, R.S. Integrated microRNA and mRNA expression profiling in a rat colon carcinogenesis model: Effect of a chemo-protective diet. *Physiol. Genomics* **2011**, *43*, 640–654. [CrossRef] [PubMed]

172. Sun, Y.; Zuo, L.; Xu, C.; Shen, T.; Pan, H.; Zhang, Z. Apoptosis and differentiation induced by sodium selenite combined with all-trans retinoic acid (ATRA) in NB4 cells. *Zhonghua Xue Ye Xue Za Zhi* **2002**, *23*, 628–630. [PubMed]

173. Terao, M.; Fratelli, M.; Kurosaki, M.; Zanetti, A.; Guarnaccia, V.; Paroni, G.; Tsykin, A.; Lupi, M.; Gianni, M.; Goodall, G.J.; *et al.* Induction of miR-21 by retinoic acid in estrogen receptor-positive breast carcinoma cells: Biological correlates and molecular targets. *J. Biol. Chem.* **2011**, *286*, 4027–4042. [CrossRef] [PubMed]

174. Wang, X.; Gocek, E.; Liu, C.G.; Studzinski, G.P. MicroRNAs181 regulate the expression of p27Kip1 in human myeloid leukemia cells induced to differentiate by 1,25-dihydroxyvitamin D3. *Cell Cycle* **2009**, *8*, 736–741. [CrossRef] [PubMed]

175. Arts, I.C.; Hollman, P.C. Polyphenols and disease risk in epidemiologic studies. *Am. J. Clin. Nutr.* **2005**, *81*, 317–325.

176. Scalbert, A.; Manach, C.; Morand, C.; Rémésy, C.; Jiménez, L. Dietary polyphenols and the prevention of diseases. *Crit. Rev. Food Sci. Nutr.* **2005**, *45*, 287–306. [CrossRef] [PubMed]

177. Schroeter, H.; Heiss, C.; Balzer, J.; Kleinbongard, P.; Keen, C.L.; Hollenberg, N.K.; Sies, H.; Kwik-Uribe, C.; Schmitz, H.H.; Kelm, M. Epicatechin mediates beneficial effects of flavanol-rich cocoa on vascular function in humans. *Proc. Natl. Acad. Sci. USA* **2006**, *103*, 1024–1029. [CrossRef] [PubMed]

178. Spencer, J.P.; Abd El Mohsen, M.M.; Minihane, A.M.; Mathers, J.C. Biomarkers of the intake of dietary polyphenols: strengths, limitations and application in nutrition research. *Br. J. Nutr.* **2008**, *99*, 12–22. [PubMed]

179. Joven, J.; Espinel, E.; Rull, A.; Aragonès, G.; Rodríguez-Gallego, E.; Camps, J.; Micol, V.; Herranz-López, M.; Menéndez, J.A.; Borrás, I.; *et al.* Plant-derived polyphenols regulate expression of miRNA paralogs miR-103/107 and miR-122 and prevent diet-induced fatty liver disease in hyperlipidemic mice. *Biochim. Biophys. Acta* **2012**, *1820*, 894–899. [CrossRef] [PubMed]

180. Sun, M.; Estrov, Z.; Ji, Y.; Coombes, K.R.; Harris, D.H.; Kurzrock, R. Curcumin (diferuloylmethane) alters the expression profiles of microRNAs in human pancreatic cancer cells. *Mol. Cancer Ther.* **2008**, *7*, 464–473. [CrossRef] [PubMed]

181. Bao, B.; Ali, S.; Kong, D.; Sarkar, S.H.; Wang, Z.; Banerjee, S.; Aboukameel, A.; Padhye, S.; Philip, P.A.; Sarkar, F.H. Anti-tumor activity of a novel compound-CDF is mediated by regulating miR-21, miR-200, and PTEN in pancreatic cancer. *PLoS ONE* **2011**, *6*, e17850. [CrossRef] [PubMed]

182. Biagi, E.; Candela, M.; Fairweather-Tait, S.; Franceschi, C.; Brigidi, P. Aging of the human metaorganism: the microbial counterpart. *Age (Dordr)* **2012**, *34*, 247–267. [CrossRef]

183. Claesson, M.J.; Cusack, S.; O'Sullivan, O.; Greene-Diniz, R.; de Weerd, H.; Flannery, E.; Marchesi, J.R.; Falush, D.; Dinan, T.; Fitzgerald, G.; *et al.* Composition, variability, and temporal stability of the intestinal microbiota of the elderly. *Proc. Natl. Acad. Sci. USA* **2011**, *108*, 4586–4591. [CrossRef] [PubMed]

184. Eckburg, P.B.; Bik, E.M.; Bernstein, C.N.; Purdom, E.; Dethlefsen, L.; Sargent, M.; Gill, S.R.; Nelson, K.E.; Relman, D.A. Diversity of the human intestinal microbial flora. *Science* **2005**, *308*, 1635–1638. [CrossRef] [PubMed]

185. Candela, M.; Biagi, E.; Brigidi, P.; O'Toole, P.W.; de Vos, W.M. Maintenance of a healthy trajectory of the intestinal microbiome during aging: A dietary approach. *Mech. Ageing Dev.* **2014**, *136–137*, 70–75. [CrossRef] [PubMed]

186. Yatsunenko, T.; Rey, F.E.; Manary, M.J.; Trehan, I.; Dominguez-Bello, M.G.; Contreras, M.; Magris, M.; Hidalgo, G.; Baldassano, R.N.; Anokhin, A.P.; *et al.* Human gut microbiome viewed across age and geography. *Nature* **2012**, *486*, 222–227. [PubMed]

187. Jeffery, I.B.; O'Toole, P.W. Diet-microbiota interactions and their implications for healthy living. *Nutrients* **2013**, *5*, 234–252. [CrossRef] [PubMed]

188. Claesson, M.J.; Jeffery, I.B.; Conde, S.; Power, S.E.; O'Connor, E.M.; Cusack, S.; Harris, H.M.; Coakley, M.; Lakshminarayanan, B.; O'Sullivan, O.; *et al.* Gut microbiota composition correlates with diet and health in the elderly. *Nature* **2012**, *488*, 178–284. [CrossRef] [PubMed]

189. Turnbaugh, P.J.; Ridaura, V.K.; Faith, J.J.; Rey, F.E.; Knight, R.; Gordon, J.I. The effect of diet on the human gut microbiome: A metagenomic analysis in humanized gnotobiotic mice. *Sci. Transl. Med.* **2009**, *1*, 6ra14. [CrossRef] [PubMed]

190. Bäckhed, F.; Ley, R.E.; Sonnenburg, J.L.; Peterson, D.A.; Gordon, J.I. Host-bacterial mutualism in the human intestine. *Science* **2005**, *307*, 1915–1920. [CrossRef] [PubMed]

191. Duncan, S.H.; Belenguer, A.; Holtrop, G.; Johnstone, A.M.; Flint, H.J.; Lobley, G.E. Reduced dietary intake of carbohydrates by obese subjects results in decreased concentrations of butyrate and butyrate-producing bacteria in feces. *Appl. Environ. Microbiol.* **2007**, *73*, 1073–1078. [CrossRef] [PubMed]

192. David, L.A.; Maurice, C.F.; Carmody, R.N.; Gootenberg, D.B.; Button, J.E.; Wolfe, B.E.; Ling, A.V.; Devlin, A.S.; Varma, Y.; Fischbach, M.A.; *et al.* Diet rapidly and reproducibly alters the human gut microbiome. *Nature* **2014**, *505*, 559–563. [CrossRef] [PubMed]

193. Biagi, E.; Nylund, L.; Candela, M.; Ostan, R.; Bucci, L.; Pini, E.; Nikkïla, J.M.; Monti, D.; Satokari, R.; Franceschi, C.; *et al.* Through aging, and beyond: gut microbiota and inflammatory status in seniors and centenarians. *PLoS ONE* **2010**, *5*, e10667. [CrossRef] [PubMed]

194. Boyle, P.; Ferlay, J. Mortality and survival in breast and colorectal cancer. *Nat. Clin. Pract. Oncol.* **2005**, *2*, 424–425. [CrossRef] [PubMed]

195. Mladenova, D.; Kohonen-Corish, M.R. Review: Mouse models of inflammatory bowel disease: insights into the mechanisms of inflammation-associated colorectal cancer. *In Vivo* **2012**, *26*, 627–646. [PubMed]

196. Nikolaki, S.; Tsiamis, G. Microbial diversity in the era of omic technologies. *Biomed. Res. Int.* **2013**, *2013*, 958719. [CrossRef] [PubMed]

197. Tjalsma, H.; Boleij, A.; Marchesi, J.R.; Dutilh, B.E. A bacterial driver-passenger model for colorectal cancer: beyond the usual suspects. *Nat. Rev. Microbiol.* **2012**, *10*, 575–582. [CrossRef] [PubMed]

198. Schwabe, R.F.; Wang, T.C. Cancer. Bacteria deliver a genotoxic hit. *Science* **2012**, *338*, 52–53. [CrossRef] [PubMed]

199. Nicholson, J.K.; Lindon, J.C. Systems biology: Metabonomics. *Nature* **2008**, *455*, 1054–1056. [CrossRef] [PubMed]

200. Wishart, D.S.; Knox, C.; Guo, A.C.; Eisner, R.; Young, N.; Gautam, B.; Hau, D.D.; Psychogios, N.; Dong, E.; Bouatra, S.; et al. HMDB: A knowledgebase for the human metabolome. Nucl. Acids Res. 2009, 37, 603–610. [CrossRef]

201. Fahy, E.; Subramaniam, S.; Murphy, R.C.; Nishijima, M.; Raetz, C.R.; Shimizu, T.; Spener, F.; van Meer, G.; Wakelam, M.J.; Dennis, E.A. Update of the LIPID MAPS comprehensive classification system for lipids. J. Lipid Res. 2009, 50, 9–14. [CrossRef]

202. Vinayavekhin, N.; Homan, E.; Saghatelian, A. Exploring disease through metabolomics. ACS Chem. Biol. 2010, 5, 91–103. [CrossRef] [PubMed]

203. Gieger, C.; Geistlinger, L.; Altmaier, E.; Hrabé de Angelis, M.; Kronenberg, F.; Meitinger, T.; Mewes, H.W.; Wichmann, H.-E.; Weinberger, K.M.; Adamski, J.; et al. Genetics meets metabolomics: A genome-wide association study of metabolite profiles in human serum. PLoS Genet 2008, 4, e1000282. [CrossRef] [PubMed]

204. Chadeau-Hyam, M.; Ebbels, T.M.; Brown, I.J.; Chan, Q.; Stamler, J.; Huang, C.C.; Daviglus, M.L.; Ueshima, H.; Zhao, L.; Holmes, E.; et al. Metabolic profiling and the metabolome-wide association study: significance level for biomarker identification. J. Proteome Res. 2010, 9, 4620–4627. [CrossRef] [PubMed]

205. Nicholson, J.K.; Holmes, E.; Elliott, P. The metabolome-wide association study: A new look at human disease risk factors. J Proteome Res 2008, 7, 3637–3638. [CrossRef] [PubMed]

206. Bictash, M.; Ebbels, T.M.; Chan, Q.; Loo, R.L.; Yap, I.K.; Brown, I.J.; de Iorio, M.; Daviglus, M.L.; Holmes, E.; Stamler, J.; et al. Opening up the "Black Box": Metabolic phenotyping and metabolome-wide association studies in epidemiology. J. Clin. Epidemiol. 2010, 63, 970–979. [CrossRef] [PubMed]

207. Watson, E.; MacNeil, L.T.; Ritter, A.D.; Yilmaz, L.S.; Rosebrock, A.P.; Caudy, A.A.; Walhout, A.J. Interspecies systems biology uncovers metabolites affecting C. elegans gene expression and life history traits. Cell 2014, 156, 759–770. [CrossRef] [PubMed]

208. Nookaew, I.; Gabrielsson, B.G.; Holmäng, A.; Sandberg, A.S.; Nielsen, J. Identifying molecular effects of diet through systems biology: Influence of herring diet on sterol metabolism and protein turnover in mice. PLoS ONE 2010, 5, e12361. [CrossRef] [PubMed]

209. Griffin, J.L.; Shockcor, J.P. Metabolic profiles of cancer cells. Nat. Rev. Cancer 2004, 4, 551–561. [CrossRef] [PubMed]

210. Spratlin, J.L.; Serkova, N.J.; Eckhardt, S.G. Clinical applications of metabolomics in oncology: A review. Clin. Cancer Res. 2009, 15, 431–440. [CrossRef] [PubMed]

211. Tieri, P.; de la Fuente, A.; Termanini, A.; Franceschi, C. Integrating Omics data for signaling pathways, interactome reconstruction, and functional analysis. Methods Mol. Biol. 2011, 719, 415–433. [PubMed]

212. Sreekumar, A.; Poisson, L.M.; Rajendiran, T.M.; Khan, A.P.; Cao, Q.; Yu, J.; Laxman, B.; Mehra, R.; Lonigro, R.J.; Li, Y.; et al. Metabolomic profiles delineate potential role for sarcosine in prostate cancer progression. Nature 2009, 457, 910–914. [CrossRef] [PubMed]

213. De Boer, N.K.H.; de Meij, T.G.; Oort, F.A.; Ben Larbi, I.; Mulder, C.J.; van Bodegraven, A.A.; van der Schee, M.P. The Scent of Colorectal Cancer: Detection by Volatile Organic Compound Analysis. Clin. Gastroenterol. Hepatol. 2014, 12, 1085–1089. [CrossRef] [PubMed]

214. Floegel, A.; Wientzek, A.; Bachlechner, U.; Jacobs, S.; Drogan, D.; Prehn, C.; Adamski, J.; Krumsiek, J.; Schulze, M.B.; Pischon, T.; et al. Linking diet, physical activity, cardiorespiratory fitness and obesity to serum metabolite networks: findings from a population-based study. Int. J. Obes. (Lond) 2014, 38, 1388–1396. [CrossRef]

215. Eurostat. Available online: http://ec.europa.eu/eurostat/help/new-eurostat-website (accessed on 7 April 2015).

216. The European Project NU-AGE (FP7,n° 266486; 2011–2016). Available online: http://www.nu-age.eu (accessed on 7 April 2015).

217. Santoro, A.; Pini, E.; Scurti, M.; Palmas, G.; Berendsen, A.; Brzozowska, A.; Pietruszka, B.; Szczecinska, A.; Cano, N.; Meunier, N.; et al. The NU-AGE Consortium. Combating inflammaging through a Mediterranean whole diet approach: the NU-AGE project's conceptual framework and design. Mech. Ageing Dev. 2014, 136–137, 3–13. [CrossRef] [PubMed]

218. Berendsen, A.; Santoro, A.; Pini, E.; Cevenini Ostan, R.; Pietruszka, B.; Rolf, K.; Cano, N.; Caille, A.; Lyon-Belgy, N.; Fairweather-Tait, S.; et al. A randomized trial on the effect of a full dietary intervention on ageing in European elderly people: Design of the NU-AGE dietary intervention study. Mech. Ageing Dev. 2013, 134, 523–530. [CrossRef] [PubMed]

219. Calçada, D.; Vianello, D.; Giampieri, E.; Sala, C.; Castellani, G.; de Graaf, A.; Kremer, B.; van Ommen, B.; Feskens, E.; Santoro, A.; *et al.* The role of low-grade inflammation and metabolic flexibility in aging and nutritional modulation thereof: a systems biology approach. *Mech. Ageing Dev.* **2014**, *136–137*, 138–147. [CrossRef] [PubMed]

220. Mediterranean diet and inflammaging in the elderly: The European project NU-AGE. *Mech. Ageing Dev.* **2014**, *136–137*. [CrossRef] [PubMed]

221. Hughes, V. Microbiome: Cultural differences. *Nature* **2012**, *492*, S14–S15. [CrossRef] [PubMed]

n-3 Polyunsaturated Fatty Acids and Mechanisms to Mitigate Inflammatory Paracrine Signaling in Obesity-Associated Breast Cancer

Jennifer M. Monk [1,2], Harmony F. Turk [3], Danyelle M. Liddle [1], Anna A. De Boer [1], Krista A. Power [1,2], David W.L. Ma [1] and Lindsay E. Robinson [1,*]

[1] Department of Human Health and Nutritional Sciences, University of Guelph, Guelph, ON N1G 2W1, Canada; jmonk02@uoguelph.ca (J.M.M.); dliddle@uoguelph.ca (D.M.L.); adeboer@uoguelph.ca (A.A.D.B.); krista.power@agr.gc.ca (K.A.P.); davidma@uoguelph.ca (D.W.L.M.)
[2] Guelph Food Research Centre, Agriculture and Agri-Food Canada, Guelph, ON N1G 5C9, Canada
[3] Institut Curie, Paris 75248, France; harmony.turk@curie.fr
*   Author to whom correspondence should be addressed; lrobinso@uoguelph.ca

Abstract: Globally, the prevalence of obesity is increasing which subsequently increases the risk of the development of obesity-related chronic diseases. Low-grade chronic inflammation and dysregulated adipose tissue inflammatory mediator/adipokine secretion are well-established in obesity, and these factors increase the risk of developing inflammation-associated cancer. Breast cancer is of particular interest given that increased inflammation within the subcutaneous mammary adipose tissue depot can alter the local tissue inflammatory microenvironment such that it resembles that of obese visceral adipose tissue. Therefore, in obese women with breast cancer, increased inflammatory mediators both locally and systemically can perpetuate inflammation-associated pro-carcinogenic signaling pathways, thereby increasing disease severity. Herein, we discuss some of these inflammation-associated pro-carcinogenic mechanisms of the combined obese breast cancer phenotype and offer evidence that dietary long chain *n*-3 polyunsaturated fatty acids (PUFA) may have utility in mitigating the severity of obesity-associated inflammation and breast cancer.

Keywords: breast cancer; inflammation; obesity; adipokines; *n*-3 polyunsaturated fatty acids; leptin; adiponectin; aromatase; lipid rafts; eicosanoids

1. Introduction

Based on body mass index (BMI), globally 1.5 billion people are overweight (BMI ≥ 25.0 kg/m^2), and 500 million of these individuals are classified as obese (BMI ≥ 30.0 kg/m^2) [1]. The clinical consequence of obesity is that it acts as an independent risk factor for several other pathologies, including cancer [1,2]. In this context, obesity is associated with increased mortality in several types of cancer, including breast cancer (BC) [3]. It is estimated that obesity contributes to 50% of all BC cases in older women [4]. Furthermore, considering the prevalence of obesity in younger populations and the projected expansion of the obese population [1], the impact on BC incidence is likely to be exacerbated in the future. Obesity increases the risk of developing the most common BC subtype, estrogen receptor (ER)-positive and progesterone receptor (PR)-positive BC (*i.e.*, hormone-sensitive form of the disease) [4–7]. Paradoxically the incidence of hormone sensitive BC increases with age, which coincides with increasing adiposity and decreasing circulating estrogen levels [8]. In fact, in postmenopausal women the majority of BC cases associated with obesity are ER-positive with a phenotype exhibiting larger and faster growing tumors that metastasize to axillary lymph nodes [4,5,9–11]. The positive association between BC development and obesity in postmenopausal women is well-established using multiple anthropometric indices of obesity including BMI, adiposity and waist:hip circumference ratio [4,5,9–12]. Interestingly, postmenopausal BC risk is increased by the degree of weight gain during adult life prior to menopause [13,14], thereby indicating that the effects of obesity during the premenopausal phase impact BC risk later in life. Conversely, in premenopausal women the link between BC risk and BMI as a measure of obesity status is more controversial [15–17]. Studies finding no association commonly normalize data to BMI alone, which is a poor discriminator of body fat and lean mass, and fails to account for visceral adiposity which is believed to be a more deleterious adipose depot compared to subcutaneous [18,19]. Premenopausal women with high BMI have been shown to develop significantly larger tumors and worse histopathological features including increased tumor vascularization and metastasis to axillary lymph nodes compared to healthy BMI BC patients [9]. Additionally, premenopausal obesity has been shown to increase the risk of developing triple negative BC (ER, PR and HER negative) [9,20] and hormone receptor-negative BC (ER and PR-negative) [21,22]. Collectively, these data indicate that independent of hormonal status, obesity increases overall BC risk, an effect that is, at least in part, attributed to inflammatory mechanisms and paracrine interactions (i.e., cross-talk) between cell types within the mammary tissue that promote tumorigenesis [4,23,24].

The connection between obesity and ER-positive BC in post-menopausal women is likely attributable to two main interrelated factors that will be a key focus of this review, including: (i) increased adipose tissue (AT) mass and the associated increase in inflammatory mediator production (both locally and systemically); and (ii) elevated AT aromatase activation, which is up-regulated by inflammatory mediators and drives aberrant estrogen production within the AT, thereby promoting BC tumorigenesis. The obesity-associated inflammatory mammary tumor microenvironment is complex and the resultant phenotype is underscored by autocrine and paracrine interactions between adipocytes, tumor infiltrating macrophages (TAM) and epithelial cells, which produce AT-derived inflammatory mediators, collectively referred to as adipokines, which will be discussed in more detail herein. The inflammatory mammary tumor microenvironment should not be confused with "inflammatory breast cancer" (IBC), a rare (1%–6% of all breast malignancies) aggressive BC subtype with higher grade metastatic hormone receptor negative tumors that has been reviewed elsewhere [25,26]. Moreover, we provide evidence that dietary long-chain (LC) n-3 polyunsaturated fatty acids (PUFA), particularly fish oil (marine)-derived eicosapentaenoic acid (EPA, 20:5n-3) and docosahexaenoic acid (DHA, 22:6n3), which have well established anti-inflammatory effects in obesity [27–41] and anti-carcinogenic effects in BC [42–56], may represent an effective complementary approach in the prevention and/or treatment of obesity-associated BC by attenuating inflammatory adipokine-mediated paracrine interactions within the mammary tumor microenvironment.

2. Obese Inflammatory Phenotype

AT is an endocrine organ that secretes greater than 50 recognized proteins including several cytokines and chemokines, both of which are included in the term adipokine (i.e., of AT origin) [57]. In the classic obese phenotype (reviewed elsewhere [2,58,59]), the tissue stress and remodeling that occurs in expanding visceral AT is associated with dysregulated adipokine secretion and a subsequent state of chronic, sub-clinical, low-grade, systemic inflammation [2,60]. The cellular source of these inflammatory mediators includes adipocytes and cells of the stromal vascular fraction (SVF) including endothelial cells, fibroblasts, macrophages and T cells [60]. These adipokines can influence whole-body metabolism, insulin sensitivity and inflammation through autocrine, paracrine and endocrine signaling. Most notably, in obesity both the local AT and circulating levels of inflammatory mediators, such as TNFα, IL-6, IL-1β, MCP-1, leptin and many others (reviewed by [58,59]), are elevated, while levels of adiponectin, an anti-inflammatory adipokine, are decreased [61]. Many of these same adipokines are up-regulated in obese BC and activate signaling pathways that drive inflammation-associated malignant transformation, and therefore, when present in the mammary tissue result in a more severe BC phenotype, as discussed in detail below.

3. *n*-3 Polyunsaturated Fatty Acids and Obesity

In obesity, marine source LC *n*-3 PUFA have been shown to modulate and improve several critical aspects of the obese phenotype, collectively reducing AT inflammation. Specifically, *n*-3 PUFA modulate the production of AT-derived adipokines by increasing anti-inflammatory adiponectin levels [27–35], while decreasing production of inflammatory mediators such as leptin [36–39] and cytokines including TNFα, IL-6 and MCP-1 [29,35,40,41]. Moreover, dietary *n*-3 PUFA have been found to reverse and/or improved obesity-associated hepatic steatosis and impairments in glucose metabolism and insulin sensitivity [27–29,35,62–64]. Collectively, these anti-inflammatory effects of *n*-3 PUFA alter the obesity-associated inflammatory microenvironment and improve the overall obese phenotype. One well-documented effect of *n*-3 PUFA is the suppression of inflammation by interfering with pro-inflammatory signaling cascades via peroxisome proliferator-activated receptor (PPAR)γ-dependent and independent mechanisms that involve up-regulation of adiponectin, in murine [65] and human adipocytes [66]. Additionally, PPARγ is involved in trans-repression of nuclear factor kappa-light-chain-enhancer of activated B cells (NFκB) transcriptional activity leading to decreased expression of NFκB responsive genes including several inflammatory cytokines (TNFα, IL-1β, IL-6 and MCP-1) [67]. In this connection, *n*-3 PUFA functioning as PPAR-receptor ligands also interfere with other transcription factors involved in inflammatory signal transduction pathways including AP-1, STAT-1 and NFAT [68].

n-3 PUFA can also perturb inflammatory signaling in obesity through PPARγ independent signaling mechanisms, most notably by acting as ligands for the G-protein coupled receptor 120 (GPR120) [69]. GPR120 has been shown to be partly responsible for the anti-inflammatory effects of DHA by using the adaptor β-arrestin2 to interfere with inflammatory mediator-stimulated NFκB activation in macrophages [69]. Additionally, EPA and DHA exert anti-inflammatory effects following their selective incorporation into the phospholipid fraction of cell membranes where they can act to decrease the signaling efficiency of protein complexes in lipid rafts [70], or serve as substrates for the synthesis of anti-inflammatory bioactive lipid mediators (*i.e.*, eicosanoids) [71,72]. Taken together, *n*-3 PUFA may beneficially modulate obesity-associated pro-inflammatory paracrine interactions between the different cell types within AT. Overall, *n*-3 PUFA utilize multiple mechanisms to suppress inflammatory signaling, thereby modulating the obesity-associated inflammatory phenotype.

4. *n*-3 Polyunsaturated Fatty Acids and Breast Cancer

Marine-derived *n*-3 PUFA have well-established anti-tumorigenic effects in chemically induced, transgenic and xenograft rodent models of BC [73]. As a point of reference, amongst high LC *n*-3 PUFA consuming populations, the typical Japanese diet contains 1%–2% of daily energy as LC *n*-3 PUFA [74,75], whereas intake levels are higher amongst the Greenland Inuit who typically consume 2.4%–6.3% of daily energy as LC *n*-3 PUFA [76,77]. Although higher levels of *n*-3 PUFA intake can be achieved through supplementation, these physiologically relevant intake levels have been recapitulated in BC rodent dietary intervention studies which demonstrate a beneficial effect of *n*-3 PUFA on the BC phenotype [42–44,46,48,49,55,78]. In this connection, *n*-3 PUFA are recognized for their potential application in reducing obesity-associated inflammation and consequent tumorigenic risk [45]. In brief, LC *n*-3 PUFA are incorporated into mammary AT and tumor tissue [46,47], thereby increasing the levels of *n*-3 PUFA-derived lipid mediators at the expense of those derived from *n*-6 PUFA (*i.e.*, arachidonic acid (AA, C20:4*n*-6)-derived eicosanoids) [42,56,78], altering adipokine secretion [54] and interrupting tumorigenic signaling pathways [79]. These chemoprotective effects of *n*-3 PUFA result in decreased cell proliferation and increased apoptosis, ultimately resulting in reduced BC tumor incidence, growth, multiplicity, and metastasis in rodent models of BC [43,44,46,48–53,55,79]. Further, in a model of obese postmenopausal BC, *n*-3 PUFA supplementation reduced mammary AT inflammation and markers of inflammatory M1 macrophage infiltration [80] which was associated with reduced tumor burden, indicating that the inflammatory microenvironment promotes tumorigenesis and that *n*-3 PUFA directly antagonize this process. Similar *n*-3 PUFA-mediated anti-tumorigenic effects have been reported in overweight humans wherein *n*-3 PUFA supplementation up-regulated the expression of several genes involved in cell cycle regulation [81]. These studies clearly demonstrate that *n*-3 PUFA can independently modulate responsiveness to cell proliferative and/or apoptotic signaling. This is further highlighted in Figure 1, which outlines the effects of *n*-3 PUFA on critical adipokine/inflammatory mediator levels that underlie the paracrine interactions within the obese mammary tumor microenvironment that ultimately impact proliferative and apoptotic signaling and will be discussed in this review.

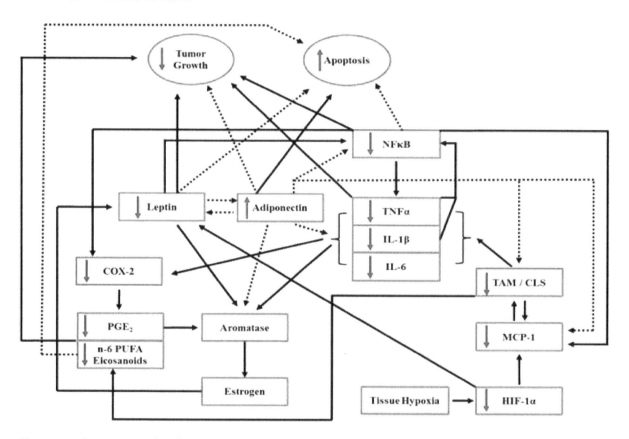

Figure 1. Summary of inflammatory mediator paracrine interactions produced within the obese mammary tissue tumor microenvironment highlighting the complex interactions mediated by adipocytes, macrophages and epithelial cells (main cellular sources of inflammatory mediators). Solid arrows denote stimulatory effects and dotted arrows denote inhibitory effects between inflammatory mediators. Red arrows indicate the effects of *n*-3 PUFA to increase or decrease inflammatory mediator levels, thereby subsequently up-regulating (adiponectin, *n*-3 PUFA-derived eicosanoids) or down-regulating (leptin, *n*-6 PUFA-derived eicosanoids, cytokines (TNFα, IL-1β, IL-6 and MCP-1) and macrophage tissue infiltration). TAM, tumor associated-macrophage; CLS, crown-like structure; HIF-1α, hypoxia induced factor-1α; COX-2, cyclooxygenase-2; PGE$_2$, prostaglandin E$_2$; TNFα, tumor necrosis factor-α; IL, interleukin; MCP-1, monocyte chemoattractant protein-1.

A recent meta-analysis that included 21 independent prospective cohort studies determined that marine source *n*-3 PUFA intake was associated with a 14% reduction in BC risk (RR = 0.86 for highest *versus* lowest category of intake (95% confidence interval 0.78–0.94)) [82]. The results were also sustained if the data was analyzed based on either reported dietary intake levels or tissue biomarker levels of *n*-3 PUFA, thereby removing concerns regarding intake compliance or accuracy in dietary recall data. In obese women, a decreased risk of BC was found to be significantly associated with both increased intake of *n*-3 PUFA and altered dietary fatty acid composition by increasing the ratio of *n*-3:*n*-6 PUFA intake, although this association was not significant in overweight or normal weight women [83]. These data suggest that obesity status may affect the association between *n*-3 PUFA intake and BC risk. To the best of our knowledge, this is the only case-control study that has specifically investigated the relationship between obesity, *n*-3 PUFA intake and BC risk. Interestingly, the chemoprotective effect of an increased ratio of *n*-3:*n*-6 PUFA intake has been reported elsewhere [84], and several case-control studies have reported an inverse association between BC risk and increased *n*-3 PUFA intake and/or increasing the *n*-3:*n*-6 PUFA ratio in breast AT [85–88]. Although obesity status was not independently assessed, some of these studies report a trend with more normal weight women in the control group and more overweight and obese women with BC [85,88]. In contrast, others have reported no association between AT *n*-3 PUFA levels and the development of BC; however, BMI was lower among these BC cases [89]. Taken together, while higher *n*-3 PUFA intake and tissue content is more often than not associated with a decreased risk of developing BC, controversy exists surrounding the associations between BC incidence, obesity status and *n*-3 PUFA intake, warranting case-control studies that investigate a relationship between all endpoints.

5. *n*-3 PUFA, Lipid Rafts and Breast Cancer

Extensive research has indicated that *n*-3 PUFA have a unique ability to broadly affect cell signaling. A ubiquitous mechanism by which *n*-3 PUFA can alter signal transduction is by modifying lipid rafts, which are heterogeneous, highly ordered membrane microdomains that facilitate several signaling events [90,91]. Lipid rafts laterally isolate their components from the bulk membrane and then are able to coalesce in response to stimuli to form signaling platforms [92,93], thereby playing an integral role in the propagation of multiple signaling events that are involved in tumor-promoting activities, including cell proliferation, survival, migration, and invasion [94]. The physical properties that facilitate the segregation of lipid raft domains from the bulk membrane is imparted by the enrichment of cholesterol, sphingolipids, and other phospholipids with saturated, long hydrocarbon chains within lipid rafts [95,96]. *n*-3 PUFA display low affinity for cholesterol due to their high degree of unsaturation [97,98]; therefore, enrichment of the membrane with *n*-3 PUFA can alter the composition and organization of raft domains. Altering the properties of lipid rafts can then have major effects on signaling events that are initiated or propagated by these integral domains.

An important property of lipid rafts is their size and number. Changes to the size of rafts can impose substantial changes on their function. It has been shown that rafts must be small and mobile for optimal activity [99]. Studies in BC cells, in addition to many other cell types, have demonstrated the ability of *n*-3 PUFA to alter the size of lipid rafts. Specifically, DHA was found to alter the size of lipid rafts in BC cells, resulting in lipid rafts of varying height [100]. The same study illustrated that DHA decreased the total amount of lipid rafts on the order of 20%–30%. This is particularly interesting because the levels of lipid rafts are elevated in some forms of cancer, including BC [101], and perturbing these domains can sensitize cells to apoptosis [102]. In addition to altering the size and number of lipid rafts, DHA was found to reduce cell surface levels of lipid rafts by enhancing their internalization [102]. These data implicate *n*-3 PUFA-induced changes in the physical properties of lipid rafts as a mechanism by which these fatty acids exert a chemoprotective effect.

The composition of raft domains is also central to their function as signaling platforms, and *n*-3 PUFA can substantially alter the contents of lipid rafts. The lipid composition of rafts endows the properties necessary for ordering and segregation. BC cells treated with a combination of EPA and DHA were demonstrated to have significantly reduced cholesterol, sphingomyelin, and diacylglycerol lipid raft content [103]. Another study demonstrated differential effects of EPA and DHA on the lipid composition of rafts [100]. EPA was shown to displace AA from raft domains, whereas DHA reduced cholesterol and sphingomyelin content. In addition to lipids, many proteins reside in lipid rafts and require localization to lipid rafts for signal transduction. Importantly, many of these proteins are established mediators of oncogenesis, and displacing these proteins can markedly reduce their signaling capacity. In MDA-MB-231 BC cells, several raft-associated proteins, including EGFR, Hsp90, Akt, and Src, are redistributed out of raft domains in response to DHA treatment [102], which induced increased BC cell apoptosis. Additionally, DHA was demonstrated to disrupt lipid rafts and reduce HER-2 signaling in mammary epithelial cells overexpressing HER-2 [104]. All of these proteins are involved in the regulation of cell survival and proliferation, and many are targets for cancer therapy. Another well-known therapeutic target for BC metastasis is the chemokine receptor, CXCR4. Treatment of BC cells with DHA or EPA caused redistribution of CXCR4 from lipid rafts to the cell surface [105], resulting in an overall reduction in cell migration. In addition to shifting proteins out of lipid rafts, n-3 PUFA can prompt the localization of some proteins into these domains. For example, CD95 (APO-1/FAS) is the transmembrane death receptor which activates the extrinsic apoptosis pathway and activation results in CD95 aggregation in the plasma membrane, followed closely by recruitment of Fas-associated death domain-containing protein (FADD) and caspase-8 to the CD95 receptor, forming the death-inducing signaling complex (DISC) [106]. EPA and DHA have been shown to induce translocation of CD95 into lipid rafts in MDA-MB-231 BC cells and this effect was accompanied by reduced cell growth [107]. Moreover, when DHA was used as a co-treatment it enhanced the chemotherapeutic effects of doxorubicin [107], an anti-neoplastic drug therapy, which has been shown to induce apoptosis and the movement of DISC to membrane rafts [108,109]. All of these data support the regulation of lipid rafts by n-3 PUFA as a mechanism by which they exert protective effects in BC and may also have utility as a complementary therapy in combination with pharmaceuticals, although further study is required.

6. Paracrine Interactions, Inflammatory Mediator Signaling and Breast Cancer

The majority of breast tissue is comprised of adipocytes, whereas epithelial cells account for only 10% of total breast cellular volume [110]. Mammary epithelial cells are embedded within the AT, which facilitates direct contact between epithelial cells and adjacent adipocytes and allows for direct functional interactions between AT and mammary tumor cells in a paracrine manner. Within the BC tumor microenvironment, these cellular interactions are further influenced by exposure to circulating AT adipokines [111,112]. Inflammation plays a role in the carcinogenic process and approximately 20% of all cancers originate in association with inflammation [113]. Given the chronic low grade-inflammatory state perpetuated in obesity [114,115], it is likely that obese AT-derived inflammatory mediator production could exacerbate inflammation-associated tumorigenic effects. Specifically, these mediators include n-6 PUFA-derived eicosanoids, and adipokines such as leptin and inflammatory cytokines (TNFα, IL-1β and IL-6) with a concomitant reduction in the anti-inflammatory adipokine, adiponectin (discussed below), which are produced in both visceral AT depots and surprisingly also within mammary AT depots, and collectively contribute to the development of a more severe BC phenotype via stimulating BC growth, invasion and metastasis. Typically in obesity-associated BC, inflammatory processes precede tumorigenesis. However, once developed, mammary tumor cells may also serve as a cellular source of inflammatory mediators and support the on-going inflammatory milieu within the mammary tumor microenvironment, thereby potentiating a feed-forward pro-tumorigenic mechanism facilitated by local inflammatory autocrine and paracrine interactions. In summary, autocrine and paracrine signaling between cell types within the mammary AT and tumor tissue are thought to play a central role in breast tumorigenesis [110,116], indicating that dysregulation of adipokines may underlie the association between obesity and BC.

One of the main cellular sources of these inflammatory mediators, apart from adipocytes, is macrophages that infiltrate obese AT and form crown-like structures (CLS) [117,118]. CLS are inflammatory lesions defined as adipocytes surrounded by an aggregation of macrophages that undergo necrosis and fuse to form a syncytium of lipid-containing giant multinucleated cells [119]. Obese mice have increased CLS formation in both visceral AT and mammary AT, which is associated with increased local inflammatory cytokine production (TNFα, IL-1β and IL-6), COX-2 induction and eicosanoid (PGE$_2$) production, as well as increased aromatase gene expression, enzyme activity and subsequent estrogen synthesis [119–122]. Therefore, CLS formation represents a tissue localization wherein largely adipocyte-macrophage-mediated paracrine interactions promote both the development and persistence of an inflammatory AT microenvironment, which through further paracrine interactions signal to the mammary epithelial cells to promote BC growth and invasion [120,121]. Transformed mammary epithelial cells and/or the BC tumor itself can further serve as a cellular source for inflammatory mediator production and amplify the on-going local production of inflammatory mediators, and spread these signals to the surrounding non-involved mammary tissue. Moreover, in obesity, mammary AT, which is a subcutaneous AT depot, is transformed to mimic the inflammatory milieu that characterizes the obese visceral AT phenotype [120,121]. The obesity-associated mammary AT phenotypic switch is significant because evidence suggests that subcutaneous AT tends to be less inflammatory compared to visceral sources [118,123] and therefore, in obese mammary AT, a typically less inflammatory depot exhibits a more pronounced inflammatory phenotype that can drive tumorigenesis. In obesity, dietary *n*-3 PUFA supplementation has been shown to reduce AT CLS formation, reduce macrophage AT infiltration by reducing MCP-1 tissue expression and improve the inflammatory secretory profile, in part, by increasing adiponectin [27,28].

The mammary AT tumor microenvironment is complex. Increased local production of inflammatory adipokines underpin the paracrine signaling that regulates the cellular interactions between adipocytes, stromal epithelial cells and infiltrating macrophages, which ultimately drive and define mammary tumor development and the end-stage phenotype (tumor size, type and inflammatory status). Up-regulated paracrine interactions (*i.e.*, cross-talk) in obesity-associated BC perpetuate the carcinogenic process by stimulating multiple, overlapping signaling pathways. These pathways converge to stimulate aromatase expression/activation that aberrantly produces local estrogen, promote cell proliferation and/or inhibit apoptosis and stimulate the production of additional inflammatory mediators within mammary tissue, all of which ultimately support tumorigenesis. The critical inflammatory mediators that are up-regulated in obesity-associated BC perpetuate the carcinogenic process and exhibit redundant effects by stimulating multiple and overlapping signaling pathways that converge to stimulate aromatase expression/activation, resulting in aberrant local estrogen production, which promotes cell proliferation and/or inhibits apoptosis, and stimulate the production of additional inflammatory mediators within mammary tissue, ultimately resulting in tumorigenesis. Since a large and diverse list of hormones, adipokines and lipid mediators are implicated in promoting obesity-associated mammary tumorigenesis, our review will focus on a critical subset that work in concert to promote estrogen production (via aromatase activation) and tumorigenesis, specifically eicosanoids, inflammatory cytokines, leptin and adiponectin; however, we recognize that other mediators play a role in this process such as insulin, insulin-like growth factors, resistin nampt/visfatin and cholesterol as reviewed elsewhere [124–126]. The specific mechanisms/pathways through which obesity-associated inflammatory adipokines exert pro-tumorigenic effects are discussed in detail below, and the complexity of these paracrine interactions are shown in Figure 1.

7. The Role of Estrogen and Aromatase Activation in BC

Circulating estrogen levels are higher in obese women compared to lean women, and increased circulating estrogen is associated with approximately a two-fold increased risk of postmenopausal BC [5,6,127–129]. Additionally, obesity, particularly abdominal adiposity, increases estradiol production and bioavailability due to a reduction in hepatic synthesis of sex hormone-binding globulin (SHBG) in postmenopausal women [6,12,127,129,130]. These hormonal changes are widely believed to play an underlying role in the increased risk of BC in obese postmenopausal women [6,12,127,131]. After menopause, the primary source of estrogen are extra-ovarian sites, primarily in the AT, and aberrant AT estrogen production is attributable to increased aromatase activity, which is present at higher levels in mammary tumors compared to normal mammary tissue [132,133]. Aromatase is the rate-limiting enzyme in the estrogen biosynthesis pathway [131] which catalyzes the peripheral conversion of androstenedione and testosterone to estrone and estradiol, respectively [110]. Downstream conversion of estrone to the biologically potent estradiol is catalyzed by 17β-hydroxysteroid dehydrogenase, which is also expressed within AT [131]. In obese individuals, aromatase expression is reported to be increased by two-fold compared to normal weight individuals [125]. Additionally, aromatase expression is four to five-fold higher within breast tumor tissue compared to non-involved tissues within the same breast [125]. Consequently, mammary tissue estrogen levels are reported to be 10–50 times higher compared to blood levels in postmenopausal healthy women, which has been shown to play a critical role in BC cell growth [134–138].

Typically, mammary tumors are located in regions of the breast with the highest aromatase expression and activity [139,140]. Furthermore, breast tissue aromatase expression is highest in the quadrant of the breast that contains the greatest proportion of adipose stromal cells, as there is little aromatase activity in mature adipocytes [141], and accordingly, aromatase expression is typically highest in the adipose stromal cells adjacent to the tumor mass [139,140,142]. Therefore, the ratio of stromal cells to adipocytes within mammary tissue may have a predictive value in potential tumor development. Moreover, mammary tumors are typically surrounded by a layer of proliferating cancer-associated fibroblasts (CAF) which have also been shown to express aromatase, thereby indicating that factors produced by the tumor may also stimulate aromatase expression in the surrounding CAF [143].

Aromatase expression and activity is strongly influenced by local inflammatory paracrine signaling within mammary tissue. For instance, malignant epithelial cells along with AT macrophages produce pro-inflammatory mediators, including the eicosanoid PGE_2, which induce aromatase activity and stimulate estrogen production in pre-adipocytes [131,143,144]. The resultant inflammatory mammary tissue microenvironment is further propagated in the obese state, thereby creating a favorable tissue microenvironment to promote the progression of BC growth [120,121]. Further, in obese human BC tissue, aromatase expression is associated with increased tissue levels of COX-2 and PGE_2 [121]. In BC tissue, COX-2 expression is induced by pro-inflammatory cytokines, notably TNFα, and the resultant increased PGE_2 levels are associated with large tumor size and high proliferation rates [131,145], due to, in part, the induction of aromatase expression via activation of cAMP-PKA and PKC-mediated signaling cascades [141,146,147]. Conversely, PGE_3, an n-3 PUFA-derived eicosanoid does not induce aromatase expression [148]. Aromatase expression is negatively regulated, in part, by AMP-activated protein kinase (AMPK), which also functions as a negative regulator of the Akt/mTOR signaling pathway that is frequently activated in BC [125]. Additionally, liver kinase B1 (LKB1) can function as a tumor suppressor and can regulate aromatase expression via directly phosphorylating and activating AMPK [149]. Therefore, LKB1 and AMPK both function as negative regulators of aromatase expression in BC. As many inflammatory and metabolic factors alter aromatase expression via effects on LKB1 and/or AMPK, this may provide a critical link between obesity, inflammation and aromatase expression in BC [125]. Leptin increases aromatase expression by decreasing LKB1 protein expression and phosphorylation, whereas adiponectin exerts the opposite effect by stimulating LKB1 and its activity, leading to decreased aromatase expression [150]. Additionally, PGE_2 down-regulates the phosphorylation of AMPK and LKB1, thereby promoting aromatase expression [150]. Inflammatory cytokines such as IL-6, IL-1β and TNFα have also been shown to stimulate aromatase activity [151–154]. TNFα induces aromatase expression through two mechanisms, (i) stimulating the binding of c-fos and c-jun transcription factors to activating protein-1 (AP-1) binding site; and (ii) activation of NFκB and MAPK signaling pathways [152,153]. Obese ovariectomized rodents exhibit increased NFκB activation and inflammatory mediator production (TNF-α, IL-1β, COX-2), which is accompanied by elevated levels of aromatase expression and activity in both the mammary gland and visceral fat [120]. Collectively, these data demonstrate that inflammatory mediator signaling in the mammary tissue microenvironment is driven by autocrine/paracrine interactions that regulate critical aspects of the mammary tissue tumor phenotype including aromatase activation and local estrogen production.

These inflammatory mediators can establish a positive feedback mechanism that stimulates cell proliferation and mammary tumor development.

8. Inflammatory and Chemopromotive Fatty Acid Derived Lipid Mediators: Differential Effects of *n*-6 *versus* *n*-3 PUFA

LC *n*-3 and *n*-6 PUFA are metabolized by the cyclooxygenase (COX), lipoxygenase (LOX) and cytochrome P450 pathways to produce eicosanoids [72]. Specifically, *n*-6 PUFA (such as AA) serves as a substrate for COX enzymes (producing two-series prostanoids such as prostaglandins (PG) and thromboxanes (TX)), LOX enzymes (producing four-series leukotrienes (LT) and hydroxyeicosatetraenoic acids (HETE), principally 5-, 12- and 15-HETE), or cytochrome P450 enzymes (producing primarily 20-HETE) [72,148,155]. The same enzymes metabolize *n*-3 PUFA to structurally different three-series prostanoids, five-series LT, and primarily 19- and 20-hydroxyeicosapentaenoic acids (HEPE) and 21- and 22-hydroxydocosahexaenoic acids (HDHE), as well as the unique lipid mediators E- and D-series resolvins and protectins [72,148,156]. Although both resolvins and protectins exert anti-inflammatory effects, resolvins can stimulate the resolution phase of inflammation to begin at an earlier point, thereby limiting the tissue exposure to inflammatory signaling [157], whereas protectins reduce inflammatory cytokine production [158]. Generally, *n*-6 PUFA-derived eicosanoids are pro-inflammatory and pro-carcinogenic, whereas *n*-3 PUFA-derived lipid mediators are less biologically active and functionally oppose the synthesis and activity *n*-6 PUFA-derived eicosanoids [72,148,159]. Excessive dietary intake of *n*-6 PUFA *versus* *n*-3 PUFA (five- to 20-fold greater amounts) results in a significantly greater proportion of eicosanoids generated from *n*-6 PUFA [72,160]. Importantly, the fatty acid profile of adipocyte, immune and tumor cell membrane phospholipids can be modified by increased intake of *n*-3 PUFA, thereby suppressing the biosynthesis of AA-derived eicosanoids in favor of EPA and DHA-derived lipid mediators [72,148,159,161].

AA has been shown to be preferentially taken up by MDA-MB-231 BC cells in comparison to EPA, especially in a pro-inflammatory microenvironment [162]. Also, COX-2 and 12-LOX enzymes are overexpressed in BC tumor tissue [131], thereby increasing production of AA-derived inflammatory eicosanoids, which have established pro-tumorigenic effects, and dominate the BC phenotype [131,163–166]. Specifically, PGE_2, LTB_4 and 5-, 12- and 15-HETE, have been shown to increase cell proliferation, down-regulate apoptotic pathways, and induce rapid growth and tumor metastasis, and these effects have been shown to be counteracted by *n*-3 PUFA [50,51,159,165–169]. Furthermore, *n*-6 PUFA-derived eicosanoid levels are elevated during obesity and have been shown to stimulate breast tumor growth, invasion, and metastasis [131], indicating that obesity perpetuates local inflammatory eicosanoid production.

EPA is the preferential substrate for LOX enzymes, and therefore, when present in comparable proportions, *n*-3 PUFA-derived eicosanoids will be produced at the expense of *n*-6 PUFA-derived eicosanoids [148]. Moreover, *n*-3 PUFA suppress COX-2 expression, which is associated with decreased mammary epithelial cell proliferation in MMTV-HER-2/neu transgenic mice [78]. Mammary tumor PGE_2 and 12- and 15-HETE concentrations are dose-dependently reduced by increased dietary *n*-3 PUFA intake in female nude mice injected with MDA-MB-231 cells [42,170], which is associated with increased apoptotic activity and decreased breast tumor cell proliferation, growth and lung metastasis. Similar *n*-3 PUFA-mediated anti-tumorigenic effects have been associated with suppressed cell proliferation and decreased expression of Bcl-2 and other carcinogenic proteins including Ki-67, Her-2/neu and c-Myc [50,51,159,167,168,171]. Taken together, *n*-6 PUFA-derived eicosanoids provide a link between obesity-associated chronic inflammation and the development of BC, and are a potential target for dietary LC *n*-3 PUFA intervention to mitigate the pro-carcinogenic effects of inflammatory *n*-6 PUFA-derived eicosanoids within the mammary tumor microenvironment.

9. Role of Inflammatory Cytokines

Inflammatory cytokines (TNFα, IL-1β, IL-6 and MCP-1) also contribute to the local mammary tissue milieu through paracrine signaling and through an autocrine positive-feedback mechanism to further their own on-going production, in part, by activating the transcription factor NFκB. Interestingly, NFκB activation underlies many aspects of BC cell proliferation, invasion and metastasis [126,172,173]. Moreover, aberrant NFκB signaling is proposed to be one of the mechanisms through which chronic inflammation leads to cancer, as NFκB activation promotes tumorigenesis by inhibiting apoptosis (via activation of Bcl2, Bcl-xL, cFLIP and other genes) and increasing cell proliferation by regulating expression of cyclinD1, cyclinE, CDK2, and c-Myc [174]. Several inflammatory mediators are up-regulated by NFκB activation; specifically, inflammatory n-6 PUFA-derived eicosanoid production is stimulated by NFκB activation of COX-2 [175]. Additionally, within chronically inflamed rodent mammary tissue, NFκB increases production of TNFα and IL-1β [120] and similar findings are reported in the mammary tissue of both pre- and postmenopausal obese women [121]. IL-1β levels are increased in patients with invasive ductal carcinoma and ductal carcinomas *in situ* compared to benign mammary tissue levels [176,177], and are overexpressed in breast carcinomas, but undetectable in normal breast tissue [178]. IL-1β levels are positively correlated with the expression of angiogenic factor expression, tumor grade and the expression of AP-1 [176–178].

IL-1β and IL-6 have been shown to stimulate BC cell proliferation in an additive manner with estrogen [154], indicative of synergy between inflammatory mediators and hormones within the mammary tumor microenvironment. TNFα, another potent inflammatory cytokine, also promotes mammary tumor development [179] and has been shown to contribute to BC cell epithelial-mesenchymal transition (EMT) by increasing matrix metalloproteinase (MMP)-9 expression, thereby enhancing migration and invasive capacity [180–182]. Additionally, the high levels of IL-6 and TNFα found in obese rodent adipocyte-conditioned media and serum have been shown to promote cancer cell EMT [183]. Interestingly, the two main cellular sources of TNFα are tumor-associated macrophages (TAM) and the BC cells themselves [131], highlighting the role of inflammatory macrophages in BC.

Macrophage infiltration into mammary tumor sites (and subsequent development of CLS) is driven, in part, by chemotactic signaling. MCP-1, also referred to as CCL2, signals to increase macrophage infiltration into the inflamed mammary tissue, thereby increasing the number of deleterious TAM that accumulate in mammary tumor tissue [184,185]. The cellular sources of MCP-1 in primary breast tumor sites are tumor cells and the TAM themselves, which indicates a feed-forward mechanism wherein macrophage accumulation/tumor recruitment is perpetuated throughout the stages of tumor growth [184,185]. Overall, TAM form CLS within the mammary AT and act as the cellular source of several inflammatory mediators/cytokines that perpetuate the local inflammatory tissue microenvironment, which, through autocrine and paracrine interactions, further promotes BC development [119–122,131]. Collectively, this highlights the critical role that macrophages play in driving tumor-associated inflammatory paracrine interactions. MCP-1 tumor expression is associated with a more advanced course of tumor progression, wherein MCP-1 promotes angiogenesis by stimulating the production of angiogenic factors (such as IL-8 and VEGF) [184,185]. In obesity, circulating and AT levels of MCP-1 are increased. This chemokine provides the main chemoattractant signal that drives visceral AT macrophage infiltration and CLS formation, up-regulating local AT inflammatory mediator production and subsequently impairing glucose metabolism [58,59]. Macrophage recruitment is also stimulated by AT hypoxia. In obesity, adipocyte hypertrophy results in decreased oxygen diffusion, leading to localized tissue AT hypoxia, as evidenced by upregulation of the hypoxia master regulator, hypoxia induced factor (HIF-1α), which stimulates MCP-1 and subsequent macrophage chemotaxis [143,186,187].

Countering these effects in obesity, n-3 PUFA have been shown to improve the hypoxic AT microenvironment by reducing adipocyte size [27] and to decrease obesity-associated expression of HIF-1α [81,188]. Furthermore, n-3 PUFA reduce visceral AT MCP-1 levels [27,28,35,189,190], thereby reducing obesity-associated AT macrophage accumulation, CLS formation and AT inflammation [27,28]. We and others have shown that *n*-3 PUFA reduce inflammatory paracrine signaling between adipocytes and macrophages by decreasing NFκB activation and subsequent secretion of TNFα, MCP-1 and IL-6 [191,192]. Moreover, independent of cellular source, *n*-3 PUFA have been shown to inhibit NFκB activation by decreasing IκB phosphorylation and activation, thereby reducing production TNFα, IL-1β and IL-6 [29,35,40,41,67,191,193,194].

10. Role of Leptin

Leptin exerts pleiotropic effects apart from regulation of energy expenditure and food intake, including effects on immunity, inflammation, cell differentiation and proliferation [124,195], all of which have direct relevance to cancer. Classically, circulating leptin levels are proportional to the amount of body fat [196] and increased leptin levels are associated with increased risk of BC development and progression [197,198]. Leptin gene expression is detected in normal healthy breast epithelial tissue [110], consistent with its endogenous role in normal mammary gland development and lactation [199]; however, it is also capable of contributing to mammary tumorigenesis [200] and is expressed in the healthy tissue that surrounds malignant ductal lesions [201]. In primary tumors and various BC cell lines, both leptin and various isoforms of the leptin receptor (ObR) including the long signaling form ObR1 are overexpressed [197,202–207]. Recently, three single nucleotide polymorphisms in the leptin receptor gene (K109R, K656N and Q223R) were identified to be associated with increased BC risk, suggesting that tumor leptin receptor signaling can directly influence tumor growth and progression [208]. Interestingly, in BC patients high intra-tumor ObR gene expression was strongly correlated with decreased relapse-free survival [209], indicating that susceptibility to leptin signaling is strongly associated with BC disease prognosis.

Leptin signaling has been shown to exert autocrine and paracrine effects, ultimately promoting cell growth and proliferation via the activation of critical signaling pathways including those mediated by PKC, c-Jun *N*-terminal kinase (JNK), p38 MAPK, Janus Kinase2/Signal Transducer and Activator of Transcription 3 (JAK2/STAT3), PI3K/Akt/mTOR, Akt/GSK3 and MAPK/extracellular signal-related kinase 1/2 (ERK1/2) pathways [116,181,195,203,210–213]. Further, leptin increases the levels of cell cycle regulators in human MCF-7 BC cells by up-regulating the expression of cyclin dependent kinase 2 (cdk2) and cyclin D1, which advances cells from the G1 to S phase of the cell cycle [214], and induces cell proliferation in ZR-75-1 BC cells via up-regulation of cyclin D1 and c-Myc [215]. Therefore, overexpression and activation of leptin within the mammary tissue microenvironment can ultimately promote tumorigenesis. Similar to obese women, rodents with high leptin levels are more likely to develop mammary tumors [216,217]. Furthermore, in animal BC models leptin antagonism has produced successful outcomes. Specifically MMTV-TGF-α mice crossed with leptin deficient mice fail to develop tumors [218,219] and treatment with a leptin antagonist decreases the growth of murine triple-negative breast tumors [220] and 4T1 mammary cancer cell growth via reducing levels of VEGF, pSTAT3 and cyclin D1 [221].

An additional role of leptin in breast carcinogenesis is to potentiate estrogen signaling, as leptin has been shown to induce aromatase expression/activity and subsequent estrogen synthesis, thereby enhancing ERα activity in BC [210,222,223]. Leptin levels positively correlate with ER expression and BC tumor size [203,205]. Further, leptin can transactivate ERα via ERK1/2 signaling [210] and enhance ERα-dependent transcription by reducing ERα ubiquitination and degradation, even in the presence of an estrogen inhibitor [223], thereby potentiating the effects of estrogen on cell proliferation. Bi-directional influences of estrogen on leptin also exist, wherein estradiol induces leptin and ObR expression, in both AT and BC cell lines [203,224–226].

Another obesity-associated factor that can contribute to the increased local production of leptin and subsequent pro-tumorigenic effects is AT hypoxia. Leptin receptor expression can also be stimulated by tissue hypoxia [226] and, therefore, local tissue leptin expression is up-regulated by HIF-1α [227,228]. Conversely, *n*-3 PUFA have been shown to improve the hypoxic AT microenvironment by reducing adipocyte size [27] and to decrease obesity-associated expression of HIF-1α [81,188], thereby providing a mechanism through which local leptin signaling responsiveness could be attenuated.

Dietary n-3 PUFA have been shown to reduce leptin AT gene expression and/or circulating levels in obese rodents [36,37] and humans [38,39], an effect that was most prominent when combined with weight loss [39]. Decreased leptin signaling represents an additional mechanism through which n-3 PUFA attenuate the effects of leptin. In a rodent obesity model, n-3 PUFA supplementation was found to decrease leptin receptor gene expression [229], thereby decreasing leptin signaling. In this connection, leptin receptors have been shown to localize to lipid rafts and downstream proliferative effects of leptin mediated through p38 MAPK signaling is lipid raft dependent [230]. Thus, n-3 PUFA antagonism of lipid raft size and composition in BC [100,103], as already discussed herein, may also antagonize leptin-mediated proliferative signaling within the mammary tumor microenvironment. Therefore, these findings add to the complex interplay of autocrine and paracrine interactions that underlie the obesity-associated BC inflammatory phenotype, and suggest dietary n-3 PUFA as an intervention that may have utility in mitigating local mammary tissue leptin production and signaling to inhibit its pro-tumorigenic effects.

11. Role of Adiponectin

Adipocytes are the primary cellular source of adiponectin, which is secreted as a monomeric protein that can be oligomerized to form both low-molecular weight and high molecular weight complexes [231]. Additionally, cleavage reactions via the action of elastase, can generate globular oligomeric complexes [232] that bind with greater affinity to the adiponectin receptor 1 (AdipoR1), whereas the AdipoR2 preferentially binds full-length and multimeric adiponectin [233].

Within the context of the tumor microenvironment, adiponectin and leptin counter-regulate each other and exert opposing effects [126]. Decreased levels of adiponectin may explain, in part, the increased risk of BC in obesity. Circulating adiponectin levels are generally inversely correlated with BMI, adiposity and visceral fat mass [234,235] and the decreased adiponectin levels in obesity [236] correlate with increased BC risk [111,237,238]. Moreover, three recent independent meta-analyses of BC observational studies confirmed the correlation of higher circulating adiponectin levels with lower BC risk in postmenopausal women [239–241]. More specifically, an increase of 3 μg/mL of circulating adiponectin corresponded to a 5% reduction in BC risk [239]. In obese postmenopausal women, hypoadiponectinemia is associated with increased BC risk, and the disease has been shown to manifest with an aggressive metastatic phenotype [235,242]. In premenopausal women, however, adiponectin levels are not associated with BC risk (95% CI -0.164 to 0.204, $p = 0.829$) [239–241]. The local breast tumor tissue mRNA and protein expression of adiponectin is low, although its receptors are still expressed, indicating that adiponectin-mediated anti-tumorigenic signaling is possible in BC [111,243,244]. In animal studies, reduced production of adiponectin is associated with earlier tumor onset and accelerated tumor growth [245], and overexpression of adiponectin results in mice with reduced mammary tumor size and weight [246]. Studies using various BC cell lines demonstrate that the anti-proliferative effect of adiponectin is mediated through AdipoR1 and AdipoR2 signaling [246–248]. There is a negative correlation between AdipoR1 expression and tumor size, which suggests that the loss of AdipoR1 signaling favours tumor growth [249]. These data are indicative of a weak autocrine/paracrine activity of this hormone within the tumor microenvironment and a loss of the beneficial anti-tumor effects of adiponectin. Despite reduced tissue levels and blunted adiponectin signaling in obesity-associated BC, treatment strategies designed to stimulate adiponectin signaling might represent a novel therapeutic approach.

Adiponectin exerts an anti-proliferative effect in BC [246,247,250–253] by impacting several signaling pathways. Specifically, adiponectin has been shown to impact the glycogen synthase kinase-3β (GSK-3β)/β-catenin signaling pathway via inhibition of phosphorylation of Akt and GSK-3β and subsequent suppression of intracellular accumulation of β-catenin and its transcriptional activities, resulting in reduced cyclin-D1 expression [246,247,251]. Additionally, adiponectin has been shown to reduce BC cell proliferation by regulating the PTEN/PI3K/mTOR and MAPK pathways [212], specifically inactivating ERK1/2, stimulating AMPK activity and decreasing Akt phosphorylation, leading to reduced mTOR activity [4,251–253]. In MCF-7 BC cells, microarray analysis demonstrated that adiponectin represses expression of multiple important genes that regulate cell cycle (MAPK3 and ATM) and apoptosis (BAG1, BAG3, and TP53), as well as potential diagnostic/prognostic markers (ACADS, CYP19A1, DEGS1, and EVL) [250]. Adiponectin has also been shown to induce BC cell apoptosis [251,253] by down-regulating Bcl2 and up-regulating p53, Bax and p21 expression [4,248, 251]; however, this outcome is dependent on the BC cell line utilized and duration of adiponectin incubation (reviewed [212]). Adiponectin also exerts anti-inflammatory effects by inhibiting the effects of leptin [126] and inhibiting $TNF\alpha$ production by macrophages and adipocytes [254]. Generally, independent of cell type, adiponectin signaling down-regulates the activation of $NF\kappa B$ and production of inflammatory cytokines ($TNF\alpha$, IL-1β, IL-6 and MCP-1) [255]. Moreover, adiponectin reduces macrophage-mediated inflammation within the tumor microenvironment by suppressing IL-6 gene expression and antagonizing $NF\kappa B$, JNK and p38 MAPK mediated signaling [255,256].

Increasing the production of adiponectin in obesity may be a beneficial strategy to mitigate inflammation. n-3 PUFA have been shown to up-regulate adiponectin secretion in both murine [65] and human adipocytes [66]. Furthermore, dietary n-3 PUFA improve the obesity-associated inflammatory secretory profile, in part, by increasing adiponectin levels [27–31,35,63]. In human clinical trials, dietary n-3 PUFA have been shown to increase adiponectin levels [32–34] in obese and overweight subjects, thereby demonstrating the potential utility of n-3 PUFA to stimulate the effects of this anti-inflammatory adipokine in obesity. Considering the anti-tumorigenic effects of adiponectin and the ability of n-3 PUFA to restore adiponectin function in obesity [27–35,63], further research initiatives should be undertaken to determine the utility of n-3 PUFA in mitigating obesity-associated BC inflammation and tumor production.

12. Conclusions

In obese women with BC, increased inflammatory adipokine production, both locally in the mammary AT depot and systemically, perpetuates inflammation-associated pro-tumorigenic signaling pathways, thereby increasing disease severity. A spectrum of inflammatory mediators/adipokines are produced by adipocytes, TAM, mammary epithelial cells and tumor cells, which collectively stimulate diverse and overlapping signaling pathways that converge to stimulate aromatase activity that aberrantly increases local estrogen production, up-regulates cell proliferation and down-regulates apoptosis. The complex nature of the obesity-associated BC inflammatory pathophysiology is not likely to be attenuated or prevented by targeting any individual inflammatory mediator and/or signaling pathway, which may explain why most drug therapies, in this context, are ineffective. Instead, a pan-anti-inflammatory approach is more likely to have success in mitigating obesity-associated mammary tissue inflammatory paracrine interactions and subsequent tumorigenesis, and in this context, n-3 PUFA may have utility. n-3 PUFA have been shown to concurrently target multiple aspects of the obese BC phenotype including reduction of macrophage AT infiltration and CLS formation and down-regulation of critical adipokine production. Collectively, increased n-3 PUFA intake could attenuate obesity-associated BC. Considering the current state of obesity world-wide, further studies in human at risk populations should be made a priority.

Acknowledgments: This work was supported by the Natural Sciences and Engineering Research Council of Canada (NSERC). Danyelle M. Liddle was supported by an Ontario Graduate Scholarship. Anna A. De Boer was supported by a NSERC graduate scholarship.

Author Contributions: All authors contributed to the writing and editing of this review. The final manuscript was approved by all authors.

References

1. Wang, Y.C.; McPherson, K.; Marsh, T.; Gortmaker, S.L.; Brown, M. Health and economic burden of the projected obesity trends in the USA and the UK. *Lancet* **2011**, *378*, 815–825. [CrossRef] [PubMed]
2. Lumeng, C.N.; Saltiel, A.R. Inflammatory links between obesity and metabolic disease. *J. Clin. Investig.* **2011**, *121*, 2111–2117. [CrossRef] [PubMed]
3. Calle, E.E.; Rodriguez, C.; Walker-Thurmond, K.; Thun, M.J. Overweight, obesity, and mortality from cancer in a prospectively studied cohort of U.S. adults. *N. Engl. J. Med.* **2003**, *348*, 1625–1638. [CrossRef] [PubMed]
4. Van Kruijsdijk, R.C.; van der Wall, E.; Visseren, F.L. Obesity and cancer: The role of dysfunctional adipose tissue. *Cancer Epidemiol. Biomark. Prev.* **2009**, *18*, 2569–2578. [CrossRef]
5. Cleary, M.P.; Grossmann, M.E. Minireview: Obesity and breast cancer: The estrogen connection. *Endocrinology* **2009**, *150*, 2537–2542. [CrossRef] [PubMed]
6. Key, T.J.; Appleby, P.N.; Reeves, G.K.; Roddam, A.; Dorgan, J.F.; Longcope, C.; Stanczyk, F.Z.; Stephenson, H.E., Jr.; Falk, R.T.; Miller, R.; *et al.* Body mass index, serum sex hormones, and breast cancer risk in postmenopausal women. *J. Natl. Cancer Inst.* **2003**, *95*, 1218–1226. [CrossRef] [PubMed]
7. van den Brandt, P.A.; Spiegelman, D.; Yaun, S.S.; Adami, H.O.; Beeson, L.; Folsom, A.R.; Fraser, G.; Goldbohm, R.A.; Graham, S.; Kushi, L.; *et al.* Pooled analysis of prospective cohort studies on height, weight, and breast cancer risk. *Am. J. Epidemiol.* **2000**, *152*, 514–527.
8. Li, C.I.; Daling, J.R.; Malone, K.E. Incidence of invasive breast cancer by hormone receptor status from 1992 to 1998. *J. Clin. Oncol.* **2003**, *21*, 28–34. [CrossRef] [PubMed]
9. Biglia, N.; Peano, E.; Sgandurra, P.; Moggio, G.; Pecchio, S.; Maggiorotto, F.; Sismondi, P. Body mass index (bmi) and breast cancer: Impact on tumor histopathologic features, cancer subtypes and recurrence rate in pre and postmenopausal women. *Gynecol. Endocrinol.* **2013**, *29*, 263–267. [CrossRef] [PubMed]
10. Garrisi, V.M.; Tufaro, A.; Trerotoli, P.; Bongarzone, I.; Quaranta, M.; Ventrella, V.; Tommasi, S.; Giannelli, G.; Paradiso, A. Body mass index and serum proteomic profile in breast cancer and healthy women: A prospective study. *PLoS One* **2012**, *7*, e49631. [CrossRef] [PubMed]
11. Kamineni, A.; Anderson, M.L.; White, E.; Taplin, S.H.; Porter, P.; Ballard-Barbash, R.; Malone, K.; Buist, D.S. Body mass index, tumor characteristics, and prognosis following diagnosis of early-stage breast cancer in a mammographically screened population. *Cancer Causes Control* **2013**, *24*, 305–312. [CrossRef] [PubMed]
12. Rinaldi, S.; Key, T.J.; Peeters, P.H.; Lahmann, P.H.; Lukanova, A.; Dossus, L.; Biessy, C.; Vineis, P.; Sacerdote, C.; Berrino, F.; *et al.* Anthropometric measures, endogenous sex steroids and breast cancer risk in postmenopausal women: A study within the epic cohort. *Int. J. Cancer* **2006**, *118*, 2832–2839. [CrossRef] [PubMed]
13. John, E.M.; Phipps, A.I.; Sangaramoorthy, M. Body size, modifying factors, and postmenopausal breast cancer risk in a multiethnic population: The San Francisco bay area breast cancer study. *SpringerPlus* **2013**, *2*, 239. [CrossRef] [PubMed]
14. Krishnan, K.; Bassett, J.K.; MacInnis, R.J.; English, D.R.; Hopper, J.L.; McLean, C.; Giles, G.G.; Baglietto, L. Associations between weight in early adulthood, change in weight, and breast cancer risk in postmenopausal women. *Cancer Epidemiol. Biomark. Prev.* **2013**, *22*, 1409–1416. [CrossRef]
15. Cheraghi, Z.; Poorolajal, J.; Hashem, T.; Esmailnasab, N.; Doosti Irani, A. Effect of body mass index on breast cancer during premenopausal and postmenopausal periods: A meta-analysis. *PLoS One* **2012**, *7*, e51446. [CrossRef] [PubMed]
16. Pierobon, M.; Frankenfeld, C.L. Obesity as a risk factor for triple-negative breast cancers: A systematic review and meta-analysis. *Breast Cancer Res. Treat.* **2013**, *137*, 307–314. [CrossRef] [PubMed]
17. Amadou, A.; Ferrari, P.; Muwonge, R.; Moskal, A.; Biessy, C.; Romieu, I.; Hainaut, P. Overweight, obesity and risk of premenopausal breast cancer according to ethnicity: A systematic review and dose-response meta-analysis. *Obes. Rev.* **2013**, *14*, 665–678. [CrossRef] [PubMed]
18. Brown, K.A. Impact of obesity on mammary gland inflammation and local estrogen production. *J. Mammary Gland Biol. Neoplasia* **2014**, *19*, 183–189. [CrossRef] [PubMed]
19. Coutinho, T.; Goel, K.; Correa de Sa, D.; Carter, R.E.; Hodge, D.O.; Kragelund, C.; Kanaya, A.M.; Zeller, M.; Park, J.S.; Kober, L.; *et al.* Combining body mass index with measures of central obesity in the assessment of mortality in subjects with coronary disease: Role of "Normal weight central obesity". *J. Am. Coll. Cardiol.* **2013**, *61*, 553–560. [CrossRef] [PubMed]

20. Kimura, K.; Tanaka, S.; Iwamoto, M.; Fujioka, H.; Takahashi, Y.; Satou, N.; Uchiyama, K. Association between body mass index and breast cancer intrinsic subtypes in Japanese women. *Exp. Ther. Med.* **2012**, *4*, 391–396. [PubMed]

21. Daling, J.R.; Malone, K.E.; Doody, D.R.; Johnson, L.G.; Gralow, J.R.; Porter, P.L. Relation of body mass index to tumor markers and survival among young women with invasive ductal breast carcinoma. *Cancer* **2001**, *92*, 720–729. [CrossRef] [PubMed]

22. Fagherazzi, G.; Chabbert-Buffet, N.; Fabre, A.; Guillas, G.; Boutron-Ruault, M.C.; Mesrine, S.; Clavel-Chapelon, F. Hip circumference is associated with the risk of premenopausal er-/pr- breast cancer. *Int. J. Obes.* **2012**, *36*, 431–439. [CrossRef]

23. Olefsky, J.M.; Glass, C.K. Macrophages, inflammation, and insulin resistance. *Annu. Rev. Physiol.* **2010**, *72*, 219–246. [CrossRef]

24. Pierce, B.L.; Ballard-Barbash, R.; Bernstein, L.; Baumgartner, R.N.; Neuhouser, M.L.; Wener, M.H.; Baumgartner, K.B.; Gilliland, F.D.; Sorensen, B.E.; McTiernan, A.; *et al.* Elevated biomarkers of inflammation are associated with reduced survival among breast cancer patients. *J. Clin. Oncol.* **2009**, *27*, 3437–3444. [CrossRef] [PubMed]

25. Woodward, W.A.; Cristofanilli, M. Inflammatory breast cancer. *Semin. Radiat. Oncol.* **2009**, *19*, 256–265. [CrossRef] [PubMed]

26. Cariati, M.; Bennett-Britton, T.M.; Pinder, S.E.; Purushotham, A.D. "Inflammatory" Breast cancer. *Surg. Oncol.* **2005**, *14*, 133–143. [CrossRef] [PubMed]

27. Rossmeisl, M.; Jilkova, Z.M.; Kuda, O.; Jelenik, T.; Medrikova, D.; Stankova, B.; Kristinsson, B.; Haraldsson, G.G.; Svensen, H.; Stoknes, I.; *et al.* Metabolic effects of *n*-3 pufa as phospholipids are superior to triglycerides in mice fed a high-fat diet: Possible role of endocannabinoids. *PLoS One* **2012**, *7*, e38834. [CrossRef] [PubMed]

28. Rossmeisl, M.; Medrikova, D.; van Schothorst, E.M.; Pavlisova, J.; Kuda, O.; Hensler, M.; Bardova, K.; Flachs, P.; Stankova, B.; Vecka, M.; *et al.* Omega-3 phospholipids from fish suppress hepatic steatosis by integrated inhibition of biosynthetic pathways in dietary obese mice. *Biochim. Biophys. Acta* **2014**, *1841*, 267–278. [CrossRef] [PubMed]

29. Kalupahana, N.S.; Claycombe, K.; Newman, S.J.; Stewart, T.; Siriwardhana, N.; Matthan, N.; Lichtenstein, A.H.; Moustaid-Moussa, N. Eicosapentaenoic acid prevents and reverses insulin resistance in high-fat diet-induced obese mice via modulation of adipose tissue inflammation. *J. Nutr.* **2010**, *140*, 1915–1922. [CrossRef] [PubMed]

30. Flachs, P.; Mohamed-Ali, V.; Horakova, O.; Rossmeisl, M.; Hosseinzadeh-Attar, M.J.; Hensler, M.; Ruzickova, J.; Kopecky, J. Polyunsaturated fatty acids of marine origin induce adiponectin in mice fed a high-fat diet. *Diabetologia* **2006**, *49*, 394–397. [CrossRef] [PubMed]

31. Neschen, S.; Morino, K.; Rossbacher, J.C.; Pongratz, R.L.; Cline, G.W.; Sono, S.; Gillum, M.; Shulman, G.I. Fish oil regulates adiponectin secretion by a peroxisome proliferator-activated receptor-gamma-dependent mechanism in mice. *Diabetes* **2006**, *55*, 924–928. [CrossRef] [PubMed]

32. Itoh, M.; Suganami, T.; Satoh, N.; Tanimoto-Koyama, K.; Yuan, X.; Tanaka, M.; Kawano, H.; Yano, T.; Aoe, S.; Takeya, M.; *et al.* Increased adiponectin secretion by highly purified eicosapentaenoic acid in rodent models of obesity and human obese subjects. *Arterioscler. Thromb. Vasc. Biol.* **2007**, *27*, 1918–1925. [CrossRef] [PubMed]

33. Nomura, S.; Shouzu, A.; Omoto, S.; Inami, N.; Ueba, T.; Urase, F.; Maeda, Y. Effects of eicosapentaenoic acid on endothelial cell-derived microparticles, angiopoietins and adiponectin in patients with type 2 diabetes. *J. Atheroscler. Thromb.* **2009**, *16*, 83–90. [CrossRef] [PubMed]

34. Gammelmark, A.; Madsen, T.; Varming, K.; Lundbye-Christensen, S.; Schmidt, E.B. Low-dose fish oil supplementation increases serum adiponectin without affecting inflammatory markers in overweight subjects. *Nutr. Res.* **2012**, *32*, 15–23. [CrossRef]

35. Todoric, J.; Loffler, M.; Huber, J.; Bilban, M.; Reimers, M.; Kadl, A.; Zeyda, M.; Waldhausl, W.; Stulnig, T.M. Adipose tissue inflammation induced by high-fat diet in obese diabetic mice is prevented by *n*-3 polyunsaturated fatty acids. *Diabetologia* **2006**, *49*, 2109–2119. [CrossRef] [PubMed]

36. Takahashi, Y.; Ide, T. Dietary *n*-3 fatty acids affect mrna level of brown adipose tissue uncoupling protein 1, and white adipose tissue leptin and glucose transporter 4 in the rat. *Br. J. Nutr.* **2000**, *84*, 175–184. [PubMed]

37. Ruzickova, J.; Rossmeisl, M.; Prazak, T.; Flachs, P.; Sponarova, J.; Veck, M.; Tvrzicka, E.; Bryhn, M.; Kopecky, J. Omega-3 pufa of marine origin limit diet-induced obesity in mice by reducing cellularity of adipose tissue. *Lipids* **2004**, *39*, 1177–1185. [CrossRef] [PubMed]

38. Winnicki, M.; Somers, V.K.; Accurso, V.; Phillips, B.G.; Puato, M.; Palatini, P.; Pauletto, P. Fish-rich diet, leptin, and body mass. *Circulation* **2002**, *106*, 289–291. [CrossRef] [PubMed]

39. Mori, T.A.; Burke, V.; Puddey, I.B.; Shaw, J.E.; Beilin, L.J. Effect of fish diets and weight loss on serum leptin concentration in overweight, treated-hypertensive subjects. *J. Hypertens.* **2004**, *22*, 1983–1990. [CrossRef] [PubMed]

40. Perez-Echarri, N.; Perez-Matute, P.; Marcos-Gomez, B.; Baena, M.J.; Marti, A.; Martinez, J.A.; Moreno-Aliaga, M.J. Differential inflammatory status in rats susceptible or resistant to diet-induced obesity: Effects of epa ethyl ester treatment. *Eur. J. Nutr.* **2008**, *47*, 380–386. [CrossRef] [PubMed]

41. Puglisi, M.J.; Hasty, A.H.; Saraswathi, V. The role of adipose tissue in mediating the beneficial effects of dietary fish oil. *J. Nutr. Biochem.* **2011**, *22*, 101–108. [CrossRef] [PubMed]

42. Connolly, J.M.; Gilhooly, E.M.; Rose, D.P. Effects of reduced dietary linoleic acid intake, alone or combined with an algal source of docosahexaenoic acid, on mda-mb-231 breast cancer cell growth and apoptosis in nude mice. *Nutr. Cancer* **1999**, *35*, 44–49. [CrossRef] [PubMed]

43. Hardman, W.E.; Munoz, J., Jr.; Cameron, I.L. Role of lipid peroxidation and antioxidant enzymes in omega 3 fatty acids induced suppression of breast cancer xenograft growth in mice. *Cancer Cell Int.* **2002**, *2*, 10. [CrossRef] [PubMed]

44. Hardman, W.E.; Sun, L.; Short, N.; Cameron, I.L. Dietary omega-3 fatty acids and ionizing irradiation on human breast cancer xenograft growth and angiogenesis. *Cancer Cell Int.* **2005**, *5*, 12. [CrossRef] [PubMed]

45. Howe, L.R.; Subbaramaiah, K.; Hudis, C.A.; Dannenberg, A.J. Molecular pathways: Adipose inflammation as a mediator of obesity-associated cancer. *Clin. Cancer Res.* **2013**, *19*, 6074–6083. [CrossRef] [PubMed]

46. Leslie, M.A.; Abdelmagid, S.A.; Perez, K.; Muller, W.J.; Ma, D.W. Mammary tumour development is dose-dependently inhibited by *n*-3 polyunsaturated fatty acids in the mmtv-neu(ndl)-yd5 transgenic mouse model. *Lipids Health Dis.* **2014**, *13*, 96. [CrossRef] [PubMed]

47. Ma, D.W.; Ngo, V.; Huot, P.S.; Kang, J.X. *n*-3 polyunsaturated fatty acids endogenously synthesized in fat-1 mice are enriched in the mammary gland. *Lipids* **2006**, *41*, 35–39. [CrossRef] [PubMed]

48. MacLennan, M.B.; Clarke, S.E.; Perez, K.; Wood, G.A.; Muller, W.J.; Kang, J.X.; Ma, D.W. Mammary tumor development is directly inhibited by lifelong *n*-3 polyunsaturated fatty acids. *J. Nutr. Biochem.* **2013**, *24*, 388–395. [CrossRef] [PubMed]

49. Mandal, C.C.; Ghosh-Choudhury, T.; Yoneda, T.; Choudhury, G.G.; Ghosh-Choudhury, N. Fish oil prevents breast cancer cell metastasis to bone. *Biochem. Biophys. Res. Commun.* **2010**, *402*, 602–607. [CrossRef] [PubMed]

50. Manna, S.; Chakraborty, T.; Ghosh, B.; Chatterjee, M.; Panda, A.; Srivastava, S.; Rana, A.; Chatterjee, M. Dietary fish oil associated with increased apoptosis and modulated expression of bax and bcl-2 during 7,12-dimethylbenz(alpha)anthracene-induced mammary carcinogenesis in rats. *Prostaglandins Leukot. Essent. Fatty Acids* **2008**, *79*, 5–14. [CrossRef] [PubMed]

51. Manna, S.; Janarthan, M.; Ghosh, B.; Rana, B.; Rana, A.; Chatterjee, M. Fish oil regulates cell proliferation, protect DNA damages and decrease her-2/neu and c-myc protein expression in rat mammary carcinogenesis. *Clin. Nutr.* **2010**, *29*, 531–537. [CrossRef] [PubMed]

52. Menendez, J.A.; Lupu, R.; Colomer, R. Exogenous supplementation with omega-3 polyunsaturated fatty acid docosahexaenoic acid (dha; 22:6*n*-3) synergistically enhances taxane cytotoxicity and downregulates her-2/neu (c-erbb-2) oncogene expression in human breast cancer cells. *Eur. J. Cancer Prev.* **2005**, *14*, 263–270. [CrossRef] [PubMed]

53. Menendez, J.A.; Vazquez-Martin, A.; Ropero, S.; Colomer, R.; Lupu, R. Her2 (erbb-2)-targeted effects of the omega-3 polyunsaturated fatty acid, alpha-linolenic acid (ala; 18:3*n*-3), in breast cancer cells: The "Fat features" Of the "Mediterranean diet" As an "Anti-her2 cocktail". *Clin. Transl. Oncol.* **2006**, *8*, 812–820. [CrossRef] [PubMed]

54. Mizuno, N.K.; Rogozina, O.P.; Seppanen, C.M.; Liao, D.J.; Cleary, M.P.; Grossmann, M.E. Combination of intermittent calorie restriction and eicosapentaenoic acid for inhibition of mammary tumors. *Cancer Prev. Res.* **2013**, *6*, 540–547. [CrossRef]

55. Yee, L.D.; Young, D.C.; Rosol, T.J.; Vanbuskirk, A.M.; Clinton, S.K. Dietary (*n*-3) polyunsaturated fatty acids inhibit her-2/neu-induced breast cancer in mice independently of the ppargamma ligand rosiglitazone. *J. Nutr.* **2005**, *135*, 983–988. [PubMed]

56. Zou, Z.; Bellenger, S.; Massey, K.A.; Nicolaou, A.; Geissler, A.; Bidu, C.; Bonnotte, B.; Pierre, A.S.; Minville-Walz, M.; Rialland, M.; *et al.* Inhibition of the her2 pathway by *n*-3 polyunsaturated fatty acids prevents breast cancer in fat-1 transgenic mice. *J. Lipid Res.* **2013**, *54*, 3453–3463. [CrossRef] [PubMed]

57. Kershaw, E.E.; Flier, J.S. Adipose tissue as an endocrine organ. *J. Clin. Endocrinol. Metab.* **2004**, *89*, 2548–2556. [CrossRef] [PubMed]

58. Trayhurn, P.; Wood, I.S. Adipokines: Inflammation and the pleiotropic role of white adipose tissue. *Br. J. Nutr.* **2004**, *92*, 347–355. [CrossRef] [PubMed]

59. Balistreri, C.R.; Caruso, C.; Candore, G. The role of adipose tissue and adipokines in obesity-related inflammatory diseases. *Mediat. Inflamm.* **2010**, *2010*, 802078. [CrossRef]

60. Surmi, B.K.; Hasty, A.H. Macrophage infiltration into adipose tissue: Initiation, propagation and remodeling. *Future Lipidol.* **2008**, *3*, 545–556. [CrossRef] [PubMed]

61. Yu, J.G.; Javorschi, S.; Hevener, A.L.; Kruszynska, Y.T.; Norman, R.A.; Sinha, M.; Olefsky, J.M. The effect of thiazolidinediones on plasma adiponectin levels in normal, obese, and type 2 diabetic subjects. *Diabetes* **2002**, *51*, 2968–2974. [CrossRef] [PubMed]

62. Peyron-Caso, E.; Fluteau-Nadler, S.; Kabir, M.; Guerre-Millo, M.; Quignard-Boulange, A.; Slama, G.; Rizkalla, S.W. Regulation of glucose transport and transporter 4 (glut-4) in muscle and adipocytes of sucrose-fed rats: Effects of *n*-3 poly- and monounsaturated fatty acids. *Horm. Metab. Res.* **2002**, *34*, 360–366. [CrossRef] [PubMed]

63. Tishinsky, J.M.; de Boer, A.A.; Dyck, D.J.; Robinson, L.E. Modulation of visceral fat adipokine secretion by dietary fatty acids and ensuing changes in skeletal muscle inflammation. *Appl. Physiol. Nutr. Metab.* **2014**, *39*, 28–37. [CrossRef] [PubMed]

64. Gonzalez-Periz, A.; Horrillo, R.; Ferre, N.; Gronert, K.; Dong, B.; Moran-Salvador, E.; Titos, E.; Martinez-Clemente, M.; Lopez-Parra, M.; Arroyo, V.; *et al.* Obesity-induced insulin resistance and hepatic steatosis are alleviated by omega-3 fatty acids: A role for resolvins and protectins. *FASEB J.* **2009**, *23*, 1946–1957. [CrossRef] [PubMed]

65. Oster, R.T.; Tishinsky, J.M.; Yuan, Z.; Robinson, L.E. Docosahexaenoic acid increases cellular adiponectin mRNA and secreted adiponectin protein, as well as ppargamma mrna, in 3t3-l1 adipocytes. *Appl. Physiol. Nutr. Metab.* **2010**, *35*, 783–789. [CrossRef] [PubMed]

66. Tishinsky, J.M.; Ma, D.W.; Robinson, L.E. Eicosapentaenoic acid and rosiglitazone increase adiponectin in an additive and ppargamma-dependent manner in human adipocytes. *Obesity* **2011**, *19*, 262–268. [CrossRef] [PubMed]

67. Glass, C.K.; Saijo, K. Nuclear receptor transrepression pathways that regulate inflammation in macrophages and t cells. *Nat. Rev. Immunol.* **2010**, *10*, 365–376. [CrossRef] [PubMed]

68. Szanto, A.; Nagy, L. The many faces of ppargamma: Anti-inflammatory by any means? *Immunobiology* **2008**, *213*, 789–803. [CrossRef]

69. Oh, D.Y.; Talukdar, S.; Bae, E.J.; Imamura, T.; Morinaga, H.; Fan, W.; Li, P.; Lu, W.J.; Watkins, S.M.; Olefsky, J.M. Gpr120 is an omega-3 fatty acid receptor mediating potent anti-inflammatory and insulin-sensitizing effects. *Cell* **2010**, *142*, 687–698. [CrossRef] [PubMed]

70. Stulnig, T.M.; Huber, J.; Leitinger, N.; Imre, E.M.; Angelisova, P.; Nowotny, P.; Waldhausl, W. Polyunsaturated eicosapentaenoic acid displaces proteins from membrane rafts by altering raft lipid composition. *J. Biol. Chem.* **2001**, *276*, 37335–37340. [CrossRef] [PubMed]

71. Calder, P.C. Feeding the immune system. *Proc. Nutr. Soc.* **2013**, *72*, 299–309. [CrossRef] [PubMed]

72. Calder, P.C. *n*-3 fatty acids, inflammation and immunity: New mechanisms to explain old actions. *Proc. Nutr. Soc.* **2013**, *72*, 326–336. [CrossRef] [PubMed]

73. Liu, J.; Ma, D.W.L. The role of *n*-3 polyunsaturated fatty acids in the prevention and treatment of breast cancer. *Nutrients* **2014**, in press.

74. Conquer, J.A.; Holub, B.J. Effect of supplementation with different doses of dha on the levels of circulating dha as non-esterified fatty acid in subjects of asian indian background. *J. Lipid Res.* **1998**, *39*, 286–292. [PubMed]

75. Kris-Etherton, P.M.; Taylor, D.S.; Yu-Poth, S.; Huth, P.; Moriarty, K.; Fishell, V.; Hargrove, R.L.; Zhao, G.; Etherton, T.D. Polyunsaturated fatty acids in the food chain in the United States. *Am. J. Clin. Nutr.* **2000**, *71*, 179S–188S. [PubMed]

76. Damsgaard, C.T.; Frokiaer, H.; Lauritzen, L. The effects of fish oil and high or low linoleic acid intake on fatty acid composition of human peripheral blood mononuclear cells. *Br. J. Nutr.* **2008**, *99*, 147–154. [CrossRef] [PubMed]

77. Feskens, E.J.; Kromhout, D. Epidemiologic studies on eskimos and fish intake. *Ann. N. Y. Acad. Sci.* **1993**, *683*, 9–15. [CrossRef] [PubMed]

78. Yee, L.D.; Agarwal, D.; Rosol, T.J.; Lehman, A.; Tian, M.; Hatton, J.; Heestand, J.; Belury, M.A.; Clinton, S.K. The inhibition of early stages of her-2/neu-mediated mammary carcinogenesis by dietary *n*-3 pufas. *Mol. Nutr. Food Res.* **2013**, *57*, 320–327. [CrossRef] [PubMed]

79. Chen, Z.; Zhang, Y.; Jia, C.; Wang, Y.; Lai, P.; Zhou, X.; Wang, Y.; Song, Q.; Lin, J.; Ren, Z.; *et al.* Mtorc1/2 targeted by *n*-3 polyunsaturated fatty acids in the prevention of mammary tumorigenesis and tumor progression. *Oncogene* **2014**, *33*, 4548–4557. [CrossRef] [PubMed]

80. Chung, H.; Lee, Y.S.; Mayoral, R.; Oh, D.Y.; Siu, J.T.; Webster, N.J.; Sears, D.D.; Olefsky, J.M.; Ellies, L.G. Omega-3 fatty acids reduce obesity-induced tumor progression independent of gpr120 in a mouse model of postmenopausal breast cancer. *Oncogene* **2014**. [CrossRef]

81. Bouwens, M.; van de Rest, O.; Dellschaft, N.; Bromhaar, M.G.; de Groot, L.C.; Geleijnse, J.M.; Muller, M.; Afman, L.A. Fish-oil supplementation induces antiinflammatory gene expression profiles in human blood mononuclear cells. *Am. J. Clin. Nutr.* **2009**, *90*, 415–424. [CrossRef] [PubMed]

82. Zheng, J.S.; Hu, X.J.; Zhao, Y.M.; Yang, J.; Li, D. Intake of fish and marine *n*-3 polyunsaturated fatty acids and risk of breast cancer: Meta-analysis of data from 21 independent prospective cohort studies. *BMJ* **2013**, *346*, f3706. [CrossRef] [PubMed]

83. Chajes, V.; Torres-Mejia, G.; Biessy, C.; Ortega-Olvera, C.; Angeles-Llerenas, A.; Ferrari, P.; Lazcano-Ponce, E.; Romieu, I. Omega-3 and omega-6 polyunsaturated fatty acid intakes and the risk of breast cancer in mexican women: Impact of obesity status. *Cancer Epidemiol. Biomark. Prev.* **2012**, *21*, 319–326. [CrossRef]

84. Goodstine, S.L.; Zheng, T.; Holford, T.R.; Ward, B.A.; Carter, D.; Owens, P.H.; Mayne, S.T. Dietary (*n*-3)/(*n*-6) fatty acid ratio: Possible relationship to premenopausal but not postmenopausal breast cancer risk in U.S. Women. *J. Nutr.* **2003**, *133*, 1409–1414. [PubMed]

85. Maillard, V.; Bougnoux, P.; Ferrari, P.; Jourdan, M.L.; Pinault, M.; Lavillonniere, F.; Body, G.; le Floch, O.; Chajes, V. *n*-3 and *n*-6 fatty acids in breast adipose tissue and relative risk of breast cancer in a case-control study in tours, France. *Int. J. Cancer* **2002**, *98*, 78–83. [CrossRef] [PubMed]

86. Bagga, D.; Anders, K.H.; Wang, H.J.; Glaspy, J.A. Long-chain *n*-3-to-*n*-6 polyunsaturated fatty acid ratios in breast adipose tissue from women with and without breast cancer. *Nutr. Cancer* **2002**, *42*, 180–185. [CrossRef] [PubMed]

87. Klein, V.; Chajes, V.; Germain, E.; Schulgen, G.; Pinault, M.; Malvy, D.; Lefrancq, T.; Fignon, A.; le Floch, O.; Lhuillery, C.; *et al.* Low alpha-linolenic acid content of adipose breast tissue is associated with an increased risk of breast cancer. *Eur. J. Cancer* **2000**, *36*, 335–340. [CrossRef] [PubMed]

88. Kim, J.; Lim, S.Y.; Shin, A.; Sung, M.K.; Ro, J.; Kang, H.S.; Lee, K.S.; Kim, S.W.; Lee, E.S. Fatty fish and fish omega-3 fatty acid intakes decrease the breast cancer risk: A case-control study. *BMC Cancer* **2009**, *9*, 216. [CrossRef] [PubMed]

89. Witt, P.M.; Christensen, J.H.; Schmidt, E.B.; Dethlefsen, C.; Tjonneland, A.; Overvad, K.; Ewertz, M. Marine *n*-3 polyunsaturated fatty acids in adipose tissue and breast cancer risk: A case-cohort study from Denmark. *Cancer Causes Control* **2009**, *20*, 1715–1721. [CrossRef] [PubMed]

90. Pike, L.J. Lipid rafts: Heterogeneity on the high seas. *Biochem. J.* **2004**, *378*, 281–292. [CrossRef] [PubMed]

91. Staubach, S.; Hanisch, F.G. Lipid rafts: Signaling and sorting platforms of cells and their roles in cancer. *Expert Rev. Proteomics* **2011**, *8*, 263–277. [CrossRef] [PubMed]

92. Hofman, E.G.; Ruonala, M.O.; Bader, A.N.; van den Heuvel, D.; Voortman, J.; Roovers, R.C.; Verkleij, A.J.; Gerritsen, H.C.; van Bergen En Henegouwen, P.M. Egf induces coalescence of different lipid rafts. *J. Cell Sci.* **2008**, *121*, 2519–2528. [CrossRef] [PubMed]

93. Lingwood, D.; Simons, K. Lipid rafts as a membrane-organizing principle. *Science* **2010**, *327*, 46–50. [CrossRef] [PubMed]

94. Patra, S.K. Dissecting lipid raft facilitated cell signaling pathways in cancer. *Biochim. Biophys. Acta* **2008**, *1785*, 182–206. [PubMed]

95. Pike, L.J.; Han, X.; Chung, K.N.; Gross, R.W. Lipid rafts are enriched in arachidonic acid and plasmenylethanolamine and their composition is independent of caveolin-1 expression: A quantitative electrospray ionization/mass spectrometric analysis. *Biochemistry* **2002**, *41*, 2075–2088. [CrossRef] [PubMed]

96. Simons, K.; Sampaio, J.L. Membrane organization and lipid rafts. *Cold Spring Harb. Perspect. Biol.* **2011**, *3*, a004697. [CrossRef] [PubMed]

97. Brzustowicz, M.R.; Cherezov, V.; Caffrey, M.; Stillwell, W.; Wassall, S.R. Molecular organization of cholesterol in polyunsaturated membranes: Microdomain formation. *Biophys. J.* **2002**, *82*, 285–298. [CrossRef] [PubMed]

98. Wassall, S.R.; Brzustowicz, M.R.; Shaikh, S.R.; Cherezov, V.; Caffrey, M.; Stillwell, W. Order from disorder, corralling cholesterol with chaotic lipids. The role of polyunsaturated lipids in membrane raft formation. *Chem. Phys. Lipids* **2004**, *132*, 79–88. [PubMed]

99. Nicolau, D.V., Jr.; Burrage, K.; Parton, R.G.; Hancock, J.F. Identifying optimal lipid raft characteristics required to promote nanoscale protein-protein interactions on the plasma membrane. *Mol. Cell. Biol.* **2006**, *26*, 313–323. [CrossRef] [PubMed]

100. Corsetto, P.A.; Cremona, A.; Montorfano, G.; Jovenitti, I.E.; Orsini, F.; Arosio, P.; Rizzo, A.M. Chemical-physical changes in cell membrane microdomains of breast cancer cells after omega-3 pufa incorporation. *Cell Biochem. Biophys.* **2012**, *64*, 45–59. [CrossRef] [PubMed]

101. Li, H.; Sugimura, K.; Kaji, Y.; Kitamura, Y.; Fujii, M.; Hara, I.; Tachibana, M. Conventional MRI capabilities in the diagnosis of prostate cancer in the transition zone. *AJR Am. J. Roentgenol.* **2006**, *186*, 729–742. [CrossRef] [PubMed]

102. Lee, E.J.; Yun, U.J.; Koo, K.H.; Sung, J.Y.; Shim, J.; Ye, S.K.; Hong, K.M.; Kim, Y.N. Down-regulation of lipid raft-associated onco-proteins via cholesterol-dependent lipid raft internalization in docosahexaenoic acid-induced apoptosis. *Biochim. Biophys. Acta* **2014**, *1841*, 190–203. [CrossRef] [PubMed]

103. Schley, P.D.; Brindley, D.N.; Field, C.J. (*n*-3) pufa alter raft lipid composition and decrease epidermal growth factor receptor levels in lipid rafts of human breast cancer cells. *J. Nutr.* **2007**, *137*, 548–553. [PubMed]

104. Ravacci, G.R.; Brentani, M.M.; Tortelli, T., Jr.; Torrinhas, R.S.; Saldanha, T.; Torres, E.A.; Waitzberg, D.L. Lipid raft disruption by docosahexaenoic acid induces apoptosis in transformed human mammary luminal epithelial cells harboring her-2 overexpression. *J. Nutr. Biochem.* **2013**, *24*, 505–515. [CrossRef] [PubMed]

105. Altenburg, J.D.; Siddiqui, R.A. Omega-3 polyunsaturated fatty acids down-modulate cxcr4 expression and function in mda-mb-231 breast cancer cells. *Mol. Cancer Res.* **2009**, *7*, 1013–1020. [CrossRef] [PubMed]

106. Fulda, S.; Strauss, G.; Meyer, E.; Debatin, K.M. Functional cd95 ligand and cd95 death-inducing signaling complex in activation-induced cell death and doxorubicin-induced apoptosis in leukemic T cells. *Blood* **2000**, *95*, 301–308. [PubMed]

107. Ewaschuk, J.B.; Newell, M.; Field, C.J. Docosahexanoic acid improves chemotherapy efficacy by inducing cd95 translocation to lipid rafts in er(-) breast cancer cells. *Lipids* **2012**, *47*, 1019–1030. [CrossRef] [PubMed]

108. Bollinger, C.R.; Teichgraber, V.; Gulbins, E. Ceramide-enriched membrane domains. *Biochim. Biophys. Acta* **2005**, *1746*, 284–294. [CrossRef] [PubMed]

109. Kim, H.S.; Lee, Y.S.; Kim, D.K. Doxorubicin exerts cytotoxic effects through cell cycle arrest and fas-mediated cell death. *Pharmacology* **2009**, *84*, 300–309. [CrossRef] [PubMed]

110. Lorincz, A.M.; Sukumar, S. Molecular links between obesity and breast cancer. *Endocr. Relat. Cancer* **2006**, *13*, 279–292. [CrossRef] [PubMed]

111. Korner, A.; Pazaitou-Panayiotou, K.; Kelesidis, T.; Kelesidis, I.; Williams, C.J.; Kaprara, A.; Bullen, J.; Neuwirth, A.; Tseleni, S.; Mitsiades, N.; *et al.* Total and high-molecular-weight adiponectin in breast cancer: *In vitro* and *in vivo* studies. *J. Clin. Endocrinol. Metab.* **2007**, *92*, 1041–1048. [CrossRef] [PubMed]

112. Iyengar, P.; Combs, T.P.; Shah, S.J.; Gouon-Evans, V.; Pollard, J.W.; Albanese, C.; Flanagan, L.; Tenniswood, M.P.; Guha, C.; Lisanti, M.P.; *et al.* Adipocyte-secreted factors synergistically promote mammary tumorigenesis through induction of anti-apoptotic transcriptional programs and proto-oncogene stabilization. *Oncogene* **2003**, *22*, 6408–6423. [CrossRef] [PubMed]

113. Grivennikov, S.I.; Karin, M. Inflammatory cytokines in cancer: Tumour necrosis factor and interleukin 6 take the stage. *Ann. Rheum. Dis.* **2011**, *70* (Suppl. 1), i104–i108. [CrossRef] [PubMed]

114. Horng, T.; Hotamisligil, G.S. Linking the inflammasome to obesity-related disease. *Nat. Med.* **2011**, *17*, 164–165. [CrossRef] [PubMed]

115. Hotamisligil, G.S. Inflammation and metabolic disorders. *Nature* **2006**, *444*, 860–867. [CrossRef] [PubMed]

116. Dalamaga, M.; Diakopoulos, K.N.; Mantzoros, C.S. The role of adiponectin in cancer: A review of current evidence. *Endocr. Rev.* **2012**, *33*, 547–594. [CrossRef] [PubMed]

117. Fain, J.N. Release of inflammatory mediators by human adipose tissue is enhanced in obesity and primarily by the nonfat cells: A review. *Mediat. Inflamm.* **2010**, *2010*, 513948. [CrossRef]

118. Fain, J.N.; Madan, A.K.; Hiler, M.L.; Cheema, P.; Bahouth, S.W. Comparison of the release of adipokines by adipose tissue, adipose tissue matrix, and adipocytes from visceral and subcutaneous abdominal adipose tissues of obese humans. *Endocrinology* **2004**, *145*, 2273–2282. [CrossRef] [PubMed]

119. Cinti, S.; Mitchell, G.; Barbatelli, G.; Murano, I.; Ceresi, E.; Faloia, E.; Wang, S.; Fortier, M.; Greenberg, A.S.; Obin, M.S. Adipocyte death defines macrophage localization and function in adipose tissue of obese mice and humans. *J. Lipid Res.* **2005**, *46*, 2347–2355. [CrossRef] [PubMed]

120. Subbaramaiah, K.; Howe, L.R.; Bhardwaj, P.; Du, B.; Gravaghi, C.; Yantiss, R.K.; Zhou, X.K.; Blaho, V.A.; Hla, T.; Yang, P.; *et al.* Obesity is associated with inflammation and elevated aromatase expression in the mouse mammary gland. *Cancer Prev. Res.* **2011**, *4*, 329–346. [CrossRef]

121. Morris, P.G.; Hudis, C.A.; Giri, D.; Morrow, M.; Falcone, D.J.; Zhou, X.K.; Du, B.; Brogi, E.; Crawford, C.B.; Kopelovich, L.; *et al.* Inflammation and increased aromatase expression occur in the breast tissue of obese women with breast cancer. *Cancer Prev. Res.* **2011**, *4*, 1021–1029. [CrossRef]

122. Bhardwaj, P.; Du, B.; Zhou, X.K.; Sue, E.; Harbus, M.D.; Falcone, D.J.; Giri, D.; Hudis, C.A.; Kopelovich, L.; Subbaramaiah, K.; *et al.* Caloric restriction reverses obesity-induced mammary gland inflammation in mice. *Cancer Prev. Res.* **2013**, *6*, 282–289. [CrossRef]

123. Ibrahim, M.M. Subcutaneous and visceral adipose tissue: Structural and functional differences. *Obes. Rev.* **2010**, *11*, 11–18. [CrossRef] [PubMed]

124. Dalamaga, M. Obesity, insulin resistance, adipocytokines and breast cancer: New biomarkers and attractive therapeutic targets. *World J. Exp. Med.* **2013**, *3*, 34–42. [PubMed]

125. Ferguson, R.D.; Gallagher, E.J.; Scheinman, E.J.; Damouni, R.; LeRoith, D. The epidemiology and molecular mechanisms linking obesity, diabetes, and cancer. *Vitam. Horm.* **2013**, *93*, 51–98. [PubMed]

126. Rose, D.P.; Vona-Davis, L. Biochemical and molecular mechanisms for the association between obesity, chronic inflammation, and breast cancer. *BioFactors* **2014**, *40*, 1–12. [CrossRef] [PubMed]

127. Baglietto, L.; English, D.R.; Hopper, J.L.; MacInnis, R.J.; Morris, H.A.; Tilley, W.D.; Krishnan, K.; Giles, G.G. Circulating steroid hormone concentrations in postmenopausal women in relation to body size and composition. *Breast Cancer Res. Treat.* **2009**, *115*, 171–179. [CrossRef] [PubMed]

128. Yager, J.D.; Davidson, N.E. Estrogen carcinogenesis in breast cancer. *N. Engl. J. Med.* **2006**, *354*, 270–282. [CrossRef] [PubMed]

129. Key, T.; Appleby, P.; Barnes, I.; Reeves, G.; Endogenous, H.; Breast Cancer Collaborative, G. Endogenous sex hormones and breast cancer in postmenopausal women: Reanalysis of nine prospective studies. *J. Natl. Cancer Inst.* **2002**, *94*, 606–616. [CrossRef] [PubMed]

130. Haffner, S.M.; Katz, M.S.; Dunn, J.F. Increased upper body and overall adiposity is associated with decreased sex hormone binding globulin in postmenopausal women. *Int. J. Obes.* **1991**, *15*, 471–478. [PubMed]

131. Vona-Davis, L.; Rose, D.P. The obesity-inflammation-eicosanoid axis in breast cancer. *J. Mammary Gland Biol. Neoplasia* **2013**, *18*, 291–307. [CrossRef] [PubMed]

132. Suzuki, T.; Miki, Y.; Ohuchi, N.; Sasano, H. Intratumoral estrogen production in breast carcinoma: Significance of aromatase. *Breast Cancer* **2008**, *15*, 270–277. [CrossRef] [PubMed]

133. Irahara, N.; Miyoshi, Y.; Taguchi, T.; Tamaki, Y.; Noguchi, S. Quantitative analysis of aromatase mRNA expression derived from various promoters (i.4, i.3, pii and i.7) and its association with expression of TNF-alpha, il-6 and cox-2 mRNAs in human breast cancer. *Int. J. Cancer* **2006**, *118*, 1915–1921. [CrossRef] [PubMed]

134. Brodie, A.; Lu, Q.; Nakamura, J. Aromatase in the normal breast and breast cancer. *J. Steroid Biochem. Mol. Biol.* **1997**, *61*, 281–286. [CrossRef] [PubMed]

135. Macaulay, V.M.; Nicholls, J.E.; Gledhill, J.; Rowlands, M.G.; Dowsett, M.; Ashworth, A. Biological effects of stable overexpression of aromatase in human hormone-dependent breast cancer cells. *Br. J. Cancer* **1994**, *69*, 77–83. [CrossRef] [PubMed]

136. Simpson, E.R.; Mahendroo, M.S.; Nichols, J.E.; Bulun, S.E. Aromatase gene expression in adipose tissue: Relationship to breast cancer. *Int. J. Fertil. Menopausal Stud.* **1994**, *39* (Suppl. 2), S75–S83.

137. Pasqualini, J.R.; Chetrite, G.S. Recent insight on the control of enzymes involved in estrogen formation and transformation in human breast cancer. *J. Steroid Biochem. Mol. Biol.* **2005**, *93*, 221–236. [CrossRef] [PubMed]

138. Simpson, E.R.; Ackerman, G.E.; Smith, M.E.; Mendelson, C.R. Estrogen formation in stromal cells of adipose tissue of women: Induction by glucocorticosteroids. *Proc. Natl. Acad. Sci. USA* **1981**, *78*, 5690–5694. [CrossRef] [PubMed]

139. O'Neill, J.S.; Elton, R.A.; Miller, W.R. Aromatase activity in adipose tissue from breast quadrants: A link with tumour site. *Br. Med. J.* **1988**, *296*, 741–743. [CrossRef]

140. Bulun, S.E.; Price, T.M.; Aitken, J.; Mahendroo, M.S.; Simpson, E.R. A link between breast cancer and local estrogen biosynthesis suggested by quantification of breast adipose tissue aromatase cytochrome p450 transcripts using competitive polymerase chain reaction after reverse transcription. *J. Clin. Endocrinol. Metab.* **1993**, *77*, 1622–1628. [PubMed]

141. Bulun, S.E.; Chen, D.; Moy, I.; Brooks, D.C.; Zhao, H. Aromatase, breast cancer and obesity: A complex interaction. *Trends Endocrinol. Metab.* **2012**, *23*, 83–89. [CrossRef] [PubMed]

142. Bulun, S.E.; Simpson, E.R. Regulation of aromatase expression in human tissues. *Breast Cancer Res. Treat.* **1994**, *30*, 19–29. [CrossRef] [PubMed]

143. Simpson, E.R.; Brown, K.A. Obesity and breast cancer: Role of inflammation and aromatase. *J. Mol. Endocrinol.* **2013**, *51*, T51–T59. [CrossRef] [PubMed]

144. Subbaramaiah, K.; Morris, P.G.; Zhou, X.K.; Morrow, M.; Du, B.; Giri, D.; Kopelovich, L.; Hudis, C.A.; Dannenberg, A.J. Increased levels of cox-2 and prostaglandin e2 contribute to elevated aromatase expression in inflamed breast tissue of obese women. *Cancer Discov.* **2012**, *2*, 356–365. [CrossRef] [PubMed]

145. Pender-Cudlip, M.C.; Krag, K.J.; Martini, D.; Yu, J.; Guidi, A.; Skinner, S.S.; Zhang, Y.; Qu, X.; He, C.; Xu, Y.; et al. Delta-6-desaturase activity and arachidonic acid synthesis are increased in human breast cancer tissue. *Cancer Sci.* **2013**, *104*, 760–764. [CrossRef] [PubMed]

146. Chen, D.; Reierstad, S.; Lin, Z.; Lu, M.; Brooks, C.; Li, N.; Innes, J.; Bulun, S.E. Prostaglandin e(2) induces breast cancer related aromatase promoters via activation of p38 and c-jun nh(2)-terminal kinase in adipose fibroblasts. *Cancer Res.* **2007**, *67*, 8914–8922. [CrossRef] [PubMed]

147. Zhao, Y.; Agarwal, V.R.; Mendelson, C.R.; Simpson, E.R. Estrogen biosynthesis proximal to a breast tumor is stimulated by pge2 via cyclic amp, leading to activation of promoter II of the cyp19 (aromatase) gene. *Endocrinology* **1996**, *137*, 5739–5742. [PubMed]

148. Larsson, S.C.; Kumlin, M.; Ingelman-Sundberg, M.; Wolk, A. Dietary long-chain *n*-3 fatty acids for the prevention of cancer: A review of potential mechanisms. *Am. J. Clin. Nutr.* **2004**, *79*, 935–945. [PubMed]

149. Shackelford, D.B.; Shaw, R.J. The lkb1-ampk pathway: Metabolism and growth control in tumour suppression. *Nat. Rev. Cancer* **2009**, *9*, 563–575. [CrossRef] [PubMed]

150. Brown, K.A.; McInnes, K.J.; Hunger, N.I.; Oakhill, J.S.; Steinberg, G.R.; Simpson, E.R. Subcellular localization of cyclic amp-responsive element binding protein-regulated transcription coactivator 2 provides a link between obesity and breast cancer in postmenopausal women. *Cancer Res.* **2009**, *69*, 5392–5399. [CrossRef] [PubMed]

151. Purohit, A.; Newman, S.P.; Reed, M.J. The role of cytokines in regulating estrogen synthesis: Implications for the etiology of breast cancer. *Breast Cancer Res.* **2002**, *4*, 65–69. [CrossRef] [PubMed]

152. Zhao, Y.; Nichols, J.E.; Valdez, R.; Mendelson, C.R.; Simpson, E.R. Tumor necrosis factor-alpha stimulates aromatase gene expression in human adipose stromal cells through use of an activating protein-1 binding site upstream of promoter 1.4. *Mol. Endocrinol.* **1996**, *10*, 1350–1357. [PubMed]

153. To, S.Q.; Knower, K.C.; Clyne, C.D. Nfkappab and mapk signalling pathways mediate tnfalpha-induced early growth response gene transcription leading to aromatase expression. *Biochem. Biophys. Res. Commun.* **2013**, *433*, 96–101. [CrossRef] [PubMed]

154. Honma, S.; Shimodaira, K.; Shimizu, Y.; Tsuchiya, N.; Saito, H.; Yanaihara, T.; Okai, T. The influence of inflammatory cytokines on estrogen production and cell proliferation in human breast cancer cells. *Endocr. J.* **2002**, *49*, 371–377. [CrossRef] [PubMed]

155. Panigrahy, D.; Kaipainen, A.; Greene, E.R.; Huang, S. Cytochrome p450-derived eicosanoids: The neglected pathway in cancer. *Cancer Metastasis Rev.* **2010**, *29*, 723–735. [CrossRef] [PubMed]

156. Arnold, C.; Konkel, A.; Fischer, R.; Schunck, W.H. Cytochrome p450-dependent metabolism of omega-6 and omega-3 long-chain polyunsaturated fatty acids. *Pharmacol. Rep.* **2010**, *62*, 536–547. [CrossRef] [PubMed]

157. Bannenberg, G.; Arita, M.; Serhan, C.N. Endogenous receptor agonists: Resolving inflammation. *Sci. World J.* **2007**, *7*, 1440–1462. [CrossRef]

158. Bannenberg, G.L.; Chiang, N.; Ariel, A.; Arita, M.; Tjonahen, E.; Gotlinger, K.H.; Hong, S.; Serhan, C.N. Molecular circuits of resolution: Formation and actions of resolvins and protectins. *J. Immunol.* **2005**, *174*, 4345–4355. [CrossRef] [PubMed]

159. Rose, D.P.; Connolly, J.M. Omega-3 fatty acids as cancer chemopreventive agents. *Pharmacol. Ther.* **1999**, *83*, 217–244. [CrossRef] [PubMed]

160. Calder, P.C. The role of marine omega-3 (*n*-3) fatty acids in inflammatory processes, atherosclerosis and plaque stability. *Mol. Nutr. Food Res.* **2012**, *56*, 1073–1080. [CrossRef] [PubMed]

161. Wei, N.; Wang, B.; Zhang, Q.Y.; Mi, M.T.; Zhu, J.D.; Yu, X.P.; Yuan, J.L.; Chen, K.; Wang, J.; Chang, H. Effects of different dietary fatty acids on the fatty acid compositions and the expression of lipid metabolic-related genes in mammary tumor tissues of rats. *Nutr. Cancer* **2008**, *60*, 810–825. [CrossRef] [PubMed]

162. Kaur, B.; Jorgensen, A.; Duttaroy, A.K. Fatty acid uptake by breast cancer cells (mda-mb-231): Effects of insulin, leptin, adiponectin, and tnfalpha. *Prostaglandins Leukot. Essent. Fatty Acids* **2009**, *80*, 93–99. [CrossRef] [PubMed]

163. Liu, X.H.; Connolly, J.M.; Rose, D.P. The 12-lipoxygenase gene-transfected mcf-7 human breast cancer cell line exhibits estrogen-independent, but estrogen and omega-6 fatty acid-stimulated proliferation *in vitro*, and enhanced growth in athymic nude mice. *Cancer Lett.* **1996**, *109*, 223–230. [CrossRef] [PubMed]

164. Connolly, J.M.; Rose, D.P. Enhanced angiogenesis and growth of 12-lipoxygenase gene-transfected mcf-7 human breast cancer cells in athymic nude mice. *Cancer Lett.* **1998**, *132*, 107–112. [CrossRef] [PubMed]

165. Avis, I.; Hong, S.H.; Martinez, A.; Moody, T.; Choi, Y.H.; Trepel, J.; Das, R.; Jett, M.; Mulshine, J.L. Five-lipoxygenase inhibitors can mediate apoptosis in human breast cancer cell lines through complex eicosanoid interactions. *FASEB J.* **2001**, *15*, 2007–2009. [PubMed]

166. Tong, W.G.; Ding, X.Z.; Adrian, T.E. The mechanisms of lipoxygenase inhibitor-induced apoptosis in human breast cancer cells. *Biochem. Biophys. Res. Commun.* **2002**, *296*, 942–948. [CrossRef] [PubMed]

167. Rose, D.P.; Connolly, J.M. Effects of fatty acids and inhibitors of eicosanoid synthesis on the growth of a human breast cancer cell line in culture. *Cancer Res.* **1990**, *50*, 7139–7144. [PubMed]

168. Navarro-Tito, N.; Soto-Guzman, A.; Castro-Sanchez, L.; Martinez-Orozco, R.; Salazar, E.P. Oleic acid promotes migration on mda-mb-231 breast cancer cells through an arachidonic acid-dependent pathway. *Int. J. Biochem. Cell Biol.* **2010**, *42*, 306–317. [CrossRef] [PubMed]

169. Hu, N.; Li, Y.; Zhao, Y.; Wang, Q.; You, J.C.; Zhang, X.D.; Ye, L.H. A novel positive feedback loop involving fasn/p-erk1/2/5-lox/ltb4/fasn sustains high growth of breast cancer cells. *Acta Pharmacol. Sin.* **2011**, *32*, 921–929. [CrossRef] [PubMed]

170. Rose, D.P.; Connolly, J.M.; Rayburn, J.; Coleman, M. Influence of diets containing eicosapentaenoic or docosahexaenoic acid on growth and metastasis of breast cancer cells in nude mice. *J. Natl. Cancer Inst.* **1995**, *87*, 587–592. [CrossRef] [PubMed]

171. Erickson, K.L.; Hubbard, N.E. Fatty acids and breast cancer: The role of stem cells. *Prostaglandins Leukot. Essent. Fatty Acids* **2010**, *82*, 237–241. [CrossRef] [PubMed]

172. Sethi, S.; Sarkar, F.H.; Ahmed, Q.; Bandyopadhyay, S.; Nahleh, Z.A.; Semaan, A.; Sakr, W.; Munkarah, A.; Ali-Fehmi, R. Molecular markers of epithelial-to-mesenchymal transition are associated with tumor aggressiveness in breast carcinoma. *Transl. Oncol.* **2011**, *4*, 222–226. [CrossRef] [PubMed]

173. Zhou, Y.; Yau, C.; Gray, J.W.; Chew, K.; Dairkee, S.H.; Moore, D.H.; Eppenberger, U.; Eppenberger-Castori, S.; Benz, C.C. Enhanced NF kappa b and ap-1 transcriptional activity associated with antiestrogen resistant breast cancer. *BMC Cancer* **2007**, *7*, 59. [CrossRef] [PubMed]

174. Naugler, W.E.; Karin, M. NF-kappab and cancer-identifying targets and mechanisms. *Curr. Opin. Genet. Dev.* **2008**, *18*, 19–26. [CrossRef] [PubMed]

175. Calder, P.C. Lipids for intravenous nutrition in hospitalised adult patients: A multiple choice of options. *Proc. Nutr. Soc.* **2013**, *72*, 263–276. [CrossRef] [PubMed]

176. Kurtzman, S.H.; Anderson, K.H.; Wang, Y.; Miller, L.J.; Renna, M.; Stankus, M.; Lindquist, R.R.; Barrows, G.; Kreutzer, D.L. Cytokines in human breast cancer: Il-1alpha and il-1beta expression. *Oncol. Rep.* **1999**, *6*, 65–70. [PubMed]

177. Pantschenko, A.G.; Pushkar, I.; Anderson, K.H.; Wang, Y.; Miller, L.J.; Kurtzman, S.H.; Barrows, G.; Kreutzer, D.L. The interleukin-1 family of cytokines and receptors in human breast cancer: Implications for tumor progression. *Int. J. Oncol.* **2003**, *23*, 269–284. [PubMed]

178. Chavey, C.; Bibeau, F.; Gourgou-Bourgade, S.; Burlinchon, S.; Boissiere, F.; Laune, D.; Roques, S.; Lazennec, G. Oestrogen receptor negative breast cancers exhibit high cytokine content. *Breast Cancer Res.* **2007**, *9*, R15. [CrossRef] [PubMed]

179. Candido, J.; Hagemann, T. Cancer-related inflammation. *J. Clin. Immunol.* **2013**, *33* (Suppl. 1), S79–S84. [CrossRef]

180. Kim, S.; Choi, J.H.; Kim, J.B.; Nam, S.J.; Yang, J.H.; Kim, J.H.; Lee, J.E. Berberine suppresses TNF-alpha-induced mmp-9 and cell invasion through inhibition of ap-1 activity in mda-mb-231 human breast cancer cells. *Molecules* **2008**, *13*, 2975–2985. [CrossRef] [PubMed]

181. Wu, Y.; Deng, J.; Rychahou, P.G.; Qiu, S.; Evers, B.M.; Zhou, B.P. Stabilization of snail by NF-kappab is required for inflammation-induced cell migration and invasion. *Cancer Cell* **2009**, *15*, 416–428. [CrossRef] [PubMed]

182. Cho, S.G.; Li, D.; Stafford, L.J.; Luo, J.; Rodriguez-Villanueva, M.; Wang, Y.; Liu, M. Kiss1 suppresses tnfalpha-induced breast cancer cell invasion via an inhibition of rhoa-mediated NF-kappab activation. *J. Cell Biochem.* **2009**, *107*, 1139–1149. [CrossRef] [PubMed]

183. Kushiro, K.; Nunez, N.P. Ob/ob serum promotes a mesenchymal cell phenotype in b16bl6 melanoma cells. *Clin. Exp. Metastasis* **2011**, *28*, 877–886. [CrossRef] [PubMed]

184. Soria, G.; Ben-Baruch, A. The inflammatory chemokines ccl2 and ccl5 in breast cancer. *Cancer Lett.* **2008**, *267*, 271–285. [CrossRef] [PubMed]

185. Ueno, T.; Toi, M.; Saji, H.; Muta, M.; Bando, H.; Kuroi, K.; Koike, M.; Inadera, H.; Matsushima, K. Significance of macrophage chemoattractant protein-1 in macrophage recruitment, angiogenesis, and survival in human breast cancer. *Clin. Cancer Res.* **2000**, *6*, 3282–3289. [PubMed]

186. Ye, J.; Gao, Z.; Yin, J.; He, Q. Hypoxia is a potential risk factor for chronic inflammation and adiponectin reduction in adipose tissue of ob/ob and dietary obese mice. *Am. J. Physiol. Endocrinol. Metab.* **2007**, *293*, E1118–E1128. [CrossRef] [PubMed]

187. Cancello, R.; Henegar, C.; Viguerie, N.; Taleb, S.; Poitou, C.; Rouault, C.; Coupaye, M.; Pelloux, V.; Hugol, D.; Bouillot, J.L.; *et al.* Reduction of macrophage infiltration and chemoattractant gene expression changes in white adipose tissue of morbidly obese subjects after surgery-induced weight loss. *Diabetes* **2005**, *54*, 2277–2286. [CrossRef] [PubMed]

188. Itariu, B.K.; Zeyda, M.; Hochbrugger, E.E.; Neuhofer, A.; Prager, G.; Schindler, K.; Bohdjalian, A.; Mascher, D.; Vangala, S.; Schranz, M.; *et al.* Long-chain *n*-3 pufas reduce adipose tissue and systemic inflammation in severely obese nondiabetic patients: A randomized controlled trial. *Am. J. Clin. Nutr.* **2012**, *96*, 1137–1149. [CrossRef] [PubMed]

189. Awada, M.; Meynier, A.; Soulage, C.O.; Hadji, L.; Geloen, A.; Viau, M.; Ribourg, L.; Benoit, B.; Debard, C.; Guichardant, M.; *et al. n*-3 pufa added to high-fat diets affect differently adiposity and inflammation when carried by phospholipids or triacylglycerols in mice. *Nutr. Metab.* **2013**, *10*, 23. [CrossRef]

190. Titos, E.; Rius, B.; Gonzalez-Periz, A.; Lopez-Vicario, C.; Moran-Salvador, E.; Martinez-Clemente, M.; Arroyo, V.; Claria, J. Resolvin d1 and its precursor docosahexaenoic acid promote resolution of adipose tissue inflammation by eliciting macrophage polarization toward an m2-like phenotype. *J. Immunol.* **2011**, *187*, 5408–5418. [CrossRef] [PubMed]

191. Oliver, E.; McGillicuddy, F.C.; Harford, K.A.; Reynolds, C.M.; Phillips, C.M.; Ferguson, J.F.; Roche, H.M. Docosahexaenoic acid attenuates macrophage-induced inflammation and improves insulin sensitivity in adipocytes-specific differential effects between lc *n*-3 pufa. *J. Nutr. Biochem.* **2012**, *23*, 1192–1200. [CrossRef] [PubMed]

192. De Boer, A.A.; Monk, J.M.; Robinson, L.E. Docosahexaenoic acid decreases pro-inflammatory mediators in an *in vitro* murine adipocyte macrophage co-culture model. *PLoS One* **2014**, *9*, e85037. [CrossRef] [PubMed]

193. Novak, T.E.; Babcock, T.A.; Jho, D.H.; Helton, W.S.; Espat, N.J. Nf-kappa b inhibition by omega-3 fatty acids modulates lps-stimulated macrophage tnf-alpha transcription. *Am. J. Physiol. Lung Cell. Mol. Physiol.* **2003**, *284*, L84–L89. [PubMed]

194. Weldon, S.M.; Mullen, A.C.; Loscher, C.E.; Hurley, L.A.; Roche, H.M. Docosahexaenoic acid induces an anti-inflammatory profile in lipopolysaccharide-stimulated human thp-1 macrophages more effectively than eicosapentaenoic acid. *J. Nutr. Biochem.* **2007**, *18*, 250–258. [CrossRef] [PubMed]

195. Moon, H.S.; Dalamaga, M.; Kim, S.Y.; Polyzos, S.A.; Hamnvik, O.P.; Magkos, F.; Paruthi, J.; Mantzoros, C.S. Leptin's role in lipodystrophic and nonlipodystrophic insulin-resistant and diabetic individuals. *Endocr. Rev.* **2013**, *34*, 377–412. [CrossRef] [PubMed]

196. Widjaja, A.; Stratton, I.M.; Horn, R.; Holman, R.R.; Turner, R.; Brabant, G. Ukpds 20: Plasma leptin, obesity, and plasma insulin in type 2 diabetic subjects. *J. Clin. Endocrinol. Metab.* **1997**, *82*, 654–657. [CrossRef] [PubMed]

197. Jarde, T.; Caldefie-Chezet, F.; Damez, M.; Mishellany, F.; Penault-Llorca, F.; Guillot, J.; Vasson, M.P. Leptin and leptin receptor involvement in cancer development: A study on human primary breast carcinoma. *Oncol. Rep.* **2008**, *19*, 905–911. [PubMed]

198. Revillion, F.; Charlier, M.; Lhotellier, V.; Hornez, L.; Giard, S.; Baranzelli, M.C.; Djiane, J.; Peyrat, J.P. Messenger RNA expression of leptin and leptin receptors and their prognostic value in 322 human primary breast cancers. *Clin. Cancer Res.* **2006**, *12*, 2088–2094. [CrossRef] [PubMed]

199. Neville, M.C.; McFadden, T.B.; Forsyth, I. Hormonal regulation of mammary differentiation and milk secretion. *J. Mammary Gland Biol. Neoplasia* **2002**, *7*, 49–66. [CrossRef] [PubMed]

200. Garofalo, C.; Surmacz, E. Leptin and cancer. *J. Cell. Physiol.* **2006**, *207*, 12–22. [CrossRef] [PubMed]

201. Caldefie-Chezet, F.; Damez, M.; de Latour, M.; Konska, G.; Mishellani, F.; Fusillier, C.; Guerry, M.; Penault-Llorca, F.; Guillot, J.; Vasson, M.P. Leptin: A proliferative factor for breast cancer? Study on human ductal carcinoma. *Biochem. Biophys. Res. Commun.* **2005**, *334*, 737–741. [CrossRef] [PubMed]

202. Dieudonne, M.N.; Machinal-Quelin, F.; Serazin-Leroy, V.; Leneveu, M.C.; Pecquery, R.; Giudicelli, Y. Leptin mediates a proliferative response in human mcf7 breast cancer cells. *Biochem. Biophys. Res. Commun.* **2002**, *293*, 622–628. [CrossRef] [PubMed]

203. Garofalo, C.; Koda, M.; Cascio, S.; Sulkowska, M.; Kanczuga-Koda, L.; Golaszewska, J.; Russo, A.; Sulkowski, S.; Surmacz, E. Increased expression of leptin and the leptin receptor as a marker of breast cancer progression: Possible role of obesity-related stimuli. *Clin. Cancer Res.* **2006**, *12*, 1447–1453. [CrossRef]

204. Hu, X.; Juneja, S.C.; Maihle, N.J.; Cleary, M.P. Leptin—A growth factor in normal and malignant breast cells and for normal mammary gland development. *J. Natl. Cancer Inst.* **2002**, *94*, 1704–1711. [CrossRef] [PubMed]

205. Ishikawa, M.; Kitayama, J.; Nagawa, H. Enhanced expression of leptin and leptin receptor (ob-r) in human breast cancer. *Clin. Cancer Res.* **2004**, *10*, 4325–4331. [CrossRef] [PubMed]

206. Laud, K.; Gourdou, I.; Pessemesse, L.; Peyrat, J.P.; Djiane, J. Identification of leptin receptors in human breast cancer: Functional activity in the t47-d breast cancer cell line. *Mol. Cell. Endocrinol.* **2002**, *188*, 219–226. [CrossRef] [PubMed]

207. Yin, N.; Wang, D.; Zhang, H.; Yi, X.; Sun, X.; Shi, B.; Wu, H.; Wu, G.; Wang, X.; Shang, Y. Molecular mechanisms involved in the growth stimulation of breast cancer cells by leptin. *Cancer Res.* **2004**, *64*, 5870–5875. [CrossRef] [PubMed]

208. Nyante, S.J.; Gammon, M.D.; Kaufman, J.S.; Bensen, J.T.; Lin, D.Y.; Barnholtz-Sloan, J.S.; Hu, Y.; He, Q.; Luo, J.; Millikan, R.C. Common genetic variation in adiponectin, leptin, and leptin receptor and association with breast cancer subtypes. *Breast Cancer Res. Treat.* **2011**, *129*, 593–606. [CrossRef] [PubMed]

209. Miyoshi, Y.; Funahashi, T.; Tanaka, S.; Taguchi, T.; Tamaki, Y.; Shimomura, I.; Noguchi, S. High expression of leptin receptor mRNA in breast cancer tissue predicts poor prognosis for patients with high, but not low, serum leptin levels. *Int. J. Cancer* **2006**, *118*, 1414–1419. [CrossRef] [PubMed]

210. Catalano, S.; Mauro, L.; Marsico, S.; Giordano, C.; Rizza, P.; Rago, V.; Montanaro, D.; Maggiolini, M.; Panno, M.L.; Ando, S. Leptin induces, via erk1/erk2 signal, functional activation of estrogen receptor alpha in mcf-7 cells. *J. Biol. Chem.* **2004**, *279*, 19908–19915. [CrossRef] [PubMed]

211. Grossmann, M.E.; Cleary, M.P. The balance between leptin and adiponectin in the control of carcinogenesis—Focus on mammary tumorigenesis. *Biochimie* **2012**, *94*, 2164–2171. [CrossRef] [PubMed]

212. Jarde, T.; Perrier, S.; Vasson, M.P.; Caldefie-Chezet, F. Molecular mechanisms of leptin and adiponectin in breast cancer. *Eur. J. Cancer* **2011**, *47*, 33–43. [CrossRef] [PubMed]

213. Ray, A. Adipokine leptin in obesity-related pathology of breast cancer. *J. Biosci.* **2012**, *37*, 289–294. [CrossRef] [PubMed]

214. Okumura, M.; Yamamoto, M.; Sakuma, H.; Kojima, T.; Maruyama, T.; Jamali, M.; Cooper, D.R.; Yasuda, K. Leptin and high glucose stimulate cell proliferation in mcf-7 human breast cancer cells: Reciprocal involvement of pkc-alpha and ppar expression. *Biochim. Biophys. Acta* **2002**, *1592*, 107–116. [PubMed]

215. Chen, C.; Chang, Y.C.; Liu, C.L.; Chang, K.J.; Guo, I.C. Leptin-induced growth of human zr-75-1 breast cancer cells is associated with up-regulation of cyclin d1 and c-myc and down-regulation of tumor suppressor p53 and p21waf1/cip1. *Breast Cancer Res. Treat.* **2006**, *98*, 121–132. [CrossRef] [PubMed]

216. Seilkop, S.K. The effect of body weight on tumor incidence and carcinogenicity testing in b6c3f1 mice and f344 rats. *Fundam. Appl. Toxicol.* **1995**, *24*, 247–259. [CrossRef] [PubMed]

217. Klurfeld, D.M.; Lloyd, L.M.; Welch, C.B.; Davis, M.J.; Tulp, O.L.; Kritchevsky, D. Reduction of enhanced mammary carcinogenesis in la/n-cp (corpulent) rats by energy restriction. *Proc. Soc. Exp. Biol. Med.* **1991**, *196*, 381–384. [CrossRef] [PubMed]

218. Cleary, M.P.; Juneja, S.C.; Phillips, F.C.; Hu, X.; Grande, J.P.; Maihle, N.J. Leptin receptor-deficient mmtv-tgf-alpha/lepr(db)lepr(db) female mice do not develop oncogene-induced mammary tumors. *Exp. Biol. Med.* **2004**, *229*, 182–193.

219. Cleary, M.P.; Phillips, F.C.; Getzin, S.C.; Jacobson, T.L.; Jacobson, M.K.; Christensen, T.A.; Juneja, S.C.; Grande, J.P.; Maihle, N.J. Genetically obese mmtv-tgf-alpha/lep(ob)lep(ob) female mice do not develop mammary tumors. *Breast Cancer Res. Treat.* **2003**, *77*, 205–215. [CrossRef] [PubMed]

220. Otvos, L., Jr.; Kovalszky, I.; Riolfi, M.; Ferla, R.; Olah, J.; Sztodola, A.; Nama, K.; Molino, A.; Piubello, Q.; Wade, J.D.; *et al.* Efficacy of a leptin receptor antagonist peptide in a mouse model of triple-negative breast cancer. *Eur. J. Cancer* **2011**, *47*, 1578–1584. [CrossRef] [PubMed]

221. Gonzalez, R.R.; Cherfils, S.; Escobar, M.; Yoo, J.H.; Carino, C.; Styer, A.K.; Sullivan, B.T.; Sakamoto, H.; Olawaiye, A.; Serikawa, T.; *et al.* Leptin signaling promotes the growth of mammary tumors and increases the expression of vascular endothelial growth factor (vegf) and its receptor type two (vegf-r2). *J. Biol. Chem.* **2006**, *281*, 26320–26328. [CrossRef] [PubMed]

222. Catalano, S.; Marsico, S.; Giordano, C.; Mauro, L.; Rizza, P.; Panno, M.L.; Ando, S. Leptin enhances, via ap-1, expression of aromatase in the mcf-7 cell line. *J. Biol. Chem.* **2003**, *278*, 28668–28676. [CrossRef] [PubMed]

223. Garofalo, C.; Sisci, D.; Surmacz, E. Leptin interferes with the effects of the antiestrogen ici 182,780 in mcf-7 breast cancer cells. *Clin. Cancer Res.* **2004**, *10*, 6466–6475. [CrossRef] [PubMed]

224. Machinal-Quelin, F.; Dieudonne, M.N.; Pecquery, R.; Leneveu, M.C.; Giudicelli, Y. Direct *in vitro* effects of androgens and estrogens on ob gene expression and leptin secretion in human adipose tissue. *Endocrine* **2002**, *18*, 179–184. [CrossRef] [PubMed]

225. O'Neil, J.S.; Burow, M.E.; Green, A.E.; McLachlan, J.A.; Henson, M.C. Effects of estrogen on leptin gene promoter activation in mcf-7 breast cancer and jeg-3 choriocarcinoma cells: Selective regulation via estrogen receptors alpha and beta. *Mol. Cell. Endocrinol.* **2001**, *176*, 67–75. [CrossRef] [PubMed]

226. Liu, X.; Wu, Y.M.; Xu, L.; Tang, C.; Zhong, Y.B. [Influence of hypoxia on leptin and leptin receptor gene expression of c57bl/6j mice]. *Zhonghua Jie He He Hu Xi Za Zhi* **2005**, *28*, 173–175. [PubMed]

227. Ambrosini, G.; Nath, A.K.; Sierra-Honigmann, M.R.; Flores-Riveros, J. Transcriptional activation of the human leptin gene in response to hypoxia. Involvement of hypoxia-inducible factor 1. *J. Biol. Chem.* **2002**, *277*, 34601–34609. [CrossRef] [PubMed]

228. Grosfeld, A.; Andre, J.; Hauguel-De Mouzon, S.; Berra, E.; Pouyssegur, J.; Guerre-Millo, M. Hypoxia-inducible factor 1 transactivates the human leptin gene promoter. *J. Biol. Chem.* **2002**, *277*, 42953–42957. [CrossRef] [PubMed]

229. Fan, C.; Liu, X.; Shen, W.; Deckelbaum, R.J.; Qi, K. The regulation of leptin, leptin receptor and pro-opiomelanocortin expression by *n*-3 pufas in diet-induced obese mice is not related to the methylation of their promoters. *Nutr. Metab.* **2011**, *8*, 31. [CrossRef]

230. Zeidan, A.; Javadov, S.; Chakrabarti, S.; Karmazyn, M. Leptin-induced cardiomyocyte hypertrophy involves selective caveolae and rhoa/rock-dependent p38 mapk translocation to nuclei. *Cardiovasc. Res.* **2008**, *77*, 64–72. [CrossRef] [PubMed]

231. Kadowaki, T.; Yamauchi, T. Adiponectin and adiponectin receptors. *Endocr. Rev.* **2005**, *26*, 439–451. [CrossRef] [PubMed]

232. Waki, H.; Yamauchi, T.; Kamon, J.; Kita, S.; Ito, Y.; Hada, Y.; Uchida, S.; Tsuchida, A.; Takekawa, S.; Kadowaki, T. Generation of globular fragment of adiponectin by leukocyte elastase secreted by monocytic cell line thp-1. *Endocrinology* **2005**, *146*, 790–796. [CrossRef] [PubMed]

233. Yamauchi, T.; Kamon, J.; Ito, Y.; Tsuchida, A.; Yokomizo, T.; Kita, S.; Sugiyama, T.; Miyagishi, M.; Hara, K.; Tsunoda, M.; *et al.* Cloning of adiponectin receptors that mediate antidiabetic metabolic effects. *Nature* **2003**, *423*, 762–769. [CrossRef] [PubMed]

234. Ryan, A.S.; Berman, D.M.; Nicklas, B.J.; Sinha, M.; Gingerich, R.L.; Meneilly, G.S.; Egan, J.M.; Elahi, D. Plasma adiponectin and leptin levels, body composition, and glucose utilization in adult women with wide ranges of age and obesity. *Diabetes Care* **2003**, *26*, 2383–2388. [CrossRef] [PubMed]

235. Vona-Davis, L.; Rose, D.P. Adipokines as endocrine, paracrine, and autocrine factors in breast cancer risk and progression. *Endocr. Relat. Cancer* **2007**, *14*, 189–206. [CrossRef] [PubMed]

236. Kern, P.A.; di Gregorio, G.B.; Lu, T.; Rassouli, N.; Ranganathan, G. Adiponectin expression from human adipose tissue: Relation to obesity, insulin resistance, and tumor necrosis factor-alpha expression. *Diabetes* **2003**, *52*, 1779–1785. [CrossRef] [PubMed]

237. Miyoshi, Y.; Funahashi, T.; Kihara, S.; Taguchi, T.; Tamaki, Y.; Matsuzawa, Y.; Noguchi, S. Association of serum adiponectin levels with breast cancer risk. *Clin. Cancer Res.* **2003**, *9*, 5699–5704. [PubMed]

238. Mantzoros, C.; Petridou, E.; Dessypris, N.; Chavelas, C.; Dalamaga, M.; Alexe, D.M.; Papadiamantis, Y.; Markopoulos, C.; Spanos, E.; Chrousos, G.; *et al.* Adiponectin and breast cancer risk. *J. Clin. Endocrinol. Metab.* **2004**, *89*, 1102–1107. [CrossRef] [PubMed]

239. Macis, D.; Guerrieri-Gonzaga, A.; Gandini, S. Circulating adiponectin and breast cancer risk: A systematic review and meta-analysis. *Int. J. Epidemiol.* **2014**, *43*, 1226–1236. [CrossRef] [PubMed]

240. Ye, J.; Jia, J.; Dong, S.; Zhang, C.; Yu, S.; Li, L.; Mao, C.; Wang, D.; Chen, J.; Yuan, G. Circulating adiponectin levels and the risk of breast cancer: A meta-analysis. *Eur. J. Cancer Prev.* **2014**, *23*, 158–165. [CrossRef] [PubMed]

241. Liu, L.Y.; Wang, M.; Ma, Z.B.; Yu, L.X.; Zhang, Q.; Gao, D.Z.; Wang, F.; Yu, Z.G. The role of adiponectin in breast cancer: A meta-analysis. *PLoS One* **2013**, *8*, e73183. [CrossRef] [PubMed]

242. Grossmann, M.E.; Ray, A.; Nkhata, K.J.; Malakhov, D.A.; Rogozina, O.P.; Dogan, S.; Cleary, M.P. Obesity and breast cancer: Status of leptin and adiponectin in pathological processes. *Cancer Metastasis Rev.* **2010**, *29*, 641–653. [CrossRef] [PubMed]

243. Takahata, C.; Miyoshi, Y.; Irahara, N.; Taguchi, T.; Tamaki, Y.; Noguchi, S. Demonstration of adiponectin receptors 1 and 2 mRNA expression in human breast cancer cells. *Cancer Lett.* **2007**, *250*, 229–236. [CrossRef] [PubMed]

244. Jarde, T.; Caldefie-Chezet, F.; Damez, M.; Mishellany, F.; Perrone, D.; Penault-Llorca, F.; Guillot, J.; Vasson, M.P. Adiponectin and leptin expression in primary ductal breast cancer and in adjacent healthy epithelial and myoepithelial tissue. *Histopathology* **2008**, *53*, 484–487. [CrossRef] [PubMed]

245. Lam, J.B.; Chow, K.H.; Xu, A.; Lam, K.S.; Liu, J.; Wong, N.S.; Moon, R.T.; Shepherd, P.R.; Cooper, G.J.; Wang, Y. Adiponectin haploinsufficiency promotes mammary tumor development in mmtv-pyvt mice by modulation of phosphatase and tensin homolog activities. *PLoS One* **2009**, *4*, e4968. [CrossRef] [PubMed]

246. Wang, Y.; Lam, J.B.; Lam, K.S.; Liu, J.; Lam, M.C.; Hoo, R.L.; Wu, D.; Cooper, G.J.; Xu, A. Adiponectin modulates the glycogen synthase kinase-3beta/beta-catenin signaling pathway and attenuates mammary tumorigenesis of mda-mb-231 cells in nude mice. *Cancer Res.* **2006**, *66*, 11462–11470. [CrossRef] [PubMed]

247. Nakayama, S.; Miyoshi, Y.; Ishihara, H.; Noguchi, S. Growth-inhibitory effect of adiponectin via adiponectin receptor 1 on human breast cancer cells through inhibition of s-phase entry without inducing apoptosis. *Breast Cancer Res. Treat.* **2008**, *112*, 405–410. [CrossRef] [PubMed]

248. Dos Santos, E.; Benaitreau, D.; Dieudonne, M.N.; Leneveu, M.C.; Serazin, V.; Giudicelli, Y.; Pecquery, R. Adiponectin mediates an antiproliferative response in human mda-mb 231 breast cancer cells. *Oncol. Rep.* **2008**, *20*, 971–977. [PubMed]

249. Pfeiler, G.; Hudelist, G.; Wulfing, P.; Mattsson, B.; Konigsberg, R.; Kubista, E.; Singer, C.F. Impact of adipor1 expression on breast cancer development. *Gynecol. Oncol.* **2010**, *117*, 134–138. [CrossRef] [PubMed]

250. Jarde, T.; Caldefie-Chezet, F.; Goncalves-Mendes, N.; Mishellany, F.; Buechler, C.; Penault-Llorca, F.; Vasson, M.P. Involvement of adiponectin and leptin in breast cancer: Clinical and *in vitro* studies. *Endocr. Relat. Cancer* **2009**, *16*, 1197–1210. [CrossRef] [PubMed]

251. Dieudonne, M.N.; Bussiere, M.; dos Santos, E.; Leneveu, M.C.; Giudicelli, Y.; Pecquery, R. Adiponectin mediates antiproliferative and apoptotic responses in human mcf7 breast cancer cells. *Biochem. Biophys. Res. Commun.* **2006**, *345*, 271–279. [CrossRef] [PubMed]

252. Taliaferro-Smith, L.; Nagalingam, A.; Zhong, D.; Zhou, W.; Saxena, N.K.; Sharma, D. Lkb1 is required for adiponectin-mediated modulation of ampk-s6k axis and inhibition of migration and invasion of breast cancer cells. *Oncogene* **2009**, *28*, 2621–2633. [CrossRef] [PubMed]

253. Nkhata, K.J.; Ray, A.; Schuster, T.F.; Grossmann, M.E.; Cleary, M.P. Effects of adiponectin and leptin co-treatment on human breast cancer cell growth. *Oncol. Rep.* **2009**, *21*, 1611–1619. [PubMed]

254. Villarreal-Molina, M.T.; Antuna-Puente, B. Adiponectin: Anti-inflammatory and cardioprotective effects. *Biochimie* **2012**, *94*, 2143–2149. [CrossRef] [PubMed]

255. Ouchi, N.; Walsh, K. Adiponectin as an anti-inflammatory factor. *Clin. Chim. Acta* **2007**, *380*, 24–30. [CrossRef] [PubMed]

256. Folco, E.J.; Rocha, V.Z.; Lopez-Ilasaca, M.; Libby, P. Adiponectin inhibits pro-inflammatory signaling in human macrophages independent of interleukin-10. *J. Biol. Chem.* **2009**, *284*, 25569–25575. [CrossRef] [PubMed]

7

Macro- and Micronutrients Consumption and the Risk for Colorectal Cancer among Jordanians

Reema F. Tayyem [1,*], Hiba A. Bawadi [2], Ihab N. Shehadah [3], Suhad S. Abu-Mweis [1], Lana M. Agraib [1], Kamal E. Bani-Hani [4], Tareq Al-Jaberi [5], Majed Al-Nusairr [6] and Dennis D. Heath [7]

[1] Department of Clinical Nutrition & Dietetic, The Hashemite University, P.O. Box 150459, Zarqa 13115, Jordan; suhad.abumweis@hu.edu.jo (S.S.A.-M.); elonafrsh2003@yahoo.com (L.M.A.)

[2] Department of Health Sciences, College of Arts and Sciences, Qatar University, P.O. Box 2713, Doha, Qatar; hbawadi@qu.edu.qa

[3] Chief Gastroenterology Division, King Hussein Cancer Center, P.O. Box 35102, Amman 11180, Jordan; ishehadeh@khcc.jo

[4] Faculty of Medicine, The Hashemite University, P.O. Box 150459, Zarqa 13115, Jordan; k_banihani@hu.edu.jo

[5] Department of General and Pediatric Surgery, Jordan University of Science and Technology, P.O. Box 3030, Irbid 22110, Jordan; tmrjaberi@hotmail.com

[6] Chief Gastroenterology Division, Prince Hamza Hospital, P.O. Box 86, Amman 11118, Jordan; jwan97@hotmail.com

[7] Cancer Prevention and Control Program, Moores Cancer Center, University of California, San Diego, La Jolla, CA 92093, USA; dheath@ucsd.edu

* Author to whom correspondence should be addressed; rtayyem@hu.edu.jo

Abstract: Objective: Diet and lifestyle have been reported to be important risk factors for the development of colorectal cancer (CRC). However, the association between total energy and nutrient intake and the risk of developing CRC has not been clearly explained. The aim of our study is to examine the relationship between total energy intake and other nutrients and the development of CRC in the Jordanian population. Research Methods and Procedures: Dietary data was collected from 169 subjects who were previously diagnosed with CRC, and 248 control subjects (matched by age, gender, occupation and marital status). These control subjects were healthy and disease free. Data was collected between January 2010 and December 2012, using interview-based questionnaires. Logistic regression was used to evaluate the association between quartiles of total energy, macro- and micronutrient intakes with the risk of developing CRC in our study population. Results: Total energy intake was associated with a higher risk of developing CRC (OR = 2.60 for the highest *versus* lowest quartile of intake; 95% CI: 1.21–5.56, p-trend = 0.03). Intakes of protein (OR = 3.62, 95% CI: 1.63–8.05, p-trend = 0.002), carbohydrates (OR = 1.41, 95% CI: 0.67–2.99, p-trend = 0.043), and percentage of energy from fat (OR = 2.10, 95% CI: 0.38–11.70, p-trend = 0.009) significantly increased the risk for the development of CRC. Saturated fat, dietary cholesterol and sodium intake showed a significant association with the risk of developing CRC (OR = 5.23, 95% CI: 2.33–11.76; OR = 2.48, 95% CI: 1.18–5.21; and OR = 3.42, 95% CI: 1.59–7.38, respectively), while vitamin E and caffeine intake were indicative of a protective effect against the development of CRC, OR = 0.002 (95% CI: 0.0003–0.011) and 0.023 (95%CI: 0.008–0.067), respectively. Conclusion: Our results suggest an increased risk for the development of CRC in subjects with high dietary intake of energy, protein, saturated fat, cholesterol, and sodium, and diets high in vitamin E and caffeine were suggestive of a protective effect against the risk of developing CRC. Impact: This is the first study in Jordan to suggest that it may be possible to reduce CRC risk by adjusting the intake of some macro-and micronutrients.

Keywords: colorectal cancer; total energy; macronutrient; micronutrients

1. Introduction

Published report suggests that colorectal cancer (CRC) is one of the three most common forms of cancer with nearly 1.4 million new cases diagnosed in the year 2012 [1]. The report noted that the Republic of Korea, followed by Slovakia and Hungary had the highest incidence of diagnosed CRC, while the lowest incidence of diagnosed CRC was in Africa and Asia [1]. The National Cancer Registry of Jordan reported 554 diagnosed cases of CRC in the year 2009. This total number of cases was calculated to be 11.9% of all newly diagnosed cancer cases in the kingdom of Jordan [2]. Cancer is described in part by an abnormal cell growth that is believed to be initiated either by internal or external (environmental) factors [3]. Diet and physical activity are external factors that may play a role in the development of CRC disease [3].

Dietary intakes of energy, macro- and micro-nutrients have been implicated in the etiology of CRC [4]. Several studies have shown that high dietary intakes of energy and energy-supplying macronutrients (fat, protein and carbohydrate) may have a positive association with the risk of developing CRC [4,5]. Additionally, fruits and vegetables as sources of dietary fiber, folate, phytoestrogens, vitamin C, selenium, carotenoids, phenols, and flavonoids could protect against the development of CRC [6,7]. Antioxidants are reported to function by trapping free radicals and reactive oxygen molecules at the cellular level, thus acting as a protective mechanism against oxidative damage [6,7]. Free radicals in the body are generally produced during metabolic processes, such as those involving digestion. For example, iron found in red meat is reported to be a source of free radicals present in the body [8]. However, evidence suggesting red meat as a possible cause of colon cancer has been questioned by Santorelli *et al.* [9] in the CRC debate. Generally, in many households, meals high in fat are usually low in fruits, vegetables and fiber. Therefore, it is unclear if this increase risk in developing CRC is attributable to the high fat intake or the low fruit, vegetable and fiber intake. Free radical-induced lipid peroxidation has been implicated in malignant transformation [10]. The formation of lipid peroxidation products is normally prevented or scavenged by host antioxidants. Low levels of antioxidant nutrients in circulation have been associated with an increased risk of cancer [10].

One local Jordanian study published by Arafa *et al.* [11], showed in descriptive terms that traditional Jordanian foods are cooked with a high quantity of saturated fats and oils, and more importantly, anecdotal evidence exists that the fruits and vegetables component of the local diet is very low, while red meat and saturated fat components are quite high. More so, in the study by Arafa *et al.* [11], difference in the dietary macro- and micronutrient intake in the traditional diets were reported. The study results were descriptive in nature and did not investigate any association between diet and the risk of developing CRC. In addition, it is important to identify risk factors that could be modified to decrease CRC incidence among Jordanians. Based on current knowledge, the risk of developing CRC in the Jordanian population should be investigated in more detail. Accordingly, the aim of the present study is to investigate the association between macro-and micronutrient intake and colorectal cancer risk using data from a case-control study conducted in Jordan.

2. Materials and Methods

2.1. Study Population and Methods

The study sample consisted of 503 participants; with 232 diagnosed CRC cases and 271 controls (262 males and 241 females). Participants were enrolled in the study from January 2010 to December 2012. Participating subjects were patients diagnosed with CRC (cases) who were recruited from five Jordanian hospitals specializing in oncology diagnosis and treatment. The hospitals included King Hussein Cancer Center (KHCC), King Abdullah University Hospital, Prince Hamzeh Hospital, Jordan University Hospital, and Al-Basheer Hospital. The control group was recruited from hospital personnel, outpatients, visitors and was matched as closely as possible for age, gender, occupation and marital status. Control subjects were excluded if any first- or second degree relatives were diagnosed with CRC. The study protocol was approved by KHCC Institutional Review Board (IRB) Committee (09 KHCC 10; May 2009) and other hospitals gave their approval accordingly. Written informed consent was obtained from all subjects before their interview. The following inclusion criteria for controls were used: Jordanian nationals aged 18 years or older, ability to communicate clearly and verbally, free of any type of diagnosed cancer, diabetes mellitus, liver disease and rheumatoid arthritis. For inclusion in the diagnosed CRC cancer group, subjects must have received their diagnosis less than 1 year prior to the time of the first interview. The exclusion criteria for this group included those who were considered "critically ill", such as an in-patient at any facility and those who were unable to communicate verbally and clearly.

2.2. Data Collection

Socio-demographic, health and dietary data were collected by trained research assistants using interview-based questionnaires. The socio-demographic data included age, marital status, household income, education (illiterate, primary and secondary, diploma and B.Sc., and postgraduate degrees), occupation and tobacco usage (current and previous smokers were categorized as smokers and those who never smoked were set as non-smokers). The comprehensive health data included the participant's full medical history to confirm that only CRC diagnosed subjects and healthy disease free subjects were included. A validated Arabic quantitative Food Frequency Questionnaire (FFQ), adapted from the Diet History Questionnaire (DHQ I) of the National Cancer Institute of the United States of America [12], was used for dietary assessment. The FFQ questions sought to obtain information on the dietary history of study participants prior to CRC diagnosis, and to confirm the dietary habits of control participants. We selected a period of one year prior to the study inception date, to account for seasonal variation in food types. We noted a fixed dietary pattern for the period, with some participants suggesting this pattern existed for at least five years. A qualified dietitian asked participants, during face-to-face interviews, how frequently, on average, during the past year they had consumed one standard serving of specific food items in nine categories (<1/month, 2–3/month, 1–2/week, 3–4/week, 5–6/week, 1/day, 2–3/day, 4–5/day, or 6/day). Food lists in the modified FFQ questions were classified based on types of foods: 21 items of vegetables; 16 items of meat such as red meat (lamb and beef), chicken, fish, cold meat, and others; 21 items of fruits and juices; nine items of milk and dairy products; eight items of cereals; four items of beans; four items of soups and sauces; five items of drinks; nine items of snacks and sweets; and 14 items of herbs and spices [12]. Food models and standard measuring tools were used to help participants estimate portion size. Responses on frequency of consumption and serving size for each food item were converted into average daily intake. Data was collected from a total of 503 participants. However, the data from 86 participants was excluded due to incomplete response to required questions ($n = 58$); over-estimation of calorie intake (>5000 kcal for male and >4000 kcal for female) ($n = 12$); and under-estimation of calorie intake (<500 kcal for females and <800 kcal for males) ($n = 16$) [13]. Dietary intakes were analyzed using dietary analysis software (ESHA Food Processor SQL version 10.1.1; ESHA, Salem, OR, USA) with additional data on foods consumed in Jordan [14].

The 7-day Physical Activity Recall (PAR), developed by Sallis et al. [15] was used to measure physical activity level. 7-Day PAR is a structured interview that depends on participant's recall of time spent engaging in physical activity over a seven day period. Our participants were asked specific and probing questions in order to obtain a complete history of their physical activities. They were asked to recall their physical activities for the previous year before their enrollment into the study. PAR covers different levels of physical activity and intensity such as aerobic exercise, work-related activities, gardening, walking, recreation, and leisure-time activities. The PAR interview focuses on collecting data on intensity, time or duration, and type of activity. The number of hours spent in different activity levels were obtained and converted into Metabolic Equivalents (METs). Average METs for walking = 3.3 METs, for moderate activity = 4.0 METs, for vigorous activity = 8.0 METs. The score expressed as MET-min/week was calculated as: (MET level × minutes of activity/day × days per week). Total Physical Activity MET-min/week is obtained by METs summation and categorized as inactive (below 600 MET-min/week), minimally active and Health Enhancing Physical Activity (HEPA) active. Minimally active category included subjects who reported a minimum of at least 600 MET-min/week. The category HEPA active included any subject who performed vigorous-intensity activity on at least 3 days a week and accumulated at least 1500 MET-min/week or who performed any combination of walking, moderate-intensity or vigorous intensity activities on 5 or more days achieving a minimum of at least 3000 MET-min/week [15].

Body weight was measured to the nearest 0.1 kg, with minimal clothing and without shoes, using a calibrated portable scale. Height was measured to the nearest 0.5 cm with participants in the full standing position without shoes using a calibrated portable measuring rod. Body mass index (BMI) was calculated as the ratio of weight in kilograms to the square of height in meters [16].

2.3. Statistical Analyses

Statistical analysis was performed with SPSS IBM-20 software. The significance level was set at $p = 0.05$. For descriptive statistics, mean $\pm$ standard deviation (SD) and percentages were used. T-tests evaluated the differences between cases and controls in continuous variables, and Chi-square was used to detect differences among categorical variables.

Because all nutrients were correlated with energy intake, variation due to energy intake and its associated measurement error was minimized by energy adjustment of the nutrients using the regression method [17]. This method of energy adjustment is computed from the residuals of the regression model with total energy intake as the independent variable and the nutrient as the dependent variable. Regression equation was used to calculate the expected mean of nutrient intake of the study population. Next, for each participant, the energy-adjusted intake was calculated by adding the expected mean nutrient intake of the study population to the residual derived from the regression analysis. Shapiro-Wilk test was used to assess the normality of the distributions of dietary intake variables. Non-normally distributed variables were log transformed [17].

Nutrient intakes were modeled using quartiles of distribution in the study population with quartile 1 being the lowest intake and quartile 4 the highest. Odds ratios (ORs) and 95% CIs (95% CIs) for CRC were calculated by using logistic regression models for quartiles of nutrient intakes, with the lowest quartile as the reference category. Confounders were selected based on known risk factors for CRC reported in the literature. Potential confounders were chosen based on previous studies [4,18] including the Cancer Prevention Study II [18]. Confounders included in data analysis included age, gender, BMI, physical activity (MET-min/week), family history (beyond the second degree) of CRC, household income, educational level, marital status and smoking. Trend tests were calculated using linear regression with nutrient intakes as continuous data.

3. Results

Table 1 shows participants' age, anthropometric measurements, socio-demographic and health characteristics, stratified by gender. Average age for controls was 51.4 ± 10.9 years and 53.8 ± 12.2 years for cases. Significant differences were found between cases and controls in male height, and in female BMI. No significant differences were detected in employment, marital status, monthly income, smoking and physical activity levels between the CRC diagnosed and control participants. However, family history (beyond the second degree) of CRC and having other health problems in female participants was significantly higher in the CRC group compared to the controls.

The mean daily intakes of total energy, macronutrients, and micronutrients appear in Table 2. The CRC group reported significantly higher intakes of total energy, protein, fat, saturated fat and cholesterol ($p < 0.05$) compared to the control group. In addition, the CRC group had significantly higher intakes of folate, Iron, selenium as well as omega-3 ($p < 0.05$) when compared to the control group, and the control group had a higher percentage of calories from carbohydrate when compared to the CRC group ($p < 0.05$).

Table 1. Age, anthropometrics measurements and selected characteristics of the study participants.

Characteristics	Males (n = 193)			Females (n = 224)		
	Control (n = 113)	Case (n = 80)	p-value	Control (n = 135)	Case (n = 89)	p-value
Age years (mean ± SD)	55.2 ± 11.6	57.9 ± 12.1	0.110	48.1 ± 8.9	50.0 ± 11.0	0.161
Height cm (mean ± SD)	164.3 ± 9.6	169.5 ± 9.2	0.001	170.1 ± 40.5	166.8 ± 10.6	0.458
Weight kg (mean ± SD)	81.3 ± 16	81.1 ± 14.6	0.092	79.9 ± 14.9	77.5 ± 16.5	0.271
BMI kg/m^2 (mean ± SD)	27.3 ± 4.8	27.8 ± 5.4	0.558	30.2 ± 6.0	27.6 ± 7.4	0.004
Age Category n (%)						
<40 years	9 (8)	10 (12.7)		22 (16.9)	14 (15.9)	
40–49 years	25 (22.1)	12 (15.2)	0.397	57 (43.8)	32 (36.4)	0.095
50–59 years	36 (31.9)	15 (19.0)		35 (26.9)	20 (22.7)	
≥60 years	43 (38.1)	42 (53.2)		16 (12.3)	22 (25.0)	
Total	113 (100.0)	79 (100.0)		130 (100.0)	88 (100.0)	
Employed (%)						
Yes	63 (55.8)	30 (37.5)		26 (19.3)	21 (23.6)	
No	50 (44.2)	50 (62.5)	0.081	109 (80.7)	68 (76.4)	0.510
Total	113 (100.0)	80 (100.0)		133 (100.0)	89 (100.0)	
Marital status n (%)						
Married	106 (93.8)	76 (95)		113 (83.7)	74 (83.2)	
Single	4 (3.5)	2 (2.6)		10 (7.4)	2 (2.2)	
Divorced	-	1 (1.3)	0.695	1 (0.7)	1 (1.1)	0.364
Widowed	3 (2.7)	1 (1.3)		11 (8.1)	12 (13.5)	
Total	113 (100.0)	80 (100.0)		135 (100.0)	89 (100.0)	
Family history (beyond the second degree) of CRC n (%)						
Yes	45 (40.2)	27 (33.8)		45 (34.1)	42 (47.7)	
No	67 (59.8)	53 (66.3)	0.475	87 (65.9)	46 (52.3)	0.016
Total	112 (100.0)	80 (100.0)		132 (100.0)	88 (100.0)	
Other health problem n (%) (excluding diabetes, liver disease, rheumatoid arthritis)						
Yes	45 (40.2)	45 (57.0)		47 (34.8)	40 (44.9)	
No	67 (59.8)	34 (43.0)	0.367	88 (65.2)	48 (53.9)	0.043
Total	112 (100.0)	79 (100.0)		135 (100.0)	88 (100.0)	
Tobacco use n (%)						
Yes	36 (34.0)	17 (23.0)		4 (3.0)	7 (8.0)	
No	70 (66.0)	57 (77.0)	0.113	131 (97.0)	81 (92.0)	0.093
Total	106 (100.0)	74 (100.0)		135 (100.0)	88 (100.0)	
Household income n (%)						
<300 USA $	10 (8.8)	6 (7.4)		15 (11.0)	5 (5.6)	
300–750 USA $	27 (23.9)	19 (23.8)	0.663	41 (30.4)	24 (27.0)	0.562
>750 USA $	65 (57.6)	36 (45.0)		44 (32.6)	24 (27.0)	
Unknown	11 (9.7)	19 (23.8)		35 (26.0)	36 (40.4)	
Total	113 (100.0)	80 (100.0)		135 (100.0)	89 (100.0)	
Physical activity levels n (%)						
Inactive *	30 (27.0)	27 (33.8)		10 (9.1)	16 (18.0)	
Minimally Active †	40 (36.0)	25 (31.3)	0.469	33 (30.0)	23 (25.8)	0.183
HEPA active ‡‡	41 (36.9)	28 (35.0)		67 (60.9)	50 (56.2)	
Total	111 (100.0)	80 (100.0)		110 (100.0)	89 (100.0)	

BMI: Body Mass Index; * Inactive: not fitting in "Minimally Active" or "HEPA active"; Significance is at $p \leq 0.05$. † Minimally Active: at least 600 MET per week; ‡‡ Health Enhancing Physical Activity: HEPA active: more than 3000 MET per week.

Table 2. Mean intake per day ± SD of nutrients for the study participants.

Nutrient	Control	Case	Difference (Case − Control)	p-value *
Energy (kcal)	3476.0 ± 1172.9	3719.4 ± 1018.1	243.4	0.029
Protein (g)	109.6 ± 42.5	120.9 ± 52.4	11.3	0.016
Protein %	12.5 ± 2.3	13 ± 3.7	0.4	NS
Carbohydrate (g)	593.9 ± 203.1	608.1 ± 164.6	14.2	NS
Carbohydrate %	68.9 ± 8.6	66.1 ± 8.4	−2.8	0.001
Fiber (g)	48.4 ± 23.3	48.1 ± 21.3	−0.3	NS
Soluble Fiber (g)	6.0 ± 4.5	5.4 ± 3.5	−0.7	NS
Insoluble Fiber (g)	14.7 ± 10.8	13.1 ± 9.1	−1.5	NS
Fat (g)	80.2 ± 39.1	93.8 ± 41.3	13.6	0.001
Fat %	20.4 ± 6.6	22.1 ± 6.5	1.7	0.009
Saturated Fat (g)	29.8 ±16.3	35.4 ± 17.1	5.6	0.001
Saturated Fat %	7.6 ± 3.2	8.4 ± 3.2	0.8	0.009
Cholesterol (mg)	340.2 ± 229.0	409.3 ± 273.7	69.1	0.005
Vitamin A (RE)	1116.5 ± 850.5	1199.8 ± 871.6	83.3	NS
Beta-carotene (μg)	6478.7 ± 5259.1	6822.6 ± 556.3	343.9	NS
Vitamin B_{12} (μg)	3.9 ± 3.5	4.5 ± 4.3	0.6	NS
Vitamin C (mg)	239.2 ± 173.1	259.7 ± 207.4	20.5	NS
Vitamin D (mg)	0.8 ± 0.7	0.9 ± 0.7	0.1	NS
Vitamin E (α-Tocopherol) (mg)	6.4 ± 3.9	6.7 ± 4.1	0.2	NS
Folate (mcg)	461.3 ± 217.2	506.3 ± 186.6	44.9	0.029
Vitamin K (μg)	193.3 ± 203.8	197.5 ± 174.3	4.1	NS
Calcium (mg)	1171.1 ± 526.9	1230.5 ± 459.2	59.4	NS
Iron (mg)	25.2 ± 9.9	27.4 ± 10.1	2.3	0.022
Sodium (mg)	4796.2 ± 2837.5	5112.0 ± 2218.6	315.8	NS
Selenium (μg)	109.3 ± 53.3	120.1 ± 48.9	10.9	0.033
Phosphate (mg)	1334.4 ± 561.7	1416.6 ± 619.5	82.2	NS
Omega-3 (mg)	0.6 ± 0.4	0.7 ± 0.5	0.1	0.014
Caffeine (mg)	3036.6 ± 2829.8	2980.7 ± 3041.8	−55.9	NS

* Significance is at $p < 0.05$.

Table 3 shows the ORs and corresponding 95% CI of the CRC group by intake quartile of associated macronutrients. After adjusting for potential confounders, increasing intakes (in the highest *versus* the lowest quartile of intake) of total energy (OR = 2.60, 95% CI: 1.22–5.56, *p*-trend = 0.030), and protein (OR = 3.62, 95% CI: 1.63–8.04, *p*-trend = 0.002) were significantly associated with CRC. A significant positive trend in risk was found for carbohydrate (p = 0.043), but none of the quartiles are different from the reference category. The odds ratios for quartiles of fat intake as g/day were not calculated due to distribution issues (the bottom quartile had only 1 participant and the top quartile only 2 control participants). As noted in Table 3, saturated fat and cholesterol intakes show significant direct associations with CRC risk (OR = 5.23, 95% CI: 2.33–11.76 and OR = 2.48, 95% CI: 1.18–5.21, respectively) in the highest *versus* the lowest quartile of intake, and the trend tests were also significant. No association for intake of total fiber with CRC was detected, (*p*-trend = 0.979, Table 3). However, the upper quartile of insoluble fiber was found to be protective against CRC (OR = 0.42, 95% CI: 0.19–0.91) but the trend test was not significant (*p*-trend = 0.162).

Table 3. Adjusted ORs [a] and CIs of CRC risk by macronutrient intake quartiles.

Nutrient	Adjusted				
	Q1	Q2	Q3	Q4	*p*-Trend
Energy (Kcal)					
No. of Cases (169)/Controls (248)	32/72	45/60	44/60	48/56	0.030
OR	1	1.51	1.83	2.60 *	
95% CI	-	0.70–3.27	0.85–3.93	1.22–5.56	
Protein (g)					
No. of Cases (169)/Controls (248)	30/74	37/67	46/58	56/48	0.002
OR	1	1.66	1.74	3.62 *	
95% CI	-	0.74–3.69	0.78–3.90	1.63–8.04	
Carbohydrate (g)					
No. of Cases (169)/Controls (248)	36/68	37/67	43/62	53/51	0.043
OR	1	0.77	1.24	1.41 *	
95% CI	-	0.36–1.64	0.58–2.64	0.68–2.99	
Fiber (g)					
No. of Cases (169)/Controls (248)	46/58	49/56	33/71	41/63	0.979
OR	1	1.29	0.48	0.57	
95% CI	-	0.62–2.69	0.22–1.04	0.27–1.21	
Soluble Fiber (g)					
No. of Cases (169)/Controls (248)	43/61	53/52	39/65	34/70	0.551
OR	1	1.86	0.85	0.58	
95% CI	-	0.84–4.15	0.39–1.84	0.26–1.27	
Insoluble Fiber (g)					
No. of Cases (169)/Controls (248)	46/58	51/54	40/64	32/72	0.162
OR	1	1.04	0.66	0.42	
95% CI		0.49–2.22	0.30–1.41	0.19–0.91	
Fat [b] (g)					
No. of Cases (169)/Controls (248)	0/104	4/100	63/42	102/2	
OR	-	-	-	-	
95% CI	-	-	-	-	
Saturated Fat (g)					
No. of Cases (169)/Controls (248)	28/76	36/69	52/52	53/51	0.009
OR	1	2.23	3.61	5.23 *	
95% CI	-	1.00–4.98	1.68–7.77	2.33–11.76	
Cholesterol (mg)					
No. of Cases (169)/Controls (248)	33/71	32/72	49/56	55/49	0.027
OR	1	0.94	1.84	2.48 *	
95% CI	-	0.43–2.05	0.87–3.91	1.18–5.21	

[a] Adjusted for total energy intake normality of the distributions of dietary intake variables was assessed by the Shapiro-Wilk test. Non-normally distributed variables were log transformed. Other potential confounders included age, gender, BMI, physical activity (METs/week), family history (beyond the second degree) of CRC, education attainment, household income, marital status and tobacco use; [b] Odds ratios were also calculated for percentage of energy from fat using the following categories: 1 ($\leq$20% of energy), 2 (20%–35% of energy), 3 ($\geq$35% of energy). The ORs for category 2 and category 3 relative to category 1 were 1.80 (95% CI: 1.07–3.04), and 2.10 (95% CI: 0.38–11.70), respectively, with *p*-trend = 0.009. * Significant different from reference category, $p \leq 0.05$.

Vitamin E intake showed significant protective effect against CRC with OR = 0.02 and 95% CI: 0.0003–0.011, (Table 4). Neither quartile analysis nor the trend test was significant for vitamins A, C, B$_{12}$, D, K, and folate, beta-carotene, phosphate, and omega-3. Calcium showed a significant risk in the top two quartiles.

Table 4. Adjusted ORs [a] and CIs of CRC risk by micronutrient intake quartiles.

Nutrient	Adjusted				
	Q1	Q2	Q3	Q4	p-Trend
Vitamin A (RAE)					
No. of Cases (169)/Controls (248)	42/62	38/67	43/61	46/58	0.769
OR	1	0.90	0.87	0.77	
95% CI	-	0.43–1.89	0.43–1.77	0.37–1.58	
Beta-carotene (µg)					
No. of Cases (169)/Controls (248)	42/62	39/66	63/41	47/57	0.575
OR	1	0.78	0.78	0.71	
95% CI	-	0.38–1.59	0.38–1.63	0.33–1.55	
Vitamin B$_{12}$ (µg)					
No. of Cases (169)/Controls (248)	45/59	31/73	40/65	53/51	0.493
OR	1	0.38	0.66	1.07	
95% CI	-	0.17–0.83	0.32–1.35	0.52–2.222	
Vitamin C (mg)					
No. of Cases (169)/Controls (248)	41/63	40/65	40/64	48/56	0.359
OR	1	0.81	0.63	0.89	
95% CI	-	0.40–1.62	0.29–1.34	0.42–1.89	
Vitamin D (mg)					
No. of Cases (169)/Controls (248)	39/68	43/59	40/64	47/57	0.163
OR	1	1.07	1.33	1.47	
95% CI	-	0.50–2.31	0.64–2.76	0.70–3.08	
Vitamin E (α-Tocopherol) (mg)					
No. of Cases (169)/Controls (248)	95/9	62/43	12/92	-/104	0.001
OR	1	0.05	0.02	-	
95% CI	-	0.01–0.23	0.0003–0.011	-	
Folate (µg)					
No. of Cases (169)/Controls (248)	33/71	41/64	46/58	49/55	0.057
OR [a]	1	1.32	1.24	1.14	
95% CI	-	0.62–2.84	0.58–2.66	0.54–2.42	
Vitamin K (µg)					
No. of Cases (169)/Controls (248)	37/67	41/63	48/57	43/61	0.612
OR	1	0.95	1.12	0.95	
95% CI	-	0.68–2.13	0.88–2.70	0.74–2.29	
Calcium (mg)					
No. of Cases (169)/Controls (248)	29/75	40/65	55/49	45/59	0.146
OR	1	1.80	3.92	2.39	
95% CI	-	0.82–3.96	1.81–8.50	1.04–5.52	

[a] Adjusted for total energy intake normality of the distributions of dietary intake variables was assessed by the Shapiro-Wilk test. Non-normally distributed variables were log transformed. Other potential confounders included age, gender, BMI, physical activity (METs/week), family history (beyond the second degree) of CRC, education attainment, household income, marital status and tobacco use.

4. Discussion

The results from of the present study provide further evidence for an association between CRC risk and diet. Generally, the results of this case-control study on CRC risk illustrate a relationship between macro- and micronutrients intake and this type of cancer among Jordanians.

As BMI was obtained at the time of interview for both patients and controls, the association between obesity and CRC in this study could not be evaluated. The lower BMI in cases may reflect the effect of chemotherapy and other therapies which cancer patients were exposed to before the interview time.

Our study revealed a direct association between total energy intake and the risk of developing CRC, as supported by several other studies [4,19]. Caloric restriction was found to reduce cancer incidence in rodents and colorectal cell proliferation in humans [20]. The potential mechanism could be through insulin growth factor-1 (IGF-1), where increasing energy could be responsible for glycemic overload and a compensatory increase of serum insulin and related IGF-1, a promoter of tumor cell growth *in vitro* [21,22]. Elevated circulating insulin and IGF level may increase CRC risk, possibly by decreasing IGF-binding proteins (IGFBP-1) and increasing the bioactivity of IGF-I [23,24]. Insulin may increase the circulating IGF-1/IGFBP-3 ratio by increasing hepatic growth hormone sensitivity which could be implicated in increasing the risk for CRC [23,24].

High carbohydrate intake may increase glycemic load, insulin levels, and IGF-1 [20,21]. A significant trend for higher intake of carbohydrate was detected among cases compared to controls. This observation is consistent with some studies [25–27] but not all [4,28]. Borugian *et al.* [26] reported a significant positive association between carbohydrate intake and risk of CRC in both men (OR = 1.7; 95% CI: 1.1–2.7) and women (OR = 2.7; 95% CI: 1.5–4.8) among Chinese in North America. While, Franceschi *et al.* [27] found a direct association between dietary glycemic load and CRC risk, with OR of 1.7 (95% CI: 1.5–2.2).

The effect of fiber on CRC incidence is inconsistent; some studies report a significant inverse association between total fiber intake and CRC risk [4,29–31], whereas other studies found no association between fiber intake and CRC incidence [27,32–34]. Although our results showed no association for the intake of total fiber with CRC, a significant protective effect of insoluble fiber on the risk of CRC development at the highest quartile has been detected [32]. A prospective cohort study of women in the United States, found that total fiber was not associated with CRC risk, with relative risk (RR) for the highest relative to lowest quintile of 0.75 (95% CI: 0.48–1.17, p-trend = 0.12). In the other two mentioned studies, significant associations in age-adjusted models disappeared after adjustment for other risk factors. In the Pooling Project analysis including data from 13 cohort studies the report showed statistically significant inverse associations for colorectal cancer in the age adjusted models (Quintile 5 *vs.* Quintile 1, RR 0.84, 95% CI: 0.77–0.92), but not after multivariable adjustment (Quintile 5 *vs.* Quintile 1, RR 0.94, 95% CI: 0.86–1.03) [33]. Similarly, in an NIH-AARP analysis the statistically significant inverse association in the age adjusted model (Quintile 5 *vs.* Quintile 1, HR 0.73, 95% CI: 0.65–0.82) disappeared after multivariable adjustment (Quintile 5 *vs.* Quintile 1, RR 0.99, 95% CI: 0.85–1.15) [34].

Similar to other studies [4,12,26,35], our study results show that total fat, saturated fat and cholesterol have a significant direct effect on CRC risk. The total consumption of fat was much higher in our CRC participants than controls, with only one control in the first quartile. Our observation on fat, saturated fat and cholesterol is in agreement with the report of Arafa *et al.* [11] who reported the daily intake from saturated, mono and polyunsaturated fats and cholesterol is significantly higher among CRC diagnosed subjects as compared to controls, ($p < 0.05$). The proposed mechanism for fat involvement in colorectal carcinogenesis appears to be complex. However, Endo *et al.* [35], showed that the molecular mechanisms underlying the promotion of colorectal carcinogenesis by a high-fat diet (HFD) is through its effect on the role of the insulin-signal pathway and the c-Jun *N*-terminal kinase (JNK) pathway, which was reported to play a crucial role in insulin resistance during colorectal carcinogenesis in the presence of hyperinsulinaemia induced by a HFD. They found that colonic cell proliferation was promoted via the JNK pathway in the presence of a HFD providing an explanation of the effect of dietary fat intake on colon carcinogenesis through the JNK pathway [35].

In our study, protein intake was found to have a significant direct association with CRC. Arafa *et al.* [11] indicated that the consumption of protein among CRC diagnosed patients was higher than intake in a control group, and they speculated that this may be associated with a higher risk for development of CRC. In contrast, one other study by Sun *et al.* [5], reported an inverse association for intake of protein (OR: 0. 85, 95% CI: 0.69–1.00, p-trend = 0.002, 4th *versus* 1st quartile). However, Egeberg *et al.* [36] reported a significant association between specific red meat subtypes intake and the risk of developing colon and rectal cancers. They found that consuming lamb meat was significantly related to risk of developing colon cancer, while consuming pork meat was significantly related to the risk of developing rectal cancer [36]. No associations were found between intake of red meat, processed meat, fish, or poultry and risk for colon cancer or rectal cancer [36]. Fifty percent of participants consumed red meat more than 1–2 times per week (results not shown) in serving size ranges from 90–120 gm. However, the majority (80%) consumed poultry more than 3–4 times weekly. This may partially explain why protein intake in this study was a CRC risk factor rather than protective. In a previous report, Tayyem *et al* [37], we reported that the Jordanian population consumes more animal proteins than plant proteins [37]. In fact, meat intake increased from 7.68 kg/year per-capita in 1961 to 35.85 kg/year per-capita in 2005 [37].

In our study, vitamin E was found to have a significant inverse association with the risk of CRC development. The remarkable effect of vitamin E consumption on protecting against CRC could be attributed to the comparative ratio of 95 case/9 control participants at the lowest quartile compared to 12 case/92 control participants at the 3rd quartile of vitamin E consumption. These results are in agreement with other studies [31,38–41]. A study of Satia-Abouta *et al.* [29], that had been conducted on African Americans, revealed that vitamin E intake was strongly and inversely associated with a 70% reduced risk for colon cancer (OR 0.3; 95% CI (0.1–0.6)). This trend of association was not demonstrated in the same study in Whites (OR 1.0; 95% CI (0.6–1.6)). This could be attributed to ethnic differences [29]. Perhaps, this may be due to genetic makeup or the influence of genes in the metabolic processes. This effect may arise from vitamin E activity as an antioxidant against free radicals and reactive oxygen molecules [39].

The association between folate intake and CRC disease state is being debated and no significant association between folate and CRC risk has been reported [26,42–45], similar to results obtained in our study. However, recent research indicates that folate may have a role in the metabolism of colon carcinogenesis, perhaps by increasing 5, 10-methylenetetrahydrofolate levels for DNA synthesis [44,45].

Iron (Fe) intake was found to have a positive weak association with CRC risk [24]. Our results are consistent with those from other studies [46–48]. In Larsson *et al.* [46] study, the RR of colon cancer, comparing extreme categories of heme iron intake, was 2.29 (95% CI: 1.25–4.21) among women who consumed at least 20 g/week of alcohol, and 1.05 (95% CI: 0.74–1.48) among women who consumed less than 20 g/week of alcohol. The molecular mechanisms of iron carcinogenesis may be explained by the actions of auto-oxidation of iron involving only $Fe^{2+} + O_2$ in oxidant formation in biological systems and its pH dependency, activation of oxidative responsive transcription factors and pro-inflammatory cytokines, and iron-induced hypoxia signaling [47,48].

In our study, the intake of selenium was found to have a significant trend for direct association with CRC risk. Other studies reported the presence of an inverse association between selenium intake and plasma levels with CRC risk [49–51]. Our results may be explained by the finding of Whanger [51] who conducted a study on the form of selenium compounds with CRC risk. His results suggested that Selenomethionine (Semet), the major seleno-compound in cereal grains and enriched yeast, may be the effective form of selenium against CRC. However, Whanger [51] found that Se-methylselenocysteine (SeMCYS), the major seleno-compound in Se-accumulator plants and some plants of economic importance such as garlic and broccoli, may be ineffective against CRC and only protect against mammary tumors. Our results suggest that the effective form of selenium that could protect against CRC disease may have been limited in our participants' diets.

Some studies have shown an association between high sodium intake and CRC development [52–54], and Zhivotovskiy *et al.* [54] have reported that the risk of CRC increased almost 3.5-fold as the dietary intake of salt increased with *p*-trend of 0.008.The results of our study is in agreement with these reports. One potential explanation for this is the presence of chemical carcinogens such as *N*-nitroso compounds in salted foods such as processed meats, dairy products and canned foods, which can be formed by the reaction of sodium nitrate or sodium nitrite in the curing process or in the body, or heterocyclic amines, which have been detected in fish or meat cooked in high temperatures, such as grilling, which is commonly used for grilled meat [54].

Regarding caffeine intake, our results are in agreement with other studies. Caffeine has been shown to have a negative association with CRC risk [55,56]. It inhibits colon cancer cell growth, by acting as antioxidant and effectively scavenging hydroxyl radicals (·OH) [55]. Additionally, caffeine can decrease insulin sensitivity, possibly as a result of elevated plasma epinephrine levels [56].

5. Study Limitation

In a study of this type we rely greatly on the ability and memory recall of participants to accurately and carefully provide information from a period when it was not necessarily important to remember the details of long digested meals, or physical activities that were undertaken. It is understandable that some individuals may have a greater recall than others, and that biases may exist in the minds of those being interviewed, and indeed, by the interviewer. Traumatic events such as the diagnosis of a life threatening disease condition may ultimately have a very significant role in the memory recall of some participants. Because of the obvious limitations placed on the recall of memory, we are using the only means currently available to us, the FFQ, which although prone to errors, is nevertheless an accepted and validated form used in many research studies.

We did not take into account the possible effects of cooking on the bioavailability of the various nutrients, and although we attempted to control for a range of potential confounders, we did not measure alcohol use (culturally discouraged). Nor did we consider the use of food dietary supplements; however, we are aware that the use of dietary supplements is not common or widespread. Finally, the one year dietary recall time frame may not be sufficient to determine an association with a disease state that may take years to develop; nevertheless, we see this study as a pointer to the need for further long term studies involving journal and diary entries of nutritional intakes along with physical activities for designated period of time, whether it be five to fifteen years.

A major strength of our study is the validated and detailed FFQ used to collect dietary data from our study population. Even though dietary data were collected at only one time, the FFQ has been reported to be an adequate instrument for measuring macro- and micronutrient intake [12]. Confirmative studies should verify and extend the presented data on Jordanian dietary habits in order to establish recommendations for people in Jordan to decrease colorectal cancer incidence.

6. Conclusions

This study, conducted in a Jordanian population group provides additional evidence that diets containing high energy, protein, total fat, saturated fat, cholesterol, and sodium intakes may increase the risk of CRC development, whereas high intakes of insoluble fiber, vitamin E, and caffeine may decrease the risk of these diseases. These results suggest that dietary changes could help to reduce the incidences of CRC in the Jordanian population.

Acknowledgments: The authors would like to thank the Higher Council of Science and Technology for sponsoring the research projects. We also would like to thank Shirley W. Flatt at University of California, San Diego for reviewing the statistical analysis of the research and editing the manuscript.

Author Contributions: Conception and design: Reema F. Tayyem. Development of methodology: Reema F. Tayyem, Hiba A. Bawadi. Acquisition of data: Ihab N. Shehadah, Tareq Al-Jaberi, Majed Al-Nusairr, Lana M. Agraib. Analysis and interpretation of data: Reema F. Tayyem, Suhad S. Abu-Mweis, Dennis D. Heath. Writing, review and/or revision of the manuscript: Reema F. Tayyem, Hiba A. Bawadi, Ihab N. Shehadah, Suhad S. Abu-Mweis, Dennis D. Heath, Tareq Al-Jaberi, Majed Al-Nusairr, Kamal E. Bani-Hani. Administrative, technical, or material support: Reema F. Tayyem, Kamal E. Bani-Hani. Study supervision: Reema F. Tayyem, Lana M. Agraib, Kamal E. Bani-Hani.

Abbreviation

CRC	Colorectal cancer
FFQ	Food Frequency Questionnaire
DHQ	Diet History Questionnaire I
PAR	7-day Physical Activity Recall
HEPA	Health Enhancing Physical Activity

METs   Metabolic Equivalents
BMI   Body mass index

References

1. World Cancer Research Fund and American Institute for Cancer Research. *Food, Nutrition, Physical Activity, and the Prevention of Cancer: A Global Perspective*; American Institute for Cancer Research: Washington, DC, USA, 2007.

2. Cancer Prevention Directorate: National Cancer Registry. *Incidence of Cancer in Jordan*; Cancer Prevention Directorate: National Cancer Registry: Amman, Jordan, 2009.

3. Georgakilas, A. Cancer Prevention—From Mechanisms to Translational Benefits. Available online: http://www.intechopen.com/books/cancer-prevention-from-mechanisms-to-translational-benefits (Accessed on 22 December 2014).

4. Harshman, M.R.; Aldoori, W. Diet and colorectal cancer: Review of the evidence. *Can. Fam. Physician* **2007**, *53*, 1913–1920. [PubMed]

5. Sun, Z.; Liu, L.; Wang, P.P.; Roebothan, B.; Zhao, J.; Dicks, E.; Cotterchio, M.; Buehler, S.; Campbell, P.T.; McLaughlin, J.R.; *et al.* Association of total energy intake and macronutrient consumption with colorectal cancer risk: Results from a large population-based case-control study in Newfoundland and Labrador and Ontario, Canada. *Nutr. J.* **2012**, *11*, 18. [CrossRef] [PubMed]

6. Millen, A.E.; Subar, A.F.; Graubard, B.I.; Peters, U.; Hayes, R.B.; Weissfeld, J.L.; Yokochi, L.A.; Ziegler, R.G.; PLCO Cancer Screening Trial Project Team. Fruit and vegetable intake and prevalence of colorectal adenoma in a cancer screening trial. *Am. J. Clin. Nutr.* **2007**, *86*, 1754–1764.

7. Sato, Y.; Tsubono, Y.; Nakaya, N.; Ogawa, K.; Kurashima, K.; Kuriyama, S.; Hozawa, A.; Nishino, Y.; Shibuya, D.; Tsuji, I. Fruit and vegetable consumption and risk of colorectal cancer in Japan: The Miyagi Cohort Study. *Public Health Nutr.* **2005**, *8*, 309–314. [CrossRef] [PubMed]

8. Kabat, G.C.; Miller, A.B.; Jain, M.; Rohan, T.E. A cohort study of dietary iron and heme iron intake and risk of colorectal cancer in women. *Br. J. Cancer* **2007**, *97*, 118–122. [CrossRef] [PubMed]

9. Santarelli, R.L.; Vendeuvre, J.L.; Naud, N.; Taché, S.; Guéraud, F.; Viau, M.; Genot, C.; Corpet, D.E.; Pierre, F.H. Meat processing and colon carcinogenesis: Cooked, nitrite-treated, and oxidized high-heme cured meat promotes mucin-depleted foci in rats. *Cancer Prev. Res. (Phila)* **2010**, *3*, 852–864. [CrossRef]

10. Gonzalez, R.A. Free radicals, oxidative stress and DNA metabolism in human cancer. *Cancer Investig.* **1999**, *17*, 376–377. [CrossRef]

11. Arafa, M.A.; Waly, M.I.; Jriesat, S.; Al Khafajei, A.; Sallam, S. Dietary and lifestyle characteristics of colorectal cancer in Jordan: A case-control study. *Asian Pac. J. Cancer Prev.* **2011**, *12*, 1931–1936. [PubMed]

12. Tayyem, R.F.; Abu-Mweis, S.S.; Bawadi, H.A.; Agraib, L.; Bani-Hani, K. Validation of a Food Frequency Questionnaire to assess macronutrient and micronutrient intake among Jordanians. *J. Acad. Nutr. Diet.* **2014**, *114*, 1046–1052. [CrossRef] [PubMed]

13. Willett, W. *Nutritional Epidemiology*, 2nd ed.; Oxford University Press: New York, NY, USA, 1998.

14. Pellet, P.; Shadarevian, S. *The Food Composition Tables for Use in the Middle East*, 2nd ed.; American University of Beirut: Beirut, Lebanon, 1970.

15. Sallis, J.F.; Haskell, W.L.; Wood, P.D. Physical activity assessment methodology in the Five-City Project. *Am. J. Epidemiol.* **1985**, *121*, 91–106. [PubMed]

16. Lee, R.D.; Nieman, D.C. *Nutritional Assessment*, 6th ed.; McGraw Hill: New York, NY, USA, 2012.

17. Willett, W.; Stampfer, M.J. Total energy intake: Implications for epidemiologic analyses. *Am. J. Epidemiol.* **1986**, *124*, 17–27. [PubMed]

18. Chao, A.; Thun, M.J.; Jacobs, E.J.; Henley, S.J.; Rodriguez, C.; Calle, E.E. Cigarette smoking and colorectal cancer mortality in the cancer prevention study II. *J. Natl. Cancer Inst.* **2000**, *92*, 1888–1896. [CrossRef] [PubMed]

19. Jarvandi, S.; Davidson, N.O.; Schootman, M. Increased risk of colorectal cancer in type 2 diabetes is independent of diet quality. *PLoS One* **2013**, *8*, e74616. [CrossRef] [PubMed]

20. Longo, V.D.; Fontana, L. Calorie restriction and cancer prevention: Metabolic and molecular mechanisms. *Trends Pharmacol. Sci.* **2010**, *31*, 89–98. [CrossRef] [PubMed]

21. Meinhold, C.L.; Dodd, K.W.; Jiao, L.; Flood, A.; Shikany, J.M.; Genkinger, J.M.; Hayes, R.B.; Stolzenberg-Solomon, R.Z. Available carbohydrates, glycemic load, and pancreatic cancer: Is there a link? *Am. J. Epidemiol.* **2010**, *171*, 1174–1182. [CrossRef] [PubMed]

22. Lin, J.K.; Shen, M.Y.; Lin, T.C.; Lan, Y.T.; Wang, H.S.; Yang, S.H.; Li, A.F.; Chang, S.C. Distribution of a single nucleotide polymorphism of insulin-like growth factor-1 in colorectal cancer patients and its association with mucinous adenocarcinoma. *Int. J. Biol. Markers* **2010**, *25*, 195–199. [PubMed]

23. Peters, G.; Gongoll, S.; Langner, C.; Mengel, M.; Piso, P.; Klempnauer, J.; Rüschoff, J.; Kreipe, H.; von Wasielewski, R. IGF-1R, IGF-1 and IGF-2 expression as potential prognostic and predictive markers in colorectal-cancer. *Virchows Arch.* **2003**, *443*, 139–145. [CrossRef]

24. Kaaks, R.; Toniolo, P.; Akhmedkhanov, A.; Lukanova, A.; Biessy, C.; Dechaud, H.; Rinaldi, S.; Zeleniuch-Jacquotte, A.; Shore, R.E.; Riboli, E. Serum C-peptide, insulin-like growth factor (IGF)-I, IGF-binding proteins, and colorectal cancer risk in women. *J. Natl. Cancer Inst.* **2000**, *92*, 1592–1600. [CrossRef] [PubMed]

25. McCarl, M.; Harnack, L.; Limburg, P.J.; Anderson, K.E.; Folsom, A.R. Incidence of colorectal cancer in relation to glycemic index and load in a cohort of women. *Cancer Epidemiol. Biomark. Prev.* **2006**, *15*, 892–896. [CrossRef]

26. Borugian, M.J.; Sheps, S.B.; Whittemore, A.S.; Wu, A.H.; Potter, J.D.; Gallagher, R.P. Carbohydrates and colorectal cancer risk among Chinese in North America. *Cancer Epidemiol. Biomark.* **2002**, *11*, 187–193.

27. Franceschi, S.; Dal Maso, L.; Augustin, L.; Negri, E.; Parpinel, M.; Boyle, P.; Jenkins, D.J.; la Vecchia, C. Dietary glycemic load and colorectal cancer risk. *Ann. Oncol.* **2001**, *12*, 173–178. [CrossRef] [PubMed]

28. Dray, X.; Boutron-Ruault, M.C.; Bertrais, S.; Sapinho, D.; Benhamiche-Bouvier, A.M.; Faivre, J. Influence of dietary factors on colorectal cancer survival. *Gut* **2003**, *52*, 868–873. [CrossRef] [PubMed]

29. Satia-Abouta, J.; Galanko, J.A.; Potter, J.D.; Ammerman, A.; Martin, C.F.; Sandler, R.S. Associations of total energy and macronutrients with colon cancer risk in African Americans and Whites: Results from the North Carolina colon cancer study. *Am. J. Epidemiol.* **2003**, *158*, 951–962. [CrossRef] [PubMed]

30. Nomura, A.M.Y.; Hankin, J.H.; Henderson, B.E.; Wilkens, L.R.; Murphy, S.P.; Pike, M.C.; le Marchand, L.; Stram, D.O.; Monroe, K.R.; Kolonel, L.N. Dietary fiber and colorectal cancer risk: The multiethnic cohort study. *Cancer Causes Control* **2007**, *18*, 753–764. [CrossRef] [PubMed]

31. Tantamango, Y.M.; Knutsen, S.F.; Beeson, L.; Fraser, G.; Sabate, J. Association between dietary fiber and incident cases of colon polyps: The adventist health study. *Gastrointest. Cancer Res.* **2011**, *4*, 161–167. [PubMed]

32. Lin, J.; Zhang, S.M.; Cook, N.R.; Rexrode, K.M.; Liu, S.; Manson, J.E.; Lee, I.M.; Buring, J.E. Dietary intakes of fruit, vegetables, and fiber, and risk of colorectal cancer in a prospective cohort of women (United States). *Cancer Causes Control* **2005**, *16*, 225–233. [CrossRef] [PubMed]

33. Park, Y.; Hunter, D.J.; Spiegelman, D.; Bergkvist, L.; Berrino, F.; van den Brandt, P.A.; Buring, J.E.; Colditz, G.A.; Freudenheim, J.L.; Fuchs, C.S.; *et al.* Dietary fiber intake and risk of colorectal cancer: A pooled analysis of prospective cohort studies. *JAMA* **2005**, *294*, 2849–2857. [CrossRef] [PubMed]

34. Schatzkin, A.; Mouw, T.; Park, Y.; Subar, A.F.; Kipnis, V.; Hollenbeck, A.; Leitzmann, M.F.; Thompson, F.E. Dietary fiber and whole-grain consumption in relation to colorectal cancer in the NIH-AARP Diet and Health Study. *Am. J. Clin. Nutr.* **2007**, *85*, 1353–1360. [PubMed]

35. Endo, H.; Hosono, K.; Fujisawa, T.; Takahashi, H.; Sugiyama, M.; Yoneda, K.; Nozaki, Y.; Fujita, K.; Yoneda, M.; Inamori, M.; *et al.* Involvement of JNK pathway in the promotion of the early stage of colorectal carcinogenesis under high-fat dietary conditions. *Gut* **2009**, *58*, 1637–1643. [CrossRef] [PubMed]

36. Egeberg, R.; Olsen, A.; Christensen, J.; Halkjær, J.; Jakobsen, M.U.; Overvad, K.; Tjønneland, A. Associations between red meat and risks for colon and rectal cancer depend on the type of red meat consumed. *J. Nutr.* **2013**, *143*, 464–472. [CrossRef] [PubMed]

37. Tayyem, R.F.; Bawadi, H.; Shawawreh, A.; Jad-Allah, H.; Abu-Oleim, S.; Khader, Y. Changes in eating pattern among Jordanians. *Dirasat Agric. Sci.* **2010**, *37*, 46–55.

38. Bostick, R.M.; Potter, J.D.; McKenzie, D.R.; Sellers, T.A.; Kushi, L.H.; Steinmetz, K.A.; Folsom, A.R. Reduced risk of colon cancer with high intake of vitamin E: The Iowa Women's Health Study. *Cancer Res.* **1993**, *53*, 4230–4237. [PubMed]

39. Ferraroni', M.; la Vecchia, C.; D'Avanzo, B.; Negri, E.; Francesc, S.; Decarli, A. Selected micronutrient intake and the risk of colorectal cancer. *Br. J. Cancer* **1994**, *70*, 1150–1155.

40. Tseng, M.; Murray, S.C.; Kupper, L.L.; Sandier, R.S. Micronutrients and the risk of colorectal adenomas. *Am. J. Epidemiol.* **1996**, *144*, 1005–1014. [CrossRef] [PubMed]

41. Williams, C.D.; Satia, J.A.; Adair, L.S.; Stevens, J.; Galanko, J.; Keku, T.O.; Sandler, R.S. Antioxidant and DNA methylation-related nutrients and risk of distal colorectal cancer. *Cancer Causes Control* **2010**, *21*, 1171–1181. [CrossRef] [PubMed]

42. De Vogel, S.; Dindore, V.; van Engeland, M.; Goldbohm, R.A.; van den Brandt, P.A.; Weijenberg, M.P. Dietary folate, methionine, riboflavin, and vitamin B-6 and risk of sporadic colorectal cancer. *J. Nutr.* **2008**, *138*, 2372–2378. [CrossRef] [PubMed]

43. Harnack, L.; Jacobs, D.R., Jr.; Nicodemus, K.; Lazovich, D.; Anderson, K.; Folsom, A.R. Relationship of folate, vitamin B-6, vitamin B-12, and methionine intake to incidence of colorectal cancers. *Nutr. Cancer* **2002**, *43*, 152–158. [CrossRef] [PubMed]

44. Ma, J.; Stampfer, M.J.; Giovannucci, E.; Artigas, C.; Hunter, D.J.; Fuchs, C.; Willett, W.C.; Selhub, J.; Hennekens, C.H.; Rozen, R. Methylenetetrahydrofolate reductase polymorphism, dietary interactions, and risk of colorectal cancer. *Cancer Res.* **1997**, *57*, 1098–1102. [PubMed]

45. Kennedy, D.A.; Stern, S.J.; Moretti, M.; Matok, I.; Sarkar, M.; Nickel, C.; Koren, G. Folate intake and the risk of colorectal cancer: A systematic review and meta-analysis. *Cancer Epidemiol.* **2011**, *35*, 2–10. [CrossRef] [PubMed]

46. Larsson, S.C.; Adami, H.O.; Giovannucci, E.; Wolk, A. Correspondence. Re: Heme iron, zinc, alcohol consumption, and risk of colon cancer. *J. Natl. Cancer Inst.* **2005**, *97*, 232–234. [CrossRef] [PubMed]

47. Sesink, A.; Termont, D.; Kleibeuker, J.H.; Meer, R.V. Red meat and colon cancer: Dietary haem, but not fat, has cytotoxic and hyperproliferative effects on rat colonic epithelium. *Carcinogenesis* **2000**, *21*, 1909–1915. [CrossRef] [PubMed]

48. Huang, X. Iron overload and its association with cancer risk in humans: Evidence for iron as a carcinogenic metal. *Mutat. Res.* **2003**, *533*, 153–171. [CrossRef] [PubMed]

49. Jacobs, E.T.; Jiang, R.; Alberts, D.S.; Greenberg, E.R.; Gunter, E.W.; Karagas, M.R.; Lanza, E.; Ratnasinghe, L.; Reid, M.E.; Schatzkin, A.; *et al.* Selenium and colorectal adenoma: Results of a pooled analysis. *J. Natl. Cancer Inst.* **2004**, *96*, 1669–1675. [CrossRef] [PubMed]

50. Me´plan, C.; Hesketh, J. The influence of selenium and selenoprotein gene variants on colorectal cancer risk. *Mutagenesis* **2012**, *27*, 177–186. [CrossRef] [PubMed]

51. Whanger, P.D. Selenium and its relationship to cancer: An update. *Br. J. Nutr.* **2004**, *91*, 11–28. [CrossRef] [PubMed]

52. Murata, A.; Fujino, Y.; Pham, T.M.; Kubo, T.; Mizoue, T.; Tokui, N.; Matsuda, S.; Yoshimura, T. Prospective cohort study evaluating the relationship between salted food intake and gastrointestinal tract cancer mortality in Japan. *Asia Pac. J. Clin. Nutr.* **2010**, *19*, 564–571. [PubMed]

53. Tuyns, A.J. Salt and gastrointestinal cancer. *Nutr. Cancer* **1988**, *11*, 229–232. [CrossRef] [PubMed]

54. Zhivotovskiy, A.S.; Kutikhin, A.G.; Azanov, A.Z.; Yuzhalin, A.E.; Magarill, Y.A.; Brusina, E.B. Colorectal cancer risk factors among the population of South-East Siberia: A case-control study. *Asian Pac. J. Cancer Prev.* **2012**, *13*, 5183–5188. [CrossRef] [PubMed]

55. Sinha, R.; Cross, A.J.; Daniel, C.R.; Graubard, B.I.; Wu, J.W.; Hollenbeck, A.R.; Gunter, M.J.; Park, Y.; Freedman, N.D. Caffeinated and decaffeinated coffee and tea intakes and risk of colorectal cancer in a large prospective study. *Am J Clin Nutr.* **2012**, *96*, 374–381. [CrossRef] [PubMed]

56. Shi, X.; Dalal, N.S.; Jain, A.C. Antioxidant behaviour of caffeine: Efficient scavenging of hydroxyl radicals. *Food Chem. Toxicol.* **1991**, *29*, 1–6. [CrossRef] [PubMed]

8

The Use of Dietary Supplements to Alleviate Androgen Deprivation Therapy Side Effects during Prostate Cancer Treatment

Andrea Dueregger [1], Isabel Heidegger [1], Philipp Ofer [1], Bernhard Perktold [2], Reinhold Ramoner [2], Helmut Klocker [1] and Iris E. Eder [1,*]

[1] Division of Experimental Urology, Department of Urology, Innsbruck Medical University, Innsbruck, A-6020 Austria; Andrea.Dueregger@student.i-med.ac.at (A.D.); Isabel-Maria.Heidegger@i-med.ac.at (I.H.); Philipp.Ofer@i-med.ac.at (P.O.); helmut.klocker@uki.at (H.K.)

[2] Department of Dietetics, University of Applied Sciences Tyrol, Innsbruck A-6020, Austria; Bernhard.perktold@fhg-tirol.ac.at (B.P.); reinhold.ramoner@fhg-tirol.ac.at (R.R.)

* Author to whom correspondence should be addressed; iris.eder@i-med.ac.at

Abstract: Prostate cancer (PCa), the most commonly diagnosed cancer and second leading cause of male cancer death in Western societies, is typically androgen-dependent, a characteristic that underlies the rationale of androgen deprivation therapy (ADT). Approximately 90% of patients initially respond to ADT strategies, however many experience side effects including hot flashes, cardiotoxicity, metabolic and musculoskeletal alterations. This review summarizes pre-clinical and clinical studies investigating the ability of dietary supplements to alleviate adverse effects arising from ADT. In particular, we focus on herbal compounds, phytoestrogens, selenium (Se), fatty acids (FA), calcium, and Vitamins D and E. Indeed, there is some evidence that calcium and Vitamin D can prevent the development of osteoporosis during ADT. On the other hand, caution should be taken with the antioxidants Se and Vitamin E until the basis underlying their respective association with type 2 diabetes mellitus and PCa tumor development has been clarified. However, many other promising supplements have not yet been subjected large-scale clinical trials making it difficult to assess their efficacy. Given the demographic trend of increased PCa diagnoses and dependence on ADT as a major therapeutic strategy, further studies are required to objectively evaluate these supplements as adjuvant for PCa patients receiving ADT.

Keywords: prostate cancer; androgen deprivation therapy; adverse effects; dietary supplements; alternative therapies

1. Introduction

Prostate Cancer (PCa) is the most commonly diagnosed male cancer and the second leading cause of cancer death among men in Western societies [1,2]. Radical prostatectomy or primary radiation therapy are the preferred treatment modalities in men with locally confined PCa. For advanced tumors or tumor recurring after primary surgery or radiation therapy the androgen receptor (AR) and its signaling network are the prime targets of therapy. The androgen receptor orchestrates crucial oncogenic factors in PCa etiology since androgens drive proliferation, differentiation, and survival of benign and malignant prostate cells [3]. Hence, upon initial diagnosis, 80%–90% of PCa are androgen-dependent [4], an observation that underlies the rationale of androgen deprivation therapy (ADT), the current mainstay systemic treatment for advanced PCa [5]. Although highly effective, ADT is associated with considerable side effects that negatively affect the patient's quality of life [6,7]. These adverse events include hot flashes [8], metabolic effects such as an induced metabolic syndrome (MetS) [9–12] including insulin resistance [13,14], cardiovascular (CV) diseases [15,16], musculoskeletal side effects characterized by reduced lean body mass and muscle strength, and osteoporosis [17–20] as well as depression and sexual dysfunction. Although several medical regimens have been developed [21], their impact on minimizing ADT side effects and improving quality of life is still under discussion. Recent statistics revealed an increasing use of complementary and alternative substances by PCa patients [22]. Indeed, approximately one in four patients with PCa uses at least one complementary or alternative method with the primary aim of ameliorating ADT-induced adverse effects [23,24].

In particular, herbal and dietary supplements appeal to patients because they are perceived as being "natural" with fewer side effects than prescription medicines. Despite the widespread use of alternatives to medical treatment options, little is known about their safety, efficacy and mechanism of action.

The limitation of clinical studies investigating this issue leads to a lack of information concerning the use of different types of alternative interventions. This article focuses on the metabolic and musculoskeletal side effects of ADT, which are not alleviated by current treatment strategies. In particular, we discuss several adjuvant dietary options including herbs, phytoestrogens, selenium (Se), fatty acids (FA), calcium, and Vitamins D and E, whose use in the treatment of ADT side effects is supported by scientific evidence derived either from cell-based models, animal models or clinical trials.

2. ADT in the Treatment of PCa

The androgenic hormones testosterone (T) and 5α-dihydrotestosterone (DHT), which mediate their action through the AR, are essential for normal prostate development but also contribute to prostate tumor growth by regulating cell proliferation and differentiation. The concept of hormonal manipulation using ADT to restrict PCa growth was first described in 1941 by Huggins and Hodges [25] and is based on the observation that 80%–90% of PCa are androgen dependent. Since then, multiple strategies have been established to reduce serum androgen levels or to interfere with their function by inhibiting the AR. Current strategies for hormonal blockade used in the treatment of PCa have been reviewed recently [26] and include bilateral orchiectomy, luteinizing hormone-releasing hormone (LHRH) agonists or antagonists and anti-androgens (Figure 1 and Table 1).

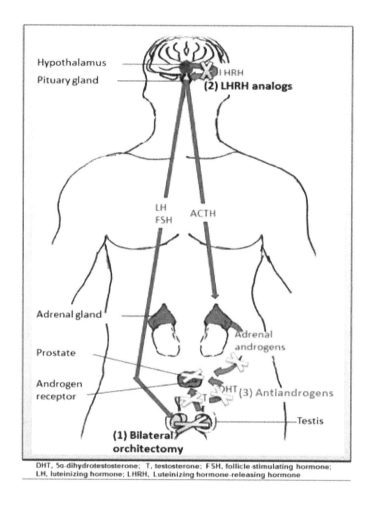

DHT, 5α-dihydrotestosterone; T, testosterone; FSH, follicle-stimulating hormone;
LH, luteinizing hormone; LHRH, Luteinizing hormone-releasing hormone

Figure 1. Mechanisms of action of androgen deprivation therapy (ADT) for blockage of the hypothalamus-pituary axis.

Current ADT strategies used in the treatment of PCa include bilateral orchiectomy (surgical castration), LHRH agonists or antagonists and anti-androgens (medical castration). (1) Bilateral orchiectomy is the surgical removal of both testicles inhibiting the production of testicular testosterone (T) and estradiol; (2) LHRH analogs reversibly decrease T production by the testis resulting in the down-regulation of LHRH receptors and thus reduced levels of luteinizing hormone (LH), follicle stimulating hormone (FSH) and T; (3) Anti-androgens (including flutamide, nilutamide, and bicalutamide) may bind competitively to the AR in cells thereby inhibiting its activation, or (abiraterone) block *de novo* androgen synthesis, both leading to apoptosis and reduced prostate tumor growth.

Table 1. Treatment options for hormone reduction.

Modality	Drug	Mechanism	Side Effects
Surgical Castration			
Bilateral Orchiectomy	-	Surgical removal of testicles, ↓T	Hot flashes, reduced muscle mass and energy, anemia and osteoporosis
Medical Castration			
LHRH Interference	*LHRH agonists* Leuproreline acetate (Trenantone®, Eligard®) Goserelin (Zoladex®) Triptorelin (Trelstar®) Histrelin (Vantas®)	LHRH receptor downregulation after initial flare, ↓LH, ↓FSH, ↓T	Hot flashes, reduced muscle mass and energy, anemia and osteoporosis, flare phenomenon, CV events, cardiotoxicity
	LHRH antagonists Degarelix (Firmagon®)	Blockade of LHRH receptor, ↓LH, ↓FSH, ↓T	Hot flashes, reduced muscle mass and energy, anemia and osteoporosis, CV events, histamine release
Antiandrogens	*Non-Steroidal* Flutamide (Eulexin®) Bicalutamide (Casodex®) Nilutamide (Nilandron®) Enzalutamide (Xtandi®)	Antagonizes AR in target tissues, ↑T	Gynecomastia, hepatotoxicity (flutamide), visual and respiratory disturbance and alcohol intolerance (nilutamide), GI problems, fatigue and hot flushes (enzalutamide)
	Steroidal Cyproterone acetate (Androcur®, Cyprostat®)	Antagonizes AR in target tissues, suppress LHRH secretion, ↓LH, ↓T	Gynecomastia, cardiovascular events, fluid retention, GI problems
	Abiraterone acetate (Zytiga®)	Inhibition of Cyp17A1 enzyme, suppresses T, estrogen and glucocorticoid biosynthesis	Vomiting, GI problems, swellings, weakness, cough, high blood pressure

LHRH, luteinizing hormone-releasing hormone; LH, luteinizing hormone; T, testosterone; AR, androgen receptor; GI, gastrointestinal; CV, cardiovascular.

Although accompanied by fewer side effects than "medical castration", the use of surgical bilateral orchiectomy is currently limited in developed countries. Rather, medical-based approaches to achieve castration levels of circulating androgens are preferred. In contrast to surgical castration, medical castration using LHRH analogs reversibly decrease T production by the testis and are therefore the preferred treatment modality. There are two different classes of LHRH analogs: LHRH agonists and antagonists. LHRH agonists stimulate the LHRH receptors in the pituitary gland resulting in a temporary increase in LH and FSH secretion, which in turn causes an initial rise in T production (the so-called "flare phenomenon [27]"). However, constant LHRH stimulation leads to a negative feedback loop resulting in the down-regulation of LHRH receptors and thus reduced levels of LH, FSH and T. In contrast to LHRH agonists, LHRH antagonists competitively bind to their receptors in the pituitary gland thereby blocking their activation by the natural ligand, inducing a rapid decrease in LH, FSH, and T levels without any flare.

Anti-androgens differ mechanistically from the above-described castration therapies as they do not alter androgen induction by direct modification of the hypothalamic-pituitary-gonadal axis in the brain. Rather, most anti-androgens (including flutamide, nilutamide, and bicalutamide) bind competitively to the AR in cells inhibiting its activation, leading to apoptosis and reduced prostate tumor growth. By contrast, abiraterone blocks *de novo* androgen synthesis via irreversible inhibition of CYP17-A1, a rate-limiting enzyme that catalyzes the conversion of cholesterol to androgen and estrogen precursors. The new-generation drugs abiraterone and enzalutamide have been developed during the past 5 years [28] and thus knowledge concerning their side effects is still limited. Since serum T and estrogen levels are maintained for all anti-androgen drugs that target the AR, hypogonadal side effects are generally less pronounced [29]. However, anti-androgens are often used in combination with LHRH analogs, thus this article will not discuss the side effect profile of anti-androgen monotherapy.

3. Adverse Effects of ADT

Frequent side effects of ADT that result in poor quality of life include hot flashes, metabolic effects such as gynacomastia as well as an increased body mass index, insulin resistance, metabolic syndrome (MetS), cardiovascular (CV) diseases, and musculoskeletal effects including reduced muscle mass, osteoporosis, and also sexual dysfunction (summarized Table 2) [1,7,30–35] Of these adverse events, metabolic and musculoskeletal effects are the most prevalent and distressing side effects reported by patients [21].

ADT targets gonadal function. Consequently, hypogonadism is prevalent in PCa patients undergoing ADT compared to those that undergo surgery and/or radiation therapy or compared to age-matched controls [7]. Thus, ADT induces a profound hypogonadism, which in turn is responsible for increased body mass index, increased fat mass, reduced lean body mass and muscle strength, and osteoporosis. Besides the desired physiological consequences of ADT in reducing serum androgens, hormonal castration is also associated with a decrease in circulating estrogens that are synthesized from androgens by peripheral aromatization (Figure 2). Despite having normal to elevated serum T levels, men with congenital aromatase deficiency (and thus, non-detectable serum estrogen levels) have a high prevalence of osteoporosis, insulin resistance and metabolic syndrome (MetS) [36], an observation that underscores the importance of estrogens in men. Moreover, it is decreased estrogen rather than T levels that are responsible for decreased bone density, accelerated rate of bone loss, and increased fracture incidence [37]. Thus, side effects induced by ADT leading to hot flashes, osteoporosis, MetS and higher CV events are related to androgen as well as estrogen deficiencies [35,38]. However, the relative contribution of T and estrogen to these adverse effects remains unclear.

ADT is associated with multiple adverse effects, many of which are related to androgen as well as estrogen deficiency that occur as a result of treatment [30,35].

Table 2. Summary of dietary supplements for the management of androgen deprivation therapy (ADT) side effects.

Side Effect	Postulated Management	Efficacy	Reference
	Herbs		
	Black cohosh	Minimal, ↓sweating symptoms, may ↓hot flashes in women.	[39,40]
Hot Flushes	Dong quai	No benefit in women or men.	[41]
	Ginseng	Minimal effects in women.	[42]
	Phyto-Estrogens		
	Soy-Isoflavons	No effect with supplements in men; possible impact with dietary source seen in women.	[43–49]
	Flaxseed	Unknown, initial studies showed impact on hormonal levels and serum lipids.	[50]
	Vitamin E	Previously recommended, but increased risk for diabetes. Might also increase the risk for PCa (SELECT trial).	[43,51–58]
	Herbs		
	Black cohosh	Potentially effective in preclinical studies (only studied in female animals).	[40,59]
Osteoporosis	**Phyto-estrogens**		
	Soy-Isoflavones	Potentially effective in preclinical studies (castrated male animals).	[60,61]
	Fatty acids		
	Omega-3 FA(CLA)	Potentially effective in preclinical studies (male and female animals).	[62–66]
	Calcium and Vitamin D	Effective in men and postmenopausal women.	[67–72]
	Herbs		
	Ginseng	No benefit.	[42]
	Garlic	Showed to reduce blood pressure.	[73,74]
	Phyto-Estrogens		
Cardiovascular Events	Soy-Isoflavones	No effect. Might reduce ↓LDL-cholesterol.	[46,75,76]
	Flaxseed	Potentially effective, reduced ↓LDL-cholesterol in postmenopausal women.	[77]
	Fatty acids		
	Omega-3 FA	No benefit. Postulated mechanism: ↓TG	[78–82]
	Selenium	No effect. Might have adverse effects on diabetes. Increased PCa risk (SELECT trial).	[24,56,58,84–90]
	Vitamin E	Negative association with CV health. Might increase PCa risk. No benefit in women.	[43,51,55,58,86,92]

CV, cardiovascular; CLA, conjugated linoleic acid; LDL, low density lipoprotein; TG, triglyceride.

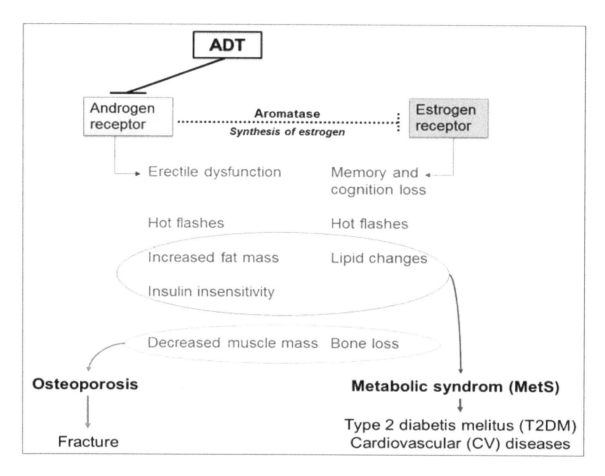

Figure 2. Side effects associated with androgen deprivation therapy (ADT).

3.1. Metabolic and Cardiovascular Side Effects

A number of prospective studies have shown that ADT increases abdominal fat and serum triglycerides (TG) and decreases insulin sensitivity [93]. Additionally, cross-sectional studies have shown that men receiving ADT are more likely to meet the diagnostic criteria of MetS [94,95]. Moreover, long term ADT therapy caused significantly higher levels of fasting insulin and glucose compared to men with PCa not on ADT as well as to age-matched controls [96]. A retrospective study involving 44 PCa patients who received ADT showed an increase in fasting blood glucose, total cholesterol, LDL cholesterol, and TG, but a decrease in HDL cholesterol in these patients [34]. In addition, longitudinal studies indicate that lower T levels in men independently predict MetS [97,98] and type 2 diabetes mellitus (T2DM) [99]. Because MetS is independently associated with CV mortality [100], it is plausible that the positive association between lower serum T levels and MetS may at least in part explain the higher CV mortality in men with PCa receiving ADT (with therapy-induced hypogonadism as the likely trigger of these events) [101]. The protective role of T on the CV system and its relationship to MetS, CV morbidity and mortality has been recently reviewed [98]. Since CV disease has become the most common cause of non-PCa-related death among this patient group [102], the potential risks of ADT with regards to CV events should be carefully weighed against the expected benefits. Moreover, since metabolic complications predominantly occur within 3–6 months after starting ADT therapy, close observation of patients especially during the first year of ADT is highly recommended [93].

3.2. Musculoskeletal Side Effects

Given that 25–40% of patients already have osteoporosis at PCa diagnosis, it must be considered that the symptoms will worsen upon administration of ADT. In general, two different forms of osteoporosis are known [103]. Whereas primary osteoporosis is caused by malnutrition and genetic predisposition, secondary osteoporosis predominantly arises in men due to hypogonadism, including that experienced by PCa patients receiving ADT [104]. Longitudinal studies report that approximately 35% of men on LHRH agonists experience at least one skeletal fracture and approximately 20% will be diagnosed as osteoporotic or osteopenic within 7 years of starting therapy [105]. The absolute excess risk of fractures ranges from 5%–7% over an average of 6 years follow-up compared to men not receiving ADT [31,106]. In particular, treatment with either LHRH analogs or orchiectomy is associated with a significant decline in bone mineral density (BMD) and increased risk of bone fractures [31,106]. In this context, it should be noted that bone fractures in men with PCa have been associated with higher mortality rates [107]. Cross-sectional studies have shown that BMD at the hip and lumbar spine decreases with the duration of continuous ADT [108]. However, BMD appears to initially decline at a fast rate. For example, greater declines of BMD were observed among recent *versus* chronic ADT users with stronger declines in both groups in contrast to ADT naïve men [109]. BMD declined at multiple sites including the lumbar spine and hip in the first year after starting ADT, however subsequent changes in the second year were much smaller and no longer statistically significant [110]. A larger study followed 618 men on ADT for up to 7 years with annual dual-energy X-ray absorptiometry (DXA) scans [111]. Whilst steady annual declines in BMD among men with normal BMD at baseline were noted, only 38 men with normal BMD at baseline still remained in the study by 3 years [111]. Thus, due to the lack of longitudinal studies, it is currently not possible to determine whether BMD loss beyond the first year of ADT is attenuated.

4. Dietary Supplements

The use of dietary supplements to alleviate side effects of ADT is an attractive approach for the majority of PCa patients. Indeed, an array of dietary supplements proposed to be useful in intervening with side effects due to declining hormone levels in men and women are promoted typically via media that lack scientific evidence. However, it should be noted that many of these supplements have been studied in the context of hormone deprivation during menopause or in the course of breast cancer therapy in women with no clinical studies carried out in men thus far (e.g., black cohosh, ginseng, garlic). Thus, it is difficult to conclude whether these dietary supplements will exhibit a similar efficacy in PCa patients receiving ADT. Of the few dietary supplement studies that have been performed in men, most were primarily aimed at reducing the risk of PCa development or reducing the risk of disease progression after initial diagnosis or first line treatment. Thus, studies in men receiving ADT are rare. Consequently, it is inappropriate to assume that beneficial (or non-beneficial) effects on PCa development or progression will similarly translate to modifying the adverse effects associated with ADT.

4.1. Herbs

Herbal supplemental approaches to manage metabolic and musculoskeletal side effects like hot flashes and osteoporosis have been extensively evaluated in breast cancer and menopausal women in small randomized trials with varying success [112,113]. Thus, it seems evident to evaluate the potential of the most promising of these herbs for the treatment of side effects in men who are being treated for PCa with ADT.

4.1.1. Black Cohosh (*Cimicifuga racemosa*)

The herbal supplement black cohosh, which is approved for the treatment of menopausal symptoms by the German health authority (Commission E), has also shown to have MetS-preventive and bone-protective properties in recent preclinical studies [59,114]. A randomized, placebo-controlled trial found no difference in the frequency of hot flashes but a significantly lower incidence of sweating in menopausal women with a history of breast cancer in the black cohosh group compared to placebo [39]. This finding is particularly pertinent given that a significant placebo effect is consistently observed in investigations of hot flashes, with the placebo effect reportedly sufficient to reduce hot flashes by up to 75% [115]. On the other hand, significant evidence of potentially beneficial effects on bone tissue was shown, although it should be noted that all clinical studies were conducted in females [59,116]. Of interest is one study that was carried out in orchidectomized male rats and showed to prevent osteoporosis *in vivo* [117].

The mechanism underlying the activity of black cohosh remains poorly understood. There is a lack of scientific evidence regarding its proposed estrogenic activity. However, it was recently shown to attenuate nucleoside uptake into cells and thus may have an impact on tumor treatment by nucleoside analogs [118]. One may speculate that its modulation of adenosine signaling may be beneficial for CV side effects of ADT [119], but this has yet to be investigated. Despite the lack of knowledge regarding the mechanism of action of black cohosh, its long history of use reveals that black cohosh is well tolerated. The use of black cohosh in PCa patients undergoing ADT may be warranted for hot flushes, CV and osteoporotic side effects. Importantly, further systematic studies assessing the safety and efficacy of black cohosh in alleviating ADT-induced side effects may be worth pursuing.

4.1.2. Dong Quai (*Angelica sinensis*)

Dong quai is a traditional Chinese herbal remedy most commonly used in the treatment of female reproductive problems. According to our knowledge, there are no pre-clinical studies addressing its effects in PCa. However, a small randomized clinical trial was conducted in men receiving ADT where dong quai was shown to be ineffective in reducing hot flashes [41]. Similarly, randomized trials in women also found no effect of dong quai on hot flashes beyond a placebo, irrespective of whether the herb was used alone or as part of a complex multi-ingredient intervention [120]. Taken together, the current evidence does not support the use of dong quai in patients undergoing ADT.

4.1.3. Ginseng (*Panax ginseng*)

Ginseng extract is widely used in traditional Chinese medicine and was reported to reduce fatigue, insomnia and depression in post-menopausal women, although there was no significant benefit on hot flashes [121]. However, a recent review of studies examining the efficacy of ginseng on menopausal symptoms highlighted the poor quality and bias of many randomized clinical trials conducted to date, raising doubt as to the usefulness of this herb in managing menopause symptoms [42]. Nonetheless, several pre-clinical and clinical studies have shown that ginseng may possess anti-cancer and hypoglycemic properties, the latter of potential benefit in ameliorating MetS in men receiving ADT [122,123].

4.1.4. Garlic (*Allium sativum*)

Garlic is frequently used as a dietary supplement for the treatment of hyperlipidemia, heart disease, and hypertension [124]. In addition, there is evidence that garlic is associated with blood pressure reduction in patients with elevated systolic blood pressure (10–12 mmHg systolic, 6–9 mmHg diastolic) but not in normotensive patients [73,74]. In this respect, it is conceivable that garlic may also reduce CV effects in PCa patients undergoing ADT. However, there is currently insufficient data to support this hypothesis and further studies that specifically address this question would be required [125].

4.2. Phytoestrogens

In the past, suppression of T was achieved using high doses of estrogens (estradiol) or selective estrogen receptor modulators [126–129]. However, these treatments were prone to severe and even fatal CV side effects [130,131]. Consequently, these treatments have been replaced by other therapeutics such as LHRH analogs. Phytoestrogens (plant estrogens) are non-steroidal naturally occurring phenolic compounds with known estrogenic effects and estrogen receptor (ER-β and/or ERα) binding properties [132–134]. Thus, these "mild" estrogens could possibly serve as natural alternatives with potentially fewer side effects. Indeed, phytoestrogens have been shown to improve metabolic health, reduce CV risk, and improve BMD and brain function [60,75,135]. There are three classes of phyto-estrogens, which are categorized according to their chemical structure as isoflavones, lignans or coumestans. Isoflavones are the largest and also the most extensively studied group of phytoestrogens, which includes genistein, daidzein and glycitein. Isoflavones are found in highest amounts in soybeans, flaxseed and legumes. Soy is stably integrated into Asian diets where daily intake is at least 40 times higher than among Western populations [136]. This is considered to be one of the factors contributing to a much lower incidence of prostate and breast cancer in Asian countries [137]. In addition, increased consumption of isoflavones has been associated with decreased incidence of diabetes and heart disease in South and East Asia [44,138]. In clinical trials, isoflavones have shown an improvement in hot flash severity, glycemic control, MetS and inflammatory profile in both men and postmenopausal women [45,76,139]. However, in a recent double-blinded, randomized, placebo-controlled pilot study, phytoestrogens failed to improve metabolic or inflammatory parameters of men with PCa during ADT [47]. This is consistent with another pilot study conducted in 33 men where high dose isoflavones showed no significant improvement in cognition, vasomotor symptoms or any other aspect of quality of life measures compared to placebo in androgen deprived men [140]. Thus, there is currently no clinical evidence for the proposed improvement of ADT-induced side effects by phytoestrogens, although limitations of these studies including small cohort sizes and short treatment durations should be taken into account.

4.3. Selenium (Se)

Se is an essential trace element, which is incorporated as selenocysteine into selenoproteins, many of which are reactive oxygen species (ROS) scavenging enzymes, such as glutathione peroxidase and thioredoxin reductase [141,142]. Thus, Se may be useful in decreasing oxidative stress and low-grade inflammation. Notably, plasma biomarkers of oxidative stress and low-grade inflammation are associated with MetS, obesity and insulin resistance, conditions that are common side effects of ADT [143]. Se was shown to have strong anti-proliferative and pro-apoptotic effects on human PCa cells and to improve severe metabolic side effects in patients [83,144]. Moreover, cancer prevention studies indicated that Se decreases ROS and is associated with decreased incidence of PCa [145,146]. Taken together, these observations provided a strong mechanistic rationale to combine ADT and Se for the treatment of PCa [5] and led to a number of epidemiological studies and clinical trials [51,83]. However, epidemiological studies have suggested that supranutritional Se intake and high plasma Se levels are not necessarily preventive against cancer, and may even be a possible risk factor for developing T2DM [83]. For example, supplementation with Se and/or Vitamin E in the large-scale Selenium and Vitamin E Cancer Prevention Trial (SELECT) did not prevent the development of PCa, rather, the incidence of newly diagnosed T2DM increased among the Se-supplemented participants [51,83]. Whilst the Nutritional Prevention of Cancer (NPC) study reported a decreased risk of PCa among Se supplemented men, an increased risk of T2DM was also observed in participants with baseline plasma Se levels in the top tertile [147]. Since then, several longitudinal studies have failed to support a causal role of Se in T2DM, although cross-sectional studies continued to find significant associations between circulating Se levels and T2DM [148]. For example, serum Se was observed to be associated with adipocytokines, such as TNF-α, VCAM-1, leptin, FABP-4, and MCP-1 [149,150] and adiponectin [151]. Although on the other hand, an analysis across randomized groups showed that Se supplementation had no effect on adiponectin levels after six months of treatment [84]. Thus, it appears likely that the reported link between Se and T2DM is due to indirect effects of Se-containing ROS scavenging enzymes, affecting the hydrogen peroxide level that in turn modulates both glucose-induced insulin secretion and insulin-induced signaling [152,153]. Moreover, Se homeostasis is modulated by factors related to carbohydrate metabolism, suggesting that low serum Se levels may themselves be a consequence of dysregulated energy metabolism in T2DM [153]. In addition, there appears to be a significant interaction between dietary intake of phytoestrogens and Se with important implications for heart disease, cancer, diabetes, and other conditions related to body weight [154].

From the current prospective—especially since to date there has been no study specifically evaluating the supplementation of Se in PCa patients receiving ADT—a combination of ADT with Se cannot be recommended given that many patients develop pre-diabetes.

4.4. Fatty Acids (FA)

The relative amounts and different types of dietary FA are thought to play critical roles in PCa associated MetS. Total FA intake and the ratio of omega-3 (ω-3) to omega-6 (ω-6) polyunsaturated FA (PUFAs) in the Western diet have increased significantly since the Industrial Revolution [155]. The effects of ω-3 PUFAs on CV disease, cancer as well as MetS have been investigated extensively [78, 156–161]. Consequently, the United States Food and Drug Administration (FDA) has approved ω-3 PUFAs for the prevention of CV adverse outcomes by the postulated mechanism of lowering serum triglyceride levels [162,163]. Additionally, three common dietary ω-3 FA—alpha-linolenic acid (ALA), eicosa-pentaenoic acid (EPA), and docosahexaenoic acid (DHA)—were proposed to exhibit anti-inflammatory properties [50,79,164]. Since inflammation is a major risk factor for the development of CV disease, these ω-3 FA may reduce the risk of CV disease [50,79,164]. Various pre-clinical, epidemiological and clinical studies have investigated the influence of ω-3 and ω-6 FA on the development and progression of PCa [80,155,158,161,165–173]. However, these studies have yielded contradictory results. In particular, dietary intake of long-chain ω-3 PUFA or its individual components (EPA, DHA, docosapentaenoic acid (DPA) and ALA) have been associated with PCa risk and progression [80,155,158,161,165–173]. On the other hand, encouraging results were obtained from clinical trials showing potential anti-inflammatory effects of ω-3 FA [77,174–177]. Other trials investigating higher doses of ω-3 FA (>1 g/day EPA and/or DHA) in populations at high risk for CV disease reported improvements (i.e., reduced concentrations) of selected inflammatory markers [81, 178,179]. However, it should be noted that in these studies the same dosage of ω-3 FA showed mixed response rates in healthy adults, and no beneficial effect in patients that received lower doses (<1 g/day) [81,174,175,178–185]. A single study has reported that very high intakes (6.6 g/day), which are well beyond the current recommendations (500 mg/day–1 g/day), may raise blood concentrations of some inflammation markers such as soluble tumor necrosis factor receptors 1 and 2 (sTNF-Rs 1 and 2) [79,185]. It is likely that differences in dosage, study population characteristics, the source of ω-3 FA, study duration, and background diet may explain the inconsistencies in these findings. In this respect, it may be noted that the majority of clinical trials have used marine sources of ω-3 FA (EPA and DHA from fish), whereas few have examined FA from plants (ALA from flax oil) and only two trials compared both sources [82,175]. The heterogeneous results from these studies might also be due to variations in measuring FA consumption of individuals and different techniques assessing their diet [186–190]. The main mechanisms underlying the purported anticancer effects of modulating dietary fat appear to be through reduced insulin-like growth factor signaling and alterations in membrane ω-6 to ω-3 FA ratios leading to suppressed COX-2-dependent PGE-2 production and reduction of inflammation via modification of the eicosanoid pathway [191–195]. Moreover, decreased PGE-2 levels are expected to decrease estrogen production and further also modify androgen production [190].

In summary, although ω-3 FA exhibits some anti-inflammatory potential, there is still a lack of consensus regarding their optimal use and dosage. Moreover, results from the aforementioned studies have to be interpreted with caution, since the metabolic conditions during ADT are different. Further research is warranted to better elucidate the mechanism of action and ideal consumption of ω-3 FA for potential CV health benefits during ADT.

4.5. Calcium and Vitamin D

Osteoporosis is a common and one of the most debilitating side effects of ADT. The most important nutritional factors contributing to osteoporosis include deficiencies in Vitamin D and calcium. Measurement of Vitamin D levels in osteoporotic males by a large multi-center study in the US (MrOs) revealed a deficiency in 26% and an insufficiency in 72% of subjects [54]. Because deterioration of BMD occurs soon after initiation of ADT therapy [67], the European Association of Urology does not specify recommendations but states that calcium supplementation is protective [196]. The National Comprehensive Cancer Network cite the National Osteoporosis foundation guidelines that recommend calcium (1000 mg daily) and Vitamin D (800–1000 IU daily) supplementation for all men aged 50 or above [197]. Notably however, data supporting this recommendation are lacking as shown in a recent systematic review [196]. One cross-sectional study suggested an association between low calcium intake and a greater likelihood of osteoporosis in men with PCa of whom 71 % were undergoing ADT. Unfortunately, Vitamin D use was not examined in this study [198]. Another trial reported a positive association of calcium and Vitamin D use (examined together) on hip and lumbar spine BMD in men on ADT [199]. Importantly, results from 12 different clinical trials revealed that the commonly recommended doses, of 500–1000 mg calcium and 200–500 IU Vitamin D per day still result in BMD loss in men receiving ADT [196]. Alibhai *et al.* examined long-term effects of calcium and Vitamin D in a prospective 3-year matched cohort study comparing PCa patients with and without ADT. This study found that Vitamin D but not calcium may be protective particularly in the first year of ADT [32]. In a multivariate analysis, it was further shown that the mean daily calcium intake in men receiving ADT was significantly lower in men who suffered from osteoporosis compared to those without osteoporosis [198].

In summary, calcium and Vitamin D supplementation is a recommended complementary therapy not only in elderly men with osteoporosis but also in men undergoing ADT even though the long-term impact of ADT on BMD and the value of calcium and Vitamin D in ameliorating negative effects remains to be elucidated more precisely.

4.6. Vitamin E

Vitamin E is a potent antioxidant, which is of interest to ameliorate hot flushes and CV associated side effects of ADT. Vitamin E has a long history in the treatment of pre-eclampsia (characterized by high blood pressure in pregnant women), premenstrual syndrome, painful periods, menopausal syndrome, hot flashes associated with breast cancer, and breast cysts even though randomized controlled clinical studies did not reveal any benefit [52,53,86,200]. Moreover, the Physicians Health Study II concluded that Vitamin E does not reduce the risk of major CV events (non-fatal myocardial infarction, non-fatal stroke, or CV disease death) [57]. Similarly, the Women's Health Study, which comprised approximately 40,000 healthy women, found that Vitamin E did not reduce the risk of death or major CV events. Interestingly however, there was a significant reduction in the secondary endpoint of CV deaths and in major CV events among a subgroup of women aged 65 or over [55]. The Women's Antioxidant Cardiovascular Study found that there were no overall effects of Vitamin E on CV events among women at high risk of CV disease [91]. Moreover, the intake of Vitamin E has been shown to increase all-cause mortality and may even have negative effects on CV health [92].

There have been a number of studies in men, which have purported a positive effect of Vitamin E on hot flushes and high blood pressure [201]. However, most of these studies have yielded inconclusive or conflicting findings or a lack of benefit for its use, illustrating the need for studies of higher quality in this area. Thus, clinical trials have failed to recapitulate the promising findings of *in vitro* and many observational studies. Possible reasons for this discrepancy may be that clinical trials are too short in duration to reverse the results of decades of oxidative stress contributing to atherosclerosis or that the antioxidants selected for study were chosen for their ease of availability rather than proven efficacy (Vitamin E) [202]. Recent evidence from the SELECT trial revealed an increased risk for PCa in the Vitamin E supplemented group. Taken together, current evidence does not support a beneficial effect for Vitamin E, and its use as a supplementary treatment is therefore not recommended [56,88].

5. Discussion

The administration of ADT is associated with a diverse set of known side effects that have a significant impact on patient quality of life, overall health, and mortality. Some of the dietary supplements discussed in this review may be beneficial for patients undergoing ADT. The value of calcium and Vitamin D supplementation remains to be elucidated more precisely; however, because of their long and safe history of usage they may be recommended in the prevention of osteoporosis during ADT. Phytoestrogens were shown to prevent hot flashes and other climacteric complaints and exert anti-osteoporotic effects in women. However, positive effects on CV health are still questionable and require further elucidation, especially with respect to their effects in PCa patients receiving ADT. In addition, further clinical trials evaluating the efficacy of isoflavones must be conducted before their use for relieving ADT-induced side effects can be advocated. We can conclude that dietary interventions with herbal substances may in fact be helpful in the treatment of adverse effects arising from ADT [43]; however, more clinical randomized studies in PCa patients on ADT are highly warranted to support these findings. The long history of use and lack of adverse effects of black cohosh in the treatment of climacteric complaints in women is particularly encouraging. Further evaluation of its proposed osteo-protective and anti-metabolic effects in conjunction with ADT in randomized and controlled clinical studies is also warranted. Recent data obtained in the large SELECT trial suggest that combined supplementation of Vitamin E and supranutritional Se may increase the risk of PCa, making this a non-recommended treatment for men receiving ADT. From the current perspective, a combination of ADT with Se, which has been associated with an increased risk for the development of T2DM, cannot be recommended given that many patients develop pre-diabetes.

6. Conclusions

In summary, dietary supplements are active compounds with as yet mostly poorly defined effects. As such, the unregulated self-prescription of active compounds such as soy, Se or Vitamin E may in some cases even prove to be harmful or negatively interfere with cancer treatment. Given the prevalent use of alternative dietary supplements in PCa patients, there is an urgent need to (1) perform rigorous research to determine the precise physiological effects of these different supplements with respect to relieving side effects of ADT; (2) conduct clinical trials of these supplements in men undergoing ADT and (3) establish more open lines of communication between patients and physicians regarding the use of dietary supplements and their integration into conventional treatment strategies.

Acknowledgments: We thank Natalie Sampson for reading the manuscript and performing English corrections. This work was supported by the Competence Center Oncotyrol (project 2.3.3) within the scope of the Austrian Competence Center for Excellent Technologies (COMET)—program conducted by the Austrian Research Promotion Agency (FFG) and a Category B research funding from ÖKH-KG/Tirol given to Andrea Dueregger. Andrea Dueregger was partly funded by autonomous province Bozen (Grant Number: 37/40.3) given to Petra Massoner.

Author Contributions: Andrea Dueregger and Iris E. Eder designed and wrote the review. Isabel Heidegger wrote parts of the manuscript. Bernhard Perktold, Reinhold Ramoner and Helmut Klocker were significantly involved in designing the review regarding its content and also in editing the manuscript.

References and Notes

1. Siegel, R.; Naishadham, D.; Jemal, A. Cancer statistics, 2012. *Cancer J. Clin.* **2012**, *62*, 10–29. [CrossRef]
2. Siegel, R.; Ma, J.; Zou, Z.; Jemal, A. Cancer statistics, 2014. *Cancer J. Clin.* **2014**, *64*, 9–29. [CrossRef]
3. Heinlein, C.A.; Chang, C. Androgen receptor in prostate cancer. *Endocr. Rev.* **2004**, *25*, 276–308. [CrossRef] [PubMed]
4. Denis, L.J. The role of active treatment in early prostate cancer. *Radiother. Oncol.* **2000**, *57*, 251–258. [CrossRef] [PubMed]
5. Lieberman, R. Androgen deprivation therapy for prostate cancer chemoprevention: Current status and future directions for agent development. *Urology* **2001**, *58*, 83–90. [CrossRef] [PubMed]
6. Molina, A.; Belldegrun, A. Novel therapeutic strategies for castration resistant prostate cancer: Inhibition of persistent androgen production and androgen receptor mediated signaling. *J. Urol.* **2011**, *185*, 787–794. [CrossRef] [PubMed]

7.   Basaria, S.; Davda, M.N.; Travison, T.G.; Ulloor, J.; Singh, R.; Bhasin, S. Risk factors associated with cardiovascular events during testosterone administration in older men with mobility limitation. *J. Gerontol. Series A Biol. Sci. Med. Sci.* **2013**, *68*, 153–160. [CrossRef]

8.   Hot flashes are a sudden wave of mild or intense body heat caused by rushes of hormonal changes resulting from decreased levels of estrogen. They can occur at any time and may last from a few seconds to half an hour. They are due to blood vessel dilation and constriction. Their frequency is increased in menopausal women and men receiving ADT.

9.   The "metabolic" or "insulin-resistance" syndrome (MetS) is a cluster of cardio-vascular (CV) risks related to insulin resistance [10,11]. Diagnosis of the syndrome is defined by the adult treatment panel III (ATP III) and the World health organization (WHO) as a combination of low HDL, increased waist circumference, increased triglycerides, increased fasting glucose and hypertension [11]. The syndrome itself is further associated with various metabolic abnormalities, including insulin resistance as well as other factors such as male hypogonadism [12].

10.   Ferrannini, E. Metabolic syndrome: A solution in search of a problem. *J. Clin. Endocrinol. Metab.* **2007**, *92*, 396–398. [CrossRef] [PubMed]

11.   Kahn, R.; Buse, J.; Ferrannini, E.; Stern, M. The metabolic syndrome: Time for a critical appraisal: Joint statement from the American Diabetes Association and the European Association for the Study of Diabetes. *Diabetes Care* **2005**, *28*, 2289–2304. [CrossRef] [PubMed]

12.   Cho, L.W. Metabolic syndrome. *Singap. Med. J.* **2011**, *52*, 779–785.

13.   Insulin resistance is defined clinically as the inability of a known quantity of exogenous or endogenous insulin to increase glucose uptake and utilization in an individual as much as it does in a normal population [14].

14.   Lebovitz, H.E. Insulin resistance: Definition and consequences. *Exp. Clin. Endocrinol. Diabetes* **2001**, *109*, 135–148. [CrossRef] [PubMed]

15.   Cardiovascular events refer to any incidents that may cause damage to the heart muscle involving the heart and/or blood vessels which include: arterial embolic or thrombotic events, hemorrhagic or ischemic cerebrovascular conditions, myocardial infarction, and other ischemic heart disease. Severe CV events include conditions such as myocardial infarction or congestive heart failure which may be fatal [16].

16.   WHO Fact Sheet—Cardiovascular diseases (CVDs). Available online: Http://www.who.int/mediacentre/factsheets/fs317/en/ (accessed on 4 September 2014).

17.   Osteoporosis is a skeletal disorder characterized by compromised bone strength predisposing to an increased risk for bone fractures. Bone strength reflects the integration of two main features: bone mineral density (BMD) and bone quality [18]. Osteoporosis is defined by the WHO as a BMD of 2.5 standard deviations or more below the mean peak bone mass (average of young, healthy adults) as measured by dual-energy X-ray absorptiometry (DXA). A BMD value allows fracture risk to be calculated using FRAX or CAROC assessment algorithms, which incorporate a group of clinical risk factors in addition to femoral neck BMD [19,20].

18.   Kilbanski, A.; Adams-Campbell, L.; Bassford, T.; Blair, S.N.; Boden, S.D.; Dickersin, K.; Gifford, D.R.; Glasse, L.; Goldring, S.R.; Hruska, K.; *et al.* Osteoporosis prevention, diagnosis, and therapy. *JAMA J. American Medical Association* **2001**, *285*, 785–795. [CrossRef]

19.   Leslie, W.D.; Lix, L.M.; Johansson, H.; Oden, A.; McCloskey, E.; Kanis, J.A. Independent clinical validation of a Canadian FRAX tool: Fracture prediction and model calibration. *J. Bone Miner. Res.* **2010**, *25*, 2350–2358. [CrossRef] [PubMed]

20.   Leslie, W.D.; Tsang, J.F.; Lix, L.M. Simplified system for absolute fracture risk assessment: Clinical validation in Canadian women. *J. Bone Miner. Res.* **2009**, *24*, 353–360. [CrossRef] [PubMed]

21.   Grossmann, M.; Zajac, J.D. Androgen deprivation therapy in men with prostate cancer: How should the side effects be monitored and treated? *Clin. Endocrinol.* **2011**, *74*, 289–293.

22.   Truant, T.L.; Porcino, A.J.; Ross, B.C.; Wong, M.E.; Hilario, C.T. Complementary and alternative medicine (CAM) use in advanced cancer: A systematic review. *J. Support. Oncol.* **2013**, *11*, 105–113. [CrossRef] [PubMed]

23.   Philippou, Y.; Hadjipavlou, M.; Khan, S.; Rane, A. Complementary and alternative medicine (CAM) in prostate and bladder cancer. *BJU Int.* **2013**, *112*, 1073–1079. [CrossRef] [PubMed]

24.   Klempner, S.J.; Bubley, G. Complementary and alternative medicines in prostate cancer: From bench to bedside? *The oncologist* **2012**, *17*, 830–837. [CrossRef]

25. Huggins, C.; Hodges, C.V. Studies on prostatic cancer: I. The effect of castration, of estrogen and of androgen injection on serum phosphatases in metastatic carcinoma of the prostate. *J. Urol.* **2002**, *168*, 9–12. [CrossRef] [PubMed]

26. Schroder, F.; Crawford, E.D.; Axcrona, K.; Payne, H.; Keane, T.E. Androgen deprivation therapy: Past, present and future. *BJU Int.* **2012**, *109*, 1–12. [CrossRef] [PubMed]

27. The initial administration of an LHRH agonist first causes an increase of LH with a corresponding rise in serum T over 1–2 weeks. This increase in T may initially stimulate and worsen the disease and related symptoms. To prevent this phenomenon, administration of an anti-androgen or estrogen for one week before and during the first few weeks of LHRH agonist therapy is often employed.

28. Rodrigues, D.N.; Butler, L.M.; Estelles, D.L.; de Bono, J.S. Molecular pathology and prostate cancer therapeutics: From biology to bedside. *J. Pathol.* **2014**, *232*, 178–184. [CrossRef] [PubMed]

29. Kolvenbag, G.J.; Iversen, P.; Newling, D.W. Antiandrogen monotherapy: A new form of treatment for patients with prostate cancer. *Urology* **2001**, *58*, 16–23. [CrossRef] [PubMed]

30. Grossmann, M.; Zajac, J.D. Management of side effects of androgen deprivation therapy. *Endocrinol. Metab. Clin. N. Am.* **2011**, *40*, 655–671. [CrossRef]

31. Alibhai, S.M.; Duong-Hua, M.; Sutradhar, R.; Fleshner, N.E.; Warde, P.; Cheung, A.M.; Paszat, L.F. Impact of androgen deprivation therapy on cardiovascular disease and diabetes. *J. Clin. Oncol.* **2009**, *27*, 3452–3458. [CrossRef] [PubMed]

32. Alibhai, S.M.; Mohamedali, H.Z.; Gulamhusein, H.; Panju, A.H.; Breunis, H.; Timilshina, N.; Fleshner, N.; Krahn, M.D.; Naglie, G.; Tannock, I.F.; *et al.* Changes in bone mineral density in men starting androgen deprivation therapy and the protective role of vitamin D. *Osteoporos. Int.* **2013**, *24*, 2571–2579. [CrossRef] [PubMed]

33. Yuan, J.Q.; Xu, T.; Zhang, X.W.; Yu, L.P.; Li, Q.; Liu, S.J.; Huang, X.B.; Wang, X.F. Metabolic syndrome and androgen deprivation therapy in metabolic complications of prostate cancer patients. *Chin. Med. J.* **2012**, *125*, 3725–3729. [PubMed]

34. Saglam, H.S.; Kose, O.; Kumsar, S.; Budak, S.; Adsan, O. Fasting blood glucose and lipid profile alterations following twelve-month androgen deprivation therapy in men with prostate cancer. *Sci. World J.* **2012**, *2012*. [CrossRef]

35. Freedland, S.J.; Eastham, J.; Shore, N. Androgen deprivation therapy and estrogen deficiency induced adverse effects in the treatment of prostate cancer. *Prostate Cancer Prostatic Dis.* **2009**, *12*, 333–338. [CrossRef] [PubMed]

36. Carani, C.; Qin, K.; Simoni, M.; Faustini-Fustini, M.; Serpente, S.; Boyd, J.; Korach, K.S.; Simpson, E.R. Effect of testosterone and estradiol in a man with aromatase deficiency. *N Engl. J. Med.* **1997**, *337*, 91–95. [CrossRef] [PubMed]

37. Khosla, S. Update in male osteoporosis. *J. Clin. Endocrinol. Metab.* **2010**, *95*, 3–10. [CrossRef] [PubMed]

38. Lee, R.J.; Saylor, P.J.; Smith, M.R. Contemporary therapeutic approaches targeting bone complications in prostate cancer. *Clin. Genitourin. Cancer* **2010**, *8*, 29–36. [CrossRef] [PubMed]

39. Jacobson, J.S.; Troxel, A.B.; Evans, J.; Klaus, L.; Vahdat, L.; Kinne, D.; Lo, K.M.; Moore, A.; Rosenman, P.J.; Kaufman, E.L.; *et al.* Randomized trial of black cohosh for the treatment of hot flashes among women with a history of breast cancer. *J. Clin. Oncol.* **2001**, *19*, 2739–2745. [PubMed]

40. Fritz, H.; Seely, D.; McGowan, J.; Skidmore, B.; Fernandes, R.; Kennedy, D.A.; Cooley, K.; Wong, R.; Sagar, S.; Balneaves, L.G.; *et al.* Black cohosh and breast cancer: A systematic review. *Integr. Cancer Ther.* **2014**, *13*, 12–29. [CrossRef] [PubMed]

41. Al-Bareeq, R.J.; Ray, A.A.; Nott, L.; Pautler, S.E.; Razvi, H. Dong Quai (*Angelica sinensis*) in the treatment of hot flashes for men on androgen deprivation therapy: Results of a randomized double-blind placebo controlled trial. *Can. Urol. Assoc. J.* **2010**, *4*, 49–53. [PubMed]

42. Kim, M.S.; Lim, H.J.; Yang, H.J.; Lee, M.S.; Shin, B.C.; Ernst, E. Ginseng for managing menopause symptoms: A systematic review of randomized clinical trials. *J. Ginseng Res.* **2013**, *37*, 30–36. [CrossRef] [PubMed]

43. Moyad, M.A. Complementary/alternative therapies for reducing hot flashes in prostate cancer patients: Reevaluating the existing indirect data from studies of breast cancer and postmenopausal women. *Urology* **2002**, *59*, 20–33. [CrossRef]

44. Zhang, X.; Shu, X.O.; Gao, Y.T.; Yang, G.; Li, Q.; Li, H.; Jin, F.; Zheng, W. Soy food consumption is associated with lower risk of coronary heart disease in Chinese women. *J. Nutr.* **2003**, *133*, 2874–2878. [PubMed]

45. Azadbakht, L.; Kimiagar, M.; Mehrabi, Y.; Esmaillzadeh, A.; Padyab, M.; Hu, F.B.; Willett, W.C. Soy inclusion in the diet improves features of the metabolic syndrome: A randomized crossover study in postmenopausal women. *Am. J. Clin. Nutr.* **2007**, *85*, 735–741. [PubMed]

46. Thelen, P.; Burfeind, P.; Schweyer, S.; Scharf, J.G.; Wuttke, W.; Ringert, R.H. Molecular principles of alternative treatment approaches for hormone-refractory prostate cancer. *Der. Urol. Ausg. A* **2007**, *46*, 1271–1274. [CrossRef]

47. Napora, J.K.; Short, R.G.; Muller, D.C.; Carlson, O.D.; Odetunde, J.O.; Xu, X.; Carducci, M.; Travison, T.G.; Maggio, M.; Egan, J.M.; *et al.* High-dose isoflavones do not improve metabolic and inflammatory parameters in androgen-deprived men with prostate cancer. *J. Androl.* **2011**, *32*, 40–48. [CrossRef] [PubMed]

48. Albertazzi, P.; Pansini, F.; Bonaccorsi, G.; Zanotti, L.; Forini, E.; de Aloysio, D. The effect of dietary soy supplementation on hot flushes. *Obstetrics Gynecol.* **1998**, *91*, 6–11. [CrossRef]

49. Charles, C.; Yuskavage, J.; Carlson, O.; John, M.; Tagalicud, A.S.; Maggio, M.; Muller, D.C.; Egan, J.; Basaria, S. Effects of high-dose isoflavones on metabolic and inflammatory markers in healthy postmenopausal women. *Menopause* **2009**, *16*, 395–400. [CrossRef] [PubMed]

50. James, M.J.; Gibson, R.A.; Cleland, L.G. Dietary polyunsaturated fatty acids and inflammatory mediator production. *Am. J. Clin. Nutr.* **2000**, *71*, 343–348.

51. Lippman, S.M.; Klein, E.A.; Goodman, P.J.; Lucia, M.S.; Thompson, I.M.; Ford, L.G.; Parnes, H.L.; Minasian, L.M.; Gaziano, J.M.; Hartline, J.A.; *et al.* Effect of selenium and vitamin E on risk of prostate cancer and other cancers: The Selenium and Vitamin E Cancer Prevention Trial (SELECT). *Jama* **2009**, *301*, 39–51. [CrossRef] [PubMed]

52. Rubenstein, B.B. Vitamin E diminishes the vasomotor symptoms of menopause. *Fed. Proc.* **1948**, *7*, 106. [PubMed]

53. Raffy, A. Menopause and vitamin E. *Ther. Hung.* **1955**, *4*, 12–14. [PubMed]

54. Orwoll, E.; Nielson, C.M.; Marshall, L.M.; Lambert, L.; Holton, K.F.; Hoffman, A.R.; Barrett-Connor, E.; Shikany, J.M.; Dam, T.; Cauley, J.A. Vitamin D deficiency in older men. *J. Clin. Endocrinol. Metab.* **2009**, *94*, 1214–1222. [CrossRef] [PubMed]

55. Liu, S.; Lee, I.M.; Song, Y.; Van Denburgh, M.; Cook, N.R.; Manson, J.E.; Buring, J.E. Vitamin E and risk of type 2 diabetes in the women's health study randomized controlled trial. *Diabetes* **2006**, *55*, 2856–2862. [CrossRef] [PubMed]

56. Klein, E.A.; Thompson, I.M., Jr.; Tangen, C.M.; Crowley, J.J.; Lucia, M.S.; Goodman, P.J.; Minasian, L.M.; Ford, L.G.; Parnes, H.L.; Gaziano, J.M.; *et al.* Vitamin E and the risk of prostate cancer: The Selenium and Vitamin E Cancer Prevention Trial (SELECT). *JAMA* **2011**, *306*, 1549–1556. [CrossRef] [PubMed]

57. Sesso, H.D.; Buring, J.E.; Christen, W.G.; Kurth, T.; Belanger, C.; MacFadyen, J.; Bubes, V.; Manson, J.E.; Glynn, R.J.; Gaziano, J.M. Vitamins E and C in the prevention of cardiovascular disease in men: The Physicians' Health Study II randomized controlled trial. *JAMA* **2008**, *300*, 2123–2133. [CrossRef] [PubMed]

58. Peters, U.; Littman, A.J.; Kristal, A.R.; Patterson, R.E.; Potter, J.D.; White, E. Vitamin E and selenium supplementation and risk of prostate cancer in the Vitamins and lifestyle (VITAL) study cohort. *Cancer Causes Control* **2008**, *19*, 75–87. [CrossRef] [PubMed]

59. Seidlova-Wuttke, D.; Stecher, G.; Kammann, M.; Haunschild, J.; Eder, N.; Stahnke, V.; Wessels, J.; Wuttke, W. Osteoprotective effects of Cimicifuga racemosa and its triterpene-saponins are responsible for reduction of bone marrow fat. *Phytomedicine* **2012**, *19*, 855–860. [CrossRef] [PubMed]

60. Kuhnle, G.G.; Ward, H.A.; Vogiatzoglou, A.; Luben, R.N.; Mulligan, A.; Wareham, N.J.; Forouhi, N.G.; Khaw, K.T. Association between dietary phyto-oestrogens and bone density in men and postmenopausal women. *Br. J. Nutr.* **2011**, *106*, 1063–1069. [CrossRef] [PubMed]

61. Soung, D.Y.; Devareddy, L.; Khalil, D.A.; Hooshmand, S.; Patade, A.; Lucas, E.A.; Arjmandi, B.H. Soy affects trabecular microarchitecture and favorably alters select bone-specific gene expressions in a male rat model of osteoporosis. *Calcif. Tissue Int.* **2006**, *78*, 385–391. [CrossRef] [PubMed]

62. Hogstrom, M.; Nordstrom, P.; Nordstrom, A. n-3 Fatty acids are positively associated with peak bone mineral density and bone accrual in healthy men: The NO2 Study. *Am. J. Clin. Nutr.* **2007**, *85*, 803–807. [PubMed]

63. Watkins, B.A.; Li, Y.; Lippman, H.E.; Seifert, M.F. Omega-3 polyunsaturated fatty acids and skeletal health. *Exp. Biol Med. (Maywood)* **2001**, *226*, 485–497.

64. Fernandes, G.; Bhattacharya, A.; Rahman, M.; Zaman, K.; Banu, J. Effects of n-3 fatty acids on autoimmunity and osteoporosis. *Front. Biosci.* **2008**, *13*, 4015–4020. [CrossRef] [PubMed]

65. Shen, C.L.; Yeh, J.K.; Rasty, J.; Chyu, M.C.; Dunn, D.M.; Li, Y.; Watkins, B.A. Improvement of bone quality in gonad-intact middle-aged male rats by long-chain n-3 polyunsaturated fatty acid. *Calcif. Tissue Int.* **2007**, *80*, 286–293. [CrossRef] [PubMed]

66. Rahman, M.M.; Bhattacharya, A.; Banu, J.; Fernandes, G. Conjugated linoleic acid protects against age-associated bone loss in C57BL/6 female mice. *J. Nutr. Biochem.* **2007**, *18*, 467–474. [CrossRef] [PubMed]

67. Tang, B.M.; Eslick, G.D.; Nowson, C.; Smith, C.; Bensoussan, A. Use of calcium or calcium in combination with vitamin D supplementation to prevent fractures and bone loss in people aged 50 years and older: A meta-analysis. *Lancet* **2007**, *370*, 657–666. [CrossRef] [PubMed]

68. Gates, B.J.; Das, S. Management of osteoporosis in elderly men. *Maturitas* **2011**, *69*, 113–119. [CrossRef] [PubMed]

69. Gielen, E.; Boonen, S.; Vanderschueren, D.; Sinnesael, M.; Verstuyf, A.; Claessens, F.; Milisen, K.; Verschueren, S. Calcium and vitamin D supplementation in men. *J. Osteoporos.* **2011**, *2011*. [CrossRef]

70. Verbrugge, F.H.; Gielen, E.; Milisen, K.; Boonen, S. Who should receive calcium and vitamin D supplementation? *Age Ageing* **2012**, *41*, 576–580. [CrossRef]

71. Cranney, A.; Horsley, T.; O'Donnell, S.; Weiler, H.; Puil, L.; Ooi, D.; Atkinson, S.; Ward, L.; Moher, D.; Hanley, D.; *et al.* Effectiveness and safety of vitamin D in relation to bone health. *Evid. Rep. Technol. Assess.* **2007**, 1–235.

72. Moyad, M.A. Complementary therapies for reducing the risk of osteoporosis in patients receiving luteinizing hormone-releasing hormone treatment/orchiectomy for prostate cancer: A review and assessment of the need for more research. *Urology* **2002**, *59*, 34–40. [CrossRef] [PubMed]

73. Stabler, S.N.; Tejani, A.M.; Huynh, F.; Fowkes, C. Garlic for the prevention of cardiovascular morbidity and mortality in hypertensive patients. *Cochrane Database Syst. Rev.* **2012**, *8*. [CrossRef]

74. Shouk, R.; Abdou, A.; Shetty, K.; Sarkar, D.; Eid, A.H. Mechanisms underlying the antihypertensive effects of garlic bioactives. *Nutr Res.* **2014**, *34*, 106–115. [CrossRef] [PubMed]

75. Clarkson, T.B. Soy, soy phytoestrogens and cardiovascular disease. *J. Nutr.* **2002**, *132*, 566–569.

76. Atteritano, M.; Marini, H.; Minutoli, L.; Polito, F.; Bitto, A.; Altavilla, D.; Mazzaferro, S.; D'Anna, R.; Cannata, M.L.; Gaudio, A.; *et al.* Effects of the phytoestrogen genistein on some predictors of cardiovascular risk in osteopenic, postmenopausal women: A two-year randomized, double-blind, placebo-controlled study. *J. Clin. Endocrinol. Metab.* **2007**, *92*, 3068–3075. [CrossRef] [PubMed]

77. Bloedon, L.T.; Balikai, S.; Chittams, J.; Cunnane, S.C.; Berlin, J.A.; Rader, D.J.; Szapary, P.O. Flaxseed and cardiovascular risk factors: Results from a double blind, randomized, controlled clinical trial. *J. Am. Coll. Nutr.* **2008**, *27*, 65–74. [CrossRef] [PubMed]

78. Jacobson, T.A. Beyond lipids: The role of omega-3 fatty acids from fish oil in the prevention of coronary heart disease. *Curr. Atheroscler. Rep.* **2007**, *9*, 145–153. [CrossRef] [PubMed]

79. Kris-Etherton, P.M.; Harris, W.S.; Appel, L.J. Fish consumption, fish oil, omega-3 fatty acids, and cardiovascular disease. *Circulation* **2002**, *106*, 2747–2757. [CrossRef] [PubMed]

80. Simopoulos, A.P. The importance of the ratio of omega-6/omega-3 essential fatty acids. *Biomed. Pharmacother.* **2002**, *56*, 365–379. [CrossRef] [PubMed]

81. Hjerkinn, E.M.; Seljeflot, I.; Ellingsen, I.; Berstad, P.; Hjermann, I.; Sandvik, L.; Arnesen, H. Influence of long-term intervention with dietary counseling, long-chain n-3 fatty acid supplements, or both on circulating markers of endothelial activation in men with long-standing hyperlipidemia. *Am. J. Clin. Nutr.* **2005**, *81*, 583–589. [PubMed]

82. Dewell, A.; Marvasti, F.F.; Harris, W.S.; Tsao, P.; Gardner, C.D. Low- and high-dose plant and marine (n-3) fatty acids do not affect plasma inflammatory markers in adults with metabolic syndrome. *J. Nutr.* **2011**, *141*, 2166–2171. [CrossRef] [PubMed]

83. Koyama, H.; Mutakin; Abdulah, R.; Yamazaki, C.; Kameo, S. Selenium supplementation trials for cancer prevention and the subsequent risk of type 2 diabetes mellitus. *Nihon Eiseigaku Zasshi* **2013**, *68*, 1–10. [CrossRef] [PubMed]

84. Rayman, M.P.; Blundell-Pound, G.; Pastor-Barriuso, R.; Guallar, E.; Steinbrenner, H.; Stranges, S. A randomized trial of selenium supplementation and risk of type-2 diabetes, as assessed by plasma adiponectin. *PLoS One* **2012**, *7*, 45269. [CrossRef]

85. Faghihi, T.; Radfar, M.; Barmal, M.; Amini, P.; Qorbani, M.; Abdollahi, M.; Larijani, B. A randomized, placebo-controlled trial of selenium supplementation in patients with type 2 diabetes: Effects on glucose homeostasis, oxidative stress, and lipid profile. *Am. J. Ther.* **2013**. [CrossRef]

86. Dennehy, C.; Tsourounis, C. A review of select vitamins and minerals used by postmenopausal women. *Maturitas* **2010**, *66*, 370–380. [CrossRef] [PubMed]

87. Algotar, A.M.; Stratton, M.S.; Stratton, S.P.; Hsu, C.H.; Ahmann, F.R. No effect of selenium supplementation on serum glucose levels in men with prostate cancer. *Am. J. Med.* **2010**, *123*, 765–768. [CrossRef] [PubMed]

88. Kristal, A.R.; Darke, A.K.; Morris, J.S.; Tangen, C.M.; Goodman, P.J.; Thompson, I.M.; Meyskens, F.L., Jr.; Goodman, G.E.; Minasian, L.M.; Parnes, H.L.; *et al.* Baseline selenium status and effects of selenium and vitamin E supplementation on prostate cancer risk. *J. Nat. Cancer Inst.* **2014**, *106*. [CrossRef] [PubMed]

89. Algotar, A.M.; Stratton, M.S.; Ahmann, F.R.; Ranger-Moore, J.; Nagle, R.B.; Thompson, P.A.; Slate, E.; Hsu, C.H.; Dalkin, B.L.; Sindhwani, P.; *et al.* Phase 3 clinical trial investigating the effect of selenium supplementation in men at high-risk for prostate cancer. *Prostate* **2013**, *73*, 328–335. [CrossRef] [PubMed]

90. b>Algotar, A.M.; Hsu, C.H.; Singh, P.; Stratton, S.P. Selenium supplementation has no effect on serum glucose levels in men at high risk for Prostate Cancer. *J. Diabetes* **2013**, *5*, 465–470. [CrossRef] [PubMed]

91. Cook, N.R.; Albert, C.M.; Gaziano, J.M.; Zaharris, E.; MacFadyen, J.; Danielson, E.; Buring, J.E.; Manson, J.E. A randomized factorial trial of vitamins C and E and beta carotene in the secondary prevention of cardiovascular events in women: Results from the Women's Antioxidant Cardiovascular Study. *Arch. Internal Med.* **2007**, *167*, 1610–1618. [CrossRef]

92. Saremi, A.; Arora, R. Vitamin E and cardiovascular disease. *Am. J. Ther.* **2010**, *17*, 56–65. [CrossRef]

93. Shahani, S.; Braga-Basaria, M.; Basaria, S. Androgen deprivation therapy in prostate cancer and metabolic risk for atherosclerosis. *J. Clin. Endocrinol. Metab.* **2008**, *93*, 2042–2049. [CrossRef] [PubMed]

94. Smith, M.R.; Lee, H.; McGovern, F.; Fallon, M.A.; Goode, M.; Zietman, A.L.; Finkelstein, J.S. Metabolic changes during gonadotropin-releasing hormone agonist therapy for prostate cancer: Differences from the classic metabolic syndrome. *Cancer* **2008**, *112*, 2188–2194. [CrossRef] [PubMed]

95. Braga-Basaria, M.; Dobs, A.S.; Muller, D.C.; Carducci, M.A.; John, M.; Egan, J.; Basaria, S. Metabolic syndrome in men with prostate cancer undergoing long-term androgen-deprivation therapy. *J. Clin. Oncol.* **2006**, *24*, 3979–3983. [CrossRef] [PubMed]

96. Basaria, S.; Muller, D.C.; Carducci, M.A.; Egan, J.; Dobs, A.S. Hyperglycemia and insulin resistance in men with prostate carcinoma who receive androgen-deprivation therapy. *Cancer* **2006**, *106*, 581–588. [CrossRef] [PubMed]

97. Laaksonen, D.E.; Niskanen, L.; Punnonen, K.; Nyyssonen, K.; Tuomainen, T.P.; Valkonen, V.P.; Salonen, R.; Salonen, J.T. Testosterone and sex hormone-binding globulin predict the metabolic syndrome and diabetes in middle-aged men. *Diabetes Care* **2004**, *27*, 1036–1041. [CrossRef] [PubMed]

98. Tirabassi, G.; Gioia, A.; Giovannini, L.; Boscaro, M.; Corona, G.; Carpi, A.; Maggi, M.; Balercia, G. Testosterone and cardiovascular risk. *Intern. Emerg. Med.* **2013**, *8*, 65–69. [CrossRef] [PubMed]

99. Stellato, R.K.; Feldman, H.A.; Hamdy, O.; Horton, E.S.; McKinlay, J.B. Testosterone, sex hormone-binding globulin, and the development of type 2 diabetes in middle-aged men: Prospective results from the Massachusetts male aging study. *Diabetes Care* **2000**, *23*, 490–494. [CrossRef] [PubMed]

100. Eckel, R.H.; Alberti, K.G.; Grundy, S.M.; Zimmet, P.Z. The metabolic syndrome. *Lancet* **2010**, *375*, 181–183. [CrossRef] [PubMed]

101. Fink, R.I.; Kolterman, O.G.; Griffin, J.; Olefsky, J.M. Mechanisms of insulin resistance in aging. *J. Clin. Investig.* **1983**, *71*, 1523–1535. [CrossRef] [PubMed]

102. Lu-Yao, G.; Stukel, T.A.; Yao, S.L. Changing patterns in competing causes of death in men with prostate cancer: A population based study. *J. Urol.* **2004**, *171*, 2285–2290. [CrossRef] [PubMed]

103. WHO Assessment of fracture risk and its application to screening for postmenopausal osteoporosis. Report of a WHO Study Group. *World Health Organ. Technical Rep. Ser.* **1994**, *843*, 1–129.

104. Lee, R.J.; Saylor, P.J.; Smith, M.R. Treatment and prevention of bone complications from prostate cancer. *Bone* **2011**, *48*, 88–95. [CrossRef] [PubMed]

105. Krupski, T.L.; Smith, M.R.; Lee, W.C.; Pashos, C.L.; Brandman, J.; Wang, Q.; Botteman, M.; Litwin, M.S. Natural history of bone complications in men with prostate carcinoma initiating androgen deprivation therapy. *Cancer* **2004**, *101*, 541–549. [CrossRef] [PubMed]

106. Shahinian, V.B.; Kuo, Y.F.; Freeman, J.L.; Goodwin, J.S. Risk of fracture after androgen deprivation for prostate cancer. *N. Engl. J. Med.* **2005**, *352*, 154–164. [CrossRef] [PubMed]

107. Oefelein, M.G.; Ricchiuti, V.; Conrad, W.; Resnick, M.I. Skeletal fractures negatively correlate with overall survival in men with prostate cancer. *J. Urol.* **2002**, *168*, 1005–1007. [CrossRef] [PubMed]

108. Kiratli, B.J.; Srinivas, S.; Perkash, I.; Terris, M.K. Progressive decrease in bone density over 10 years of androgen deprivation therapy in patients with prostate cancer. *Urology* **2001**, *57*, 127–132. [CrossRef] [PubMed]

109. Greenspan, S.L.; Coates, P.; Sereika, S.M.; Nelson, J.B.; Trump, D.L.; Resnick, N.M. Bone loss after initiation of androgen deprivation therapy in patients with prostate cancer. *J. Clin. Endocrinol. Metab.* **2005**, *90*, 6410–6417. [CrossRef] [PubMed]

110. Morote, J.; Orsola, A.; Abascal, J.M.; Planas, J.; Trilla, E.; Raventos, C.X.; Cecchini, L.; Encabo, G.; Reventos, J. Bone mineral density changes in patients with prostate cancer during the first 2 years of androgen suppression. *J. Urol.* **2006**, *175*, 1679–1683. [CrossRef] [PubMed]

111. Wadhwa, V.K.; Weston, R.; Mistry, R.; Parr, N.J. Long-term changes in bone mineral density and predicted fracture risk in patients receiving androgen-deprivation therapy for prostate cancer, with stratification of treatment based on presenting values. *BJU Int.* **2009**, *104*, 800–805. [CrossRef] [PubMed]

112. Lloyd, K.B.; Hornsby, L.B. Complementary and alternative medications for women's health issues. *Nutr. Clin. Prac.* **2009**, *24*, 589–608. [CrossRef]

113. Dennehy, C.E. The use of herbs and dietary supplements in gynecology: An evidence-based review. *J. Midwifery Women's Health* **2006**, *51*, 402–409. [CrossRef]

114. Seidlova-Wuttke, D.; Eder, N.; Stahnke, V.; Kammann, M.; Stecher, G.; Haunschild, J.; Wessels, J.T.; Wuttke, W. Cimicifuga racemosa and its triterpene-saponins prevent the Metabolic Syndrome and deterioration of cartilage in the knee joint of ovariectomized rats by similar mechanisms. *Phytomedicine* **2012**, *19*, 846–853. [CrossRef]

115. Mahon, S.M.; Kaplan, M. Placebo effect in hot flush research. *Lancet Oncol.* **2012**, *13*, 188. [CrossRef]

116. Wuttke, W.; Gorkow, C.; Seidlova-Wuttke, D. Effects of black cohosh (*Cimicifuga racemosa*) on bone turnover, vaginal mucosa, and various blood parameters in postmenopausal women: A double-blind, placebo-controlled, and conjugated estrogens-controlled study. *Menopause* **2006**, *13*, 185–196. [CrossRef]

117. Seidlova-Wuttke, D.; Jarry, H.; Pitzel, L.; Wuttke, W. Effects of estradiol-17beta, testosterone and a black cohosh preparation on bone and prostate in orchidectomized rats. *Maturitas* **2005**, *51*, 177–186. [CrossRef]

118. Dueregger, A.; Guggenberger, F.; Barthelmes, J.; Stecher, G.; Schuh, M.; Intelmann, D.; Abel, G.; Haunschild, J.; Klocker, H.; Ramoner, R.; *et al.* Attenuation of nucleoside and anti-cancer nucleoside analog drug uptake in prostate cancer cells by Cimicifuga racemosa extract BNO-1055. *Phytomedicine* **2013**, *20*, 1306–1314. [CrossRef]

119. Molina-Arcas, M.; Casado, F.J.; Pastor-Anglada, M. Nucleoside transporter proteins. *Curr. Vasc. Pharmacol.* **2009**, *7*, 426–434. [CrossRef]

120. Cheema, D.; Coomarasamy, A.; El-Toukhy, T. Non-hormonal therapy of post-menopausal vasomotor symptoms: A structured evidence-based review. *Arch. Gynecol. Obstet.* **2007**, *276*, 463–469. [CrossRef]

121. Wiklund, I.K.; Mattsson, L.A.; Lindgren, R.; Limoni, C. Effects of a standardized ginseng extract on quality of life and physiological parameters in symptomatic postmenopausal women: A double-blind, placebo-controlled trial. Swedish Alternative Medicine Group. *Int. J. Clin. Pharmacol. Res.* **1999**, *19*, 89–99.

122. Nag, S.A.; Qin, J.J.; Wang, W.; Wang, M.H.; Wang, H.; Zhang, R. Ginsenosides as Anticancer Agents: *In vitro* and *in vivo* Activities, Structure-Activity Relationships, and Molecular Mechanisms of Action. *Front. Pharmacol.* **2012**, *3*, 25. [CrossRef]

123. Wang, Z.; Wang, J.; Chan, P. Treating type 2 diabetes mellitus with traditional chinese and Indian medicinal herbs. *Evid. Based Complement. Altern. Med.* **2013**, *2013*. [CrossRef]

124. Rahman, K.; Lowe, G.M. Garlic and cardiovascular disease: A critical review. *J. Nutr.* **2006**, *136*, 736–740.

125. Rabito, M.J.; Kaye, A.D. Complementary and alternative medicine and cardiovascular disease: An evidence-based review. *Evid. Based Complement. Altern. Med.* **2013**, *2013*. [CrossRef]

126. Smith, M.R.; Malkowicz, S.B.; Chu, F.; Forrest, J.; Sieber, P.; Barnette, K.G.; Rodriquez, D.; Steiner, M.S. Toremifene improves lipid profiles in men receiving androgen-deprivation therapy for prostate cancer: Interim analysis of a multicenter phase III study. *J. Clin. Oncol.* **2008**, *26*, 1824–1829. [CrossRef]

127. Smith, M.R.; Morton, R.A.; Barnette, K.G.; Sieber, P.R.; Malkowicz, S.B.; Rodriguez, D.; Hancock, M.L.; Steiner, M.S. Toremifene to reduce fracture risk in men receiving androgen deprivation therapy for prostate cancer. *J. Urol.* **2013**, *189*, 45–50. [CrossRef]

128. Kearns, A.E.; Northfelt, D.W.; Dueck, A.C.; Atherton, P.J.; Dakhil, S.R.; Rowland, K.M., Jr.; Fuloria, J.; Flynn, P.J.; Dentchev, T.; Loprinzi, C.L. Osteoporosis prevention in prostate cancer patients receiving androgen ablation therapy: Placebo-controlled double-blind study of estradiol and risedronate: N01C8. *Support. Care Cancer* **2010**, *18*, 321–328. [CrossRef]

129. Wibowo, E.; Schellhammer, P.; Wassersug, R.J. Role of estrogen in normal male function: Clinical implications for patients with prostate cancer on androgen deprivation therapy. *J. Urol.* **2011**, *185*, 17–23. [CrossRef]

130. Treatment and survival of patients with cancer of the prostate. The Veterans Administration Co-operative Urological Research Group. *Surg. Gynecol. Obstet.* **1967**, *124*, 1011–1017.

131. Byar, D.P.; Corle, D.K. Hormone therapy for prostate cancer: Results of the Veterans Administration Cooperative Urological Research Group studies. *NCI Monographs* **1987**, *7*, 165–170.

132. Murkies, A.L.; Wilcox, G.; Davis, S.R. Clinical review 92: Phytoestrogens. *J. Clin. Endocrinol. Metab.* **1998**, *83*, 297–303.

133. Turner, J.V.; Agatonovic-Kustrin, S.; Glass, B.D. Molecular aspects of phytoestrogen selective binding at estrogen receptors. *J. Pharm. Sci.* **2007**, *96*, 1879–1885. [CrossRef]

134. Dahlman-Wright, K.; Cavailles, V.; Fuqua, S.A.; Jordan, V.C.; Katzenellenbogen, J.A.; Korach, K.S.; Maggi, A.; Muramatsu, M.; Parker, M.G.; Gustafsson, J.A. International Union of Pharmacology. LXIV. Estrogen receptors. *Pharmacol. Rev.* **2006**, *58*, 773–781. [CrossRef]

135. Khosla, S.; Melton, L.J.; Riggs, B.L. The unitary model for estrogen deficiency and the pathogenesis of osteoporosis: Is a revision needed? *J. Bone Miner. Res.* **2011**, *26*, 441–451. [CrossRef]

136. De Kleijn, M.J.; van der Schouw, Y.T.; Wilson, P.W.; Adlercreutz, H.; Mazur, W.; Grobbee, D.E.; Jacques, P.F. Intake of dietary phytoestrogens is low in postmenopausal women in the United States: The Framingham study(1–4). *J. Nutr.* **2001**, *131*, 1826–1832.

137. Jemal, A.; Siegel, R.; Ward, E.; Hao, Y.; Xu, J.; Murray, T.; Thun, M.J. Cancer statistics, 2008. *Cancer J. Clin.* **2008**, *58*, 71–96. [CrossRef]

138. Villegas, R.; Gao, Y.T.; Yang, G.; Li, H.L.; Elasy, T.A.; Zheng, W.; Shu, X.O. Legume and soy food intake and the incidence of type 2 diabetes in the Shanghai Women's Health Study. *Am. J. Clin. Nutr.* **2008**, *87*, 162–167.

139. Huang, Y.; Cao, S.; Nagamani, M.; Anderson, K.E.; Grady, J.J.; Lu, L.J. Decreased circulating levels of tumor necrosis factor-alpha in postmenopausal women during consumption of soy-containing isoflavones. *J. Clin. Endocrinol. Metab.* **2005**, *90*, 3956–3962. [CrossRef]

140. Sharma, P.; Wisniewski, A.; Braga-Basaria, M.; Xu, X.; Yep, M.; Denmeade, S.; Dobs, A.S.; DeWeese, T.; Carducci, M.; Basaria, S. Lack of an effect of high dose isoflavones in men with prostate cancer undergoing androgen deprivation therapy. *J. Urol.* **2009**, *182*, 2265–2272. [CrossRef]

141. Fairweather-Tait, S.J.; Bao, Y.; Broadley, M.R.; Collings, R.; Ford, D.; Hesketh, J.E.; Hurst, R. Selenium in human health and disease. *Antioxid. Redox signal.* **2011**, *14*, 1337–1383. [CrossRef]

142. Steinbrenner, H.; Sies, H. Protection against reactive oxygen species by selenoproteins. *Biochim. Biophys. Acta* **2009**, *1790*, 1478–1485. [CrossRef]

143. Holvoet, P. Relations between metabolic syndrome, oxidative stress and inflammation and cardiovascular disease. *Verhandelingen* **2008**, *70*, 193–219.

144. Yang, M.; Sytkowski, A.J. Differential expression and androgen regulation of the human selenium-binding protein gene hSP56 in prostate cancer cells. *Cancer Res.* **1998**, *58*, 3150–3153.

145. Clark, L.C.; Dalkin, B.; Krongrad, A.; Combs G.F., Jr.; Turnbull, B.W.; Slate, E.H.; Witherington, R.; Herlong, J.H.; Janosko, E.; Carpenter, D.; et al. Decreased incidence of prostate cancer with selenium supplementation: Results of a double-blind cancer prevention trial. *Br. J. Urol.* **1998**, *81*, 730–734. [CrossRef]

146. Yoshizawa, K.; Willett, W.C.; Morris, S.J.; Stampfer, M.J.; Spiegelman, D.; Rimm, E.B.; Giovannucci, E. Study of prediagnostic selenium level in toenails and the risk of advanced prostate cancer. *J. Nat. Cancer Inst.* **1998**, *90*, 1219–1224. [CrossRef]

147. Duffield-Lillico, A.J.; Dalkin, B.L.; Reid, M.E.; Turnbull, B.W.; Slate, E.H.; Jacobs, E.T.; Marshall, J.R.; Clark, L.C. Selenium supplementation, baseline plasma selenium status and incidence of prostate cancer: An analysis of the complete treatment period of the Nutritional Prevention of Cancer Trial. *BJU Int.* **2003**, *91*, 608–612. [CrossRef]

148. Rayman, M.P.; Stranges, S. Epidemiology of selenium and type 2 diabetes: Can we make sense of it? *Free Radic. Biol. Med.* **2013**, *65*, 1557–1564.

149. Savini, I.; Catani, M.V.; Evangelista, D.; Gasperi, V.; Avigliano, L. Obesity-associated oxidative stress: Strategies finalized to improve redox state. *Int J. Mol. Sci.* **2013**, *14*, 10497–10538. [CrossRef]

150. Hassanzadeh, M.; Faridhosseini, R.; Mahini, M.; Faridhosseini, F.; Ranjbar, A. Serum Levels of TNF-, IL-6, and Selenium in Patients with Acute and Chronic Coronary Artery Disease. *Iran. J. Immunol.* **2006**, *3*, 142–145.

151. Zhang, Y.; Chen, X. Reducing selenoprotein P expression suppresses adipocyte differentiation as a result of increased preadipocyte inflammation. *Am. J. Physiol. Endocrinol. Metab.* **2011**, *300*, 77–85. [CrossRef]

152. Steinbrenner, H.; Speckmann, B.; Pinto, A.; Sies, H. High selenium intake and increased diabetes risk: Experimental evidence for interplay between selenium and carbohydrate metabolism. *J. Clin. Biochem. Nutr.* **2011**, *48*, 40–45. [CrossRef]

153. Steinbrenner, H. Interference of selenium and selenoproteins with the insulin-regulated carbohydrate and lipid metabolism. *Free Radic. Biol. Med.* **2013**, *65*, 1538–1547. [CrossRef]

154. Quiner, T.E.; Nakken, H.L.; Mason, B.A.; Lephart, E.D.; Hancock, C.R.; Christensen, M.J. Soy content of basal diets determines the effects of supplemental selenium in male mice. *J. Nutr.* **2011**, *141*, 2159–2165. [CrossRef]

155. Simopoulos, A.P. Essential fatty acids in health and chronic disease. *Am. J. Clin. Nutr.* **1999**, *70*, 560–569.

156. Nettleton, J.A. *Omega-3 Fatty Acids and Health*; Springer US: New York, NY, USA, 1995; pp. 64–76.

157. Heinze, V.M.; Actis, A.B. Dietary conjugated linoleic acid and long-chain *n*-3 fatty acids in mammary and prostate cancer protection: A review. *Int. J. Food Sci. Nutr.* **2012**, *63*, 66–78. [CrossRef]

158. Tziomalos, K.; Athyros, V.G.; Mikhailidis, D.P. Fish oils and vascular disease prevention: An update. *Curr. Med. Chem.* **2007**, *14*, 2622–2628. [CrossRef]

159. Carpentier, Y.A.; Portois, L.; Malaisse, W.J. n-3 fatty acids and the metabolic syndrome. *Am. J. Clin. Nutr.* **2006**, *83*, 1499–1504.

160. Barre, D.E. The role of consumption of alpha-linolenic, eicosapentaenoic and docosahexaenoic acids in human metabolic syndrome and type 2 diabetes–a mini-review. *J. Oleo Sci.* **2007**, *56*, 319–325. [CrossRef]

161. Chen, Y.Q.; Edwards, I.J.; Kridel, S.J.; Thornburg, T.; Berquin, I.M. Dietary fat-gene interactions in cancer. *Cancer Metastasis Rev.* **2007**, *26*, 535–551. [CrossRef]

162. Ballantyne, C.M.; Bays, H.E.; Kastelein, J.J.; Stein, E.; Isaacsohn, J.L.; Braeckman, R.A.; Soni, P.N. Efficacy and safety of eicosapentaenoic acid ethyl ester (AMR101) therapy in statin-treated patients with persistent high triglycerides (from the ANCHOR study). *Am. J. Cardiol.* **2012**, *110*, 984–992. [CrossRef]

163. Bays, H.E.; Ballantyne, C.M.; Kastelein, J.J.; Isaacsohn, J.L.; Braeckman, R.A.; Soni, P.N. Eicosapentaenoic acid ethyl ester (AMR101) therapy in patients with very high triglyceride levels (from the Multi-center, plAcebo-controlled, Randomized, double-blINd, 12-week study with an open-label Extension [MARINE] trial). *Am. J. Cardiol.* **2011**, *108*, 682–690. [CrossRef]

164. Connor, W.E. Importance of *n*-3 fatty acids in health and disease. *Am. J. Clin. Nutr.* **2000**, *71*, 171–175.

165. Wang, S.; Wu, J.; Suburu, J.; Gu, Z.; Cai, J.; Axanova, L.S.; Cramer, S.D.; Thomas, M.J.; Perry, D.L.; Edwards, I.J.; *et al.* Effect of dietary polyunsaturated fatty acids on castration-resistant Pten-null prostate cancer. *Carcinogenesis* **2012**, *33*, 404–412. [CrossRef]

166. Friedrichs, W.; Ruparel, S.B.; Marciniak, R.A.; deGraffenried, L. Omega-3 fatty acid inhibition of prostate cancer progression to hormone independence is associated with suppression of mTOR signaling and androgen receptor expression. *Nutr. Cancer* **2011**, *63*, 771–777. [CrossRef]

167. Cavazos, D.A.; Price, R.S.; Apte, S.S.; deGraffenried, L.A. Docosahexaenoic acid selectively induces human prostate cancer cell sensitivity to oxidative stress through modulation of NF-kappaB. *Prostate* **2011**, *71*, 1420–1428. [CrossRef]

168. McEntee, M.F.; Ziegler, C.; Reel, D.; Tomer, K.; Shoieb, A.; Ray, M.; Li, X.; Neilsen, N.; Lih, F.B.; O'Rourke, D.; Whelan, J. Dietary n-3 polyunsaturated fatty acids enhance hormone ablation therapy in androgen-dependent prostate cancer. *Am. J. Pathol.* **2008**, *173*, 229–241. [CrossRef]

169. Epstein, M.M.; Kasperzyk, J.L.; Mucci, L.A.; Giovannucci, E.; Price, A.; Wolk, A.; Hakansson, N.; Fall, K.; Andersson, S.O.; Andren, O. Dietary fatty acid intake and prostate cancer survival in Orebro County, Sweden. *Am. J. Epidemiol.* **2012**, *176*, 240–252. [CrossRef]

170. Aronson, W.J.; Kobayashi, N.; Barnard, R.J.; Henning, S.; Huang, M.; Jardack, P.M.; Liu, B.; Gray, A.; Wan, J.; Konijeti, R.; *et al.* Phase II prospective randomized trial of a low-fat diet with fish oil supplementation in men undergoing radical prostatectomy. *Cancer Prev Res. (Phila)* **2011**, *4*, 2062–2071. [CrossRef]

171. Fradet, V.; Cheng, I.; Casey, G.; Witte, J.S. Dietary omega-3 fatty acids, cyclooxygenase-2 genetic variation, and aggressive prostate cancer risk. *Clin. Cancer Res.* **2009**, *15*, 2559–2566. [CrossRef]

172. Berquin, I.M.; Edwards, I.J.; Chen, Y.Q. Multi-targeted therapy of cancer by omega-3 fatty acids. *Cancer Lett.* **2008**, *269*, 363–377. [CrossRef]

173. Szymanski, K.M.; Wheeler, D.C.; Mucci, L.A. Fish consumption and prostate cancer risk: A review and meta-analysis. *Am. J. Clin. Nutr.* **2010**, *92*, 1223–1233. [CrossRef]

174. Nelson, T.L.; Stevens, J.R.; Hickey, M.S. Inflammatory markers are not altered by an eight week dietary alpha-linolenic acid intervention in healthy abdominally obese adult males and females. *Cytokine* **2007**, *38*, 101–106. [CrossRef]

175. Thies, F.; Miles, E.A.; Nebe-von-Caron, G.; Powell, J.R.; Hurst, T.L.; Newsholme, E.A.; Calder, P.C. Influence of dietary supplementation with long-chain *n*-3 or *n*-6 polyunsaturated fatty acids on blood inflammatory cell populations and functions and on plasma soluble adhesion molecules in healthy adults. *Lipids* **2001**, *36*, 1183–1193. [CrossRef]

176. Zhao, G.; Etherton, T.D.; Martin, K.R.; West, S.G.; Gillies, P.J.; Kris-Etherton, P.M. Dietary alpha-linolenic acid reduces inflammatory and lipid cardiovascular risk factors in hypercholesterolemic men and women. *J. Nutr.* **2004**, *134*, 2991–2997.

177. Pot, G.K.; Geelen, A.; Majsak-Newman, G.; Harvey, L.J.; Nagengast, F.M.; Witteman, B.J.; van de Meeberg, P.C.; Hart, A.R.; Schaafsma, G.; Lund, E.K.; *et al.* Increased consumption of fatty and lean fish reduces serum C-reactive protein concentrations but not inflammation markers in feces and in colonic biopsies. *J. Nutr.* **2010**, *140*, 371–376. [CrossRef]

178. Micallef, M.A.; Garg, M.L. Anti-inflammatory and cardioprotective effects of n-3 polyunsaturated fatty acids and plant sterols in hyperlipidemic individuals. *Atherosclerosis* **2009**, *204*, 476–482. [CrossRef]

179. Kelley, D.S.; Siegel, D.; Fedor, D.M.; Adkins, Y.; Mackey, B.E. DHA supplementation decreases serum C-reactive protein and other markers of inflammation in hypertriglyceridemic men. *J. Nutr.* **2009**, *139*, 495–501. [CrossRef]

180. Geelen, A.; Brouwer, I.A.; Schouten, E.G.; Kluft, C.; Katan, M.B.; Zock, P.L. Intake of n-3 fatty acids from fish does not lower serum concentrations of C-reactive protein in healthy subjects. *Eur. J. Clin. Nutr.* **2004**, *58*, 1440–1442. [CrossRef]

181. Vega-Lopez, S.; Kaul, N.; Devaraj, S.; Cai, R.Y.; German, B.; Jialal, I. Supplementation with omega3 polyunsaturated fatty acids and all-rac alpha-tocopherol alone and in combination failed to exert an anti-inflammatory effect in human volunteers. *Metabolism* **2004**, *53*, 236–240. [CrossRef]

182. Damsgaard, C.T.; Frokiaer, H.; Andersen, A.D.; Lauritzen, L. Fish oil in combination with high or low intakes of linoleic acid lowers plasma triacylglycerols but does not affect other cardiovascular risk markers in healthy men. *J. Nutr.* **2008**, *138*, 1061–1066.

183. Yusof, H.M.; Miles, E.A.; Calder, P. Influence of very long-chain *n-3* fatty acids on plasma markers of inflammation in middle-aged men. *Prostaglandins Leukot Essent Fatty Acids* **2008**, *78*, 219–228. [CrossRef]

184. Pot, G.K.; Brouwer, I.A.; Enneman, A.; Rijkers, G.T.; Kampman, E.; Geelen, A. No effect of fish oil supplementation on serum inflammatory markers and their interrelationships: A randomized controlled trial in healthy, middle-aged individuals. *Eur. J. Clin. Nutr.* **2009**, *63*, 1353–1359. [CrossRef]

185. Fujioka, S.; Hamazaki, K.; Itomura, M.; Huan, M.; Nishizawa, H.; Sawazaki, S.; Kitajima, I.; Hamazaki, T. The effects of eicosapentaenoic acid-fortified food on inflammatory markers in healthy subjects—A randomized, placebo-controlled, double-blind study. *J. Nutr. Sci. Vitaminol.* **2006**, *52*, 261–265. [CrossRef]

186. Carayol, M.; Grosclaude, P.; Delpierre, C. Prospective studies of dietary alpha-linolenic acid intake and prostate cancer risk: A meta-analysis. *Cancer Causes Control* **2010**, *21*, 347–355. [CrossRef]

187. Ma, R.W.; Chapman, K. A systematic review of the effect of diet in prostate cancer prevention and treatment. *J. Hum. Nutr Diet.* **2009**, *22*, 187–199. [CrossRef]

188. Chua, M.E.; Sio, M.C.; Sorongon, M.C.; Dy, J.S. Relationship of dietary intake of omega-3 and omega-6 Fatty acids with risk of prostate cancer development: A meta-analysis of prospective studies and review of literature. *Prostate Cancer* **2012**, *2012*. [CrossRef]

189. Chua, M.E.; Sio, M.C.; Sorongon, M.C.; Morales, M.L., Jr. The relevance of serum levels of long chain omega-3 polyunsaturated fatty acids and prostate cancer risk: A meta-analysis. *Can.Urol. Assoc. J.* **2013**, *7*, 333–343.

190. Larsson, S.C.; Kumlin, M.; Ingelman-Sundberg, M.; Wolk, A. Dietary long-chain *n*-3 fatty acids for the prevention of cancer: A review of potential mechanisms. *Am. J. Clin. Nutr.* **2004**, *79*, 935–945.

191. Ngo, T.H.; Barnard, R.J.; Cohen, P.; Freedland, S.; Tran, C.; deGregorio, F.; Elshimali, Y.I.; Heber, D.; Aronson, W.J. Effect of isocaloric low-fat diet on human LAPC-4 prostate cancer xenografts in severe combined immunodeficient mice and the insulin-like growth factor axis. *Clin. Cancer Res.* **2003**, *9*, 2734–2743.

192. Kobayashi, N.; Barnard, R.J.; Said, J.; Hong-Gonzalez, J.; Corman, D.M.; Ku, M.; Doan, N.B.; Gui, D.; Elashoff, D.; Cohen, P.; *et al.* Effect of low-fat diet on development of prostate cancer and Akt phosphorylation in the Hi-Myc transgenic mouse model. *Cancer Res.* **2008**, *68*, 3066–3073. [CrossRef]

193. Berquin, I.M.; Min, Y.; Wu, R.; Wu, J.; Perry, D.; Cline, J.M.; Thomas, M.J.; Thornburg, T.; Kulik, G.; Smith, A.; *et al.* Modulation of prostate cancer genetic risk by omega-3 and omega-6 fatty acids. *J. Clin. Investig.* **2007**, *117*, 1866–1875. [CrossRef]

194. De Marzo, A.M.; Platz, E.A.; Sutcliffe, S.; Xu, J.; Gronberg, H.; Drake, C.G.; Nakai, Y.; Isaacs, W.B.; Nelson, W.G. Inflammation in prostate carcinogenesis. *Nat. Rev. Cancer* **2007**, *7*, 256–269. [CrossRef]

195. Chan, J.M.; Gann, P.H.; Giovannucci, E.L. Role of diet in prostate cancer development and progression. *J. Clin. Oncol.* **2005**, *23*, 8152–8160. [CrossRef]

196. Datta, M.; Schwartz, G.G. Calcium and vitamin D supplementation during androgen deprivation therapy for prostate cancer: A critical review. *Oncologist* **2012**, *17*, 1171–1179. [CrossRef]

197. Cosman, F.; de Beur, S.J.; LeBoff, M.S.; Lewiecki, E.M.; Tanner, B.; Randall, S.; Lindsay, R. Clinician's Guide to Prevention and Treatment of Osteoporosis. *Osteoporos. Int.* **2014**, *25*, 2359–2381. [CrossRef]

198. Planas, J.; Morote, J.; Orsola, A.; Salvador, C.; Trilla, E.; Cecchini, L.; Raventos, C.X. The relationship between daily calcium intake and bone mineral density in men with prostate cancer. *BJU Int.* **2007**, *99*, 812–816. [CrossRef]

199. Ryan, C.W.; Huo, D.; Stallings, J.W.; Davis, R.L.; Beer, T.M.; McWhorter, L.T. Lifestyle factors and duration of androgen deprivation affect bone mineral density of patients with prostate cancer during first year of therapy. *Urology* **2007**, *70*, 122–126. [CrossRef]

200. Mata-Granados, J.M.; Cuenca-Acebedo, R.; Luque de Castro, M.D.; Quesada Gomez, J.M. Lower vitamin E serum levels are associated with osteoporosis in early postmenopausal women: A cross-sectional study. *J. Bone Miner. Metab.* **2013**, *31*, 455–460. [CrossRef]

201. Nieman, L.K. Management of surgically hypogonadal patients unable to take sex hormone replacement therapy. *Endocrinol. Metab. Clin. N. Am.* **2003**, *32*, 325–336. [CrossRef]

202. Steinhubl, S.R. Why have antioxidants failed in clinical trials? *Am. J. Cardiol.* **2008**, *101*, 14–19. [CrossRef]

9

The Role of Dietary Fat throughout the Prostate Cancer Trajectory

Katie M. Di Sebastiano and Marina Mourtzakis *

Department of Kinesiology, University of Waterloo, 200 University Avenue W., Waterloo, ON N2L 3G1, Canada; kmdiseba@uwaterloo.ca
* Author to whom correspondence should be addressed; mmourtzakis@uwaterloo.ca

Abstract: Prostate cancer is the second most common cancer diagnosed world-wide; however, patients demonstrate exceptionally high survival rates. Many lifestyle factors, including obesity and diet, are considered risk factors for advanced prostate cancer. Dietary fat is a fundamental contributor to obesity and may be specifically important for prostate cancer patients. Prostate cancer treatment can result in changes in body composition, affecting quality of life for survivors by increasing the risk of co-morbidities, like cardiovascular disease and diabetes. We aim to examine dietary fat throughout the prostate cancer treatment trajectory, including risk, cancer development and survivorship. Focusing on one specific nutrient throughout the prostate cancer trajectory provides a unique perspective of dietary fat in prostate cancer and the mechanisms that may exacerbate prostate cancer risk, progression and recurrence. Through this approach, we noted that high intake of dietary fat, especially, high intake of animal and saturated fats, may be associated with increased prostate cancer risk. In contrast, a low-fat diet, specifically low in saturated fat, may be beneficial for prostate cancer survivors by reducing tumor angiogenesis and cancer recurrence. The insulin-like growth factor (IGF)/Akt signaling pathway appears to be the key pathway moderating dietary fat intake and prostate cancer development and progression.

Keywords: risk; progression; survivorship; IGF signaling; saturated fatty acids; monounsaturated fatty acids; polyunsaturated fatty acids; trans fatty acids

1. Introduction

Prostate cancer is the second most commonly diagnosed malignancy in men worldwide. Prostate cancer diagnoses accounts for 15% of all male cancer diagnoses, second to only lung cancer [1,2]. In 2012, more than 1.1 million prostate cancer cases were diagnosed worldwide [1,2]; however, prostate cancer mortality rates are exceptionally low, with only 307,000 prostate cancer deaths estimated in 2012, accounting for only 6.6% of male deaths. [1]. This remarkably low mortality rate is attributed to the wide-spread use of prostate-specific antigen (PSA) screening in most developed countries where the incidence of prostate cancer is higher. PSA screening allows the detection of smaller and earlier stage tumors that may or may not progress to more advanced cancer. Because of the growing incidence of prostate cancer and the low death rates, prevention of prostate cancer and, specifically, aggressive and advanced prostate cancer is of the utmost importance. Many lifestyle factors, such as obesity, diet, physical activity levels and smoking, are considered risk factors in the development of prostate cancer. Consequently, a large body of literature endeavours to elucidate the role of lifestyle factors, including obesity, in prostate cancer risk, development of the tumour and successful survivorship.

Obesity and prostate cancer endure a complex relationship. Obesity is associated with increased incidence of high-risk or aggressive prostate cancer [3]. Additionally, it is associated with increased incidence of prostate cancer recurrence [4], which may be attributed to increased adiposity and reduced muscularity in prostate cancer patients who undergo androgen deprivation therapy (ADT) [5]. One of the potential factors thought to link obesity and prostate cancer is dietary fat intake. Dietary fat is a fundamental contributor to obesity [6] and may help explain the complicated relationship between obesity and prostate cancer. For prostate cancer patients, obesity is not only a potential risk factor, but changes in body composition may affect the quality of life of prostate cancer survivors by increasing the risk of co-morbidities, like cardiovascular disease [7], and by decreasing functional outcomes [8]. Changes in dietary fat intake may help ameliorate some of the negative outcomes associated with changes in body composition in the prostate cancer survivor. Thus, many studies have looked at diet and exercise manipulation to counter the expected increase in adiposity and the loss of muscle. Further consideration into the role of obesity, dietary fat and the prostate cancer trajectory is warranted to help clarify this complex relationship.

The aim of this manuscript is to review the literature examining dietary fat throughout the prostate cancer trajectory, including risk, development and survivorship. The majority of reviews that examine the role of dietary fat in prostate cancer consider many nutrients at one particular time point during the prostate cancer trajectory (*i.e.*, the role of diet in prostate cancer risk). This narrative review will examine and summarize the role of dietary fat in prostate cancer throughout the trajectory to provide a unique and comparative perspective across the time-course of the disease. We also aim to investigate the mechanisms that exacerbate prostate cancer risk, progression and recurrence and how they may be related. Saturated fat, *n*-3 fatty acids and trans-fatty acids will be given special considerations, as these types of dietary fat may be of particular importance for the prostate cancer patient. The perspectives described in this review will facilitate the identification of gaps in the literature and will aid future studies to advance this discipline.

2. Dietary Fat and Prostate Cancer Risk

There are numerous nutritional factors associated with obesity and prostate cancer risk, including positive energy balance [9], red meat and dairy intake [10], saturated fat [11], trans fatty acid intake [12] and total dietary fat intake [11]. Conversely, *n*-3 fatty acids have been identified as having a potentially protective effect against prostate cancer [11]. The earliest identification of dietary fat as a potential risk factor for prostate cancer stems from correlations and case-controls studies; however, the results were mixed, with studies demonstrating positive, negative and no associations between dietary fat and the risk of prostate cancer. These studies are based on the principle that participants moving from countries where the risk of prostate cancer is low, such as Japan, had a significant increase in the risk of developing prostate cancer upon moving to North America [13,14]. These studies hypothesized that increased dietary fat consumption may be driving this relationship [15]; however, they did not quantify dietary fat, nor did they control for confounders, which may affect the association with prostate cancer. Early case-control studies examining dietary fat as a risk factor for prostate cancer also demonstrated mixed results [16–23]. Some of these case-control studies demonstrated positive associations between both dietary and saturated fat intake [16–19], while others found no association between dietary fat intake and prostate cancer diagnosis [20–23]. Early prospective cohort studies also demonstrated mixed results, with some demonstrating no association between high meat and dairy products [24–26] and prostate cancer risk, while animal product intake was positively associated with the risk of prostate cancer, though these associations were weak (relative risk: 1.3–1.5; $p > 0.1$ [27]; relative risk: 1.38, 95% CI: 0.89–2.16) [27,28]. These studies were also limited by the methods used to assess dietary intake. It was not until Giovannucci and colleagues [29] published their prospective analysis of dietary fat and prostate cancer risk using the Health Professionals follow-up study that the relationship between dietary fat and prostate cancer risk began to become clearer. Giovannucci *et al.* [29] used a semi-quantitative food frequency questionnaire to assess dietary fat in these men. They concluded that total fat consumption was related to the risk of advanced cancer and that this relationship was primarily related to animal fat consumption (relative risk: 1.79; 95% CI: 1.04–3.07).

Fat from dairy products, with the exception of butter, appeared to be unrelated to advanced prostate cancer risk.

These early studies formed the basis for much of the current work that has evaluated dietary fat intake as a potential risk factor for prostate cancer. A systematic review by Ma and Chapman [30] indicated that based on the Oxford Centre for Evidenced-Based Medicine Levels of Evidence, there is Level 2b evidence to suggest that dietary fat, and in particular, high intake of animal and saturated fats (~40% total fat intake; [31]), is associated with the increased risk of prostate cancer. Most of the studies evaluated in the systematic review were primarily Level 4 studies (Case series), but also including some Level 2 (prospective comparative) and 3 (retrospective cohort and case-control) studies. Ma and Chapman [30] examined numerous types of fat and identified that there is suggestive evidence to support total fat intake, animal and saturated fat intake, monounsaturated fatty acids and α-linoleic acid as being associated with the increased risk of prostate cancer, while there was not enough evidence to draw conclusions about polyunsaturated fatty acid intake, as well as eicosapentaenoic acid (EPA).

Gathirua-Mwangi and Zhang [32] evaluated the relationship between dietary fat intake and the risk of advanced cancer. Despite the limited number of studies, their conclusions were similar to Ma and Chapman [30], indicating that total fat intake (odds ratios: 1.25–1.80; 95% CI: 0.75–2.91) and, specifically, saturated fat intake are significantly associated with the increased risk of advanced prostate cancer (odds ratios: 1.44–1.80; 95% CI: 0.82–5.20) [32]. When they evaluated the classification of fatty acids, they concluded that monounsaturated and polyunsaturated fatty acids were not associated with the risk of advanced prostate cancer, nor were linoleic and linolenic acids. They also noted that higher animal fat intake was also associated with advanced prostate cancer, and a borderline inverse relationship was noted for total vegetable fat intake and advanced prostate cancer risk. The most recent evidence for this relationship comes from Pelser and colleagues [11]. They suggested that a dichotomous relationship between dietary fat consumption and prostate cancer risk exists. Using data from the NIH-AARP Diet and Health Study, they demonstrated that total fat intake and mono- and poly-unsaturated fats were not associated with the incidence of prostate cancer, but saturated fat increased the risk of advanced prostate cancer (hazards ratio: 1.21; 95% CI: 1.00–1.46) and prostate cancer death (hazards ratio: 1.47; 95% CI: 1.01–2.15). They also noted that EPA was associated with decreased risk of fatal prostate cancer (hazards ratio: 0.82; 95% CI: 0.64–1.04).

Despite the limited number of studies, the systematic reviews cited here indicated some evidence for the increased risk of prostate cancer and, specifically, advanced or fatal prostate cancer with increased dietary fat intake. When evaluating specific categories of fats, saturated and animal fats appear to pose the greatest risk for prostate cancer development, while EPA may have a protective effect. However, more evidence is needed to understand the potential mechanisms that drive the relationship between fat intake and prostate cancer development.

3. Effects of Dietary Fat on Prostate Cancer Development

A number of potential mechanisms have been identified that may mediate the effects of dietary fat on prostate cancer development and progression. These include changes in the insulin-like growth factor (IGF)-Akt pathway, androgen signaling and alterations in cell proliferation and angiogenesis.

3.1. The IGF Signaling Pathway

The IGF signaling pathway is one of the main regulating pathways in which dietary fat can promote prostate cancer development and progression. Dietary fat intake is positively correlated with circulating levels of IGF-1, which may ultimately result in increased signaling through the IGF signaling pathway [33,34]. Fat intake is also negatively correlated with insulin-like growth factor binding protein-3 (IGFBP-3), the major binding protein of IGF-1 in plasma [33,34], which is also independently associated with the risk of prostate cancer [35]. Thus, increases in circulating levels of IGF-1 and decreases in IFGBP-3 can increase the stimulation of the IGF signaling cascade, which becomes disrupted in malignant cells. Given that perturbations in the IGF system play a critical role in cell proliferation, differentiation, apoptosis and transformation, understanding the function of IGF signaling is key to determining the mechanisms of dietary fat in prostate cancer development and proliferation.

In non-malignant cells, IGF-1 binds to one of two receptors, IGF-1R and IGF-2R, with a preference for IGF-1R [36]. IGF-1R is a type 2 tyrosine kinase receptor that, under normal conditions, is involved in proliferation and differentiation; however, in transformed malignant cells, IGF-1R plays a key role in the establishment and progression of cancerous cells [36]. Cells lines without IGF-1R have an impaired ability to transform into malignant cells, though the exact mechanism is unknown [37]. In contrast, the presence of IGF-1R may also contribute to the ability of malignant cells to metastasize [36]. The primary role of IGF-1R cell growth is mediated through the IGF-1R/insulin receptor substrate (IRS)-1 axis. Numerous reviews on the role of the IGF-1R/IRS-1 axis and its role in cancer are available [36–41]. Briefly, when a ligand binds to IGF-1R, it activates the tyrosine kinase of the cytoplasmic domain of the receptor [36]. This results in the phosphorylation of the numerous IGF-1R substrates—IRS-1 and -2 Src- and collagen-homology (SHC) and growth factor receptor protein 2 (Grb2) [38–41]. The phosphorylated IRS and SHC in combination with Grb2 activate the mitogen-activated protein kinase (MAPK) cascade, resulting in cell growth and proliferation [38–41]. IRS-1 also phosphorylates phosphatidylinositol 3′-kinase (PI3K) and the Akt complex, which blocks Bad and Caspase 9, which are key pro-apoptotic proteins [38–41]. These pathways help regulate the metabolic and anti-apoptotic signal of IGF-1 [38–41]. Akt can also activate the transcription of nuclear factor-κB (NFκB) and mammalian target of rapamycin (mTOR). When NFκB is active in healthy cells, it functions as a regulator for many genes that control proliferation and cell survival; in cancerous cells, it is dysregulated, resulting in decreased cell death [38–41]. Akt activation promotes signaling in the IGF-1R/IRS-1 axis, which contributes to the dysregulation of NFκB and, ultimately, cancer cell growth. The IGF-1R/IRS-1 axis also indirectly increases mTOR activity [38–41]. mTOR then promotes cell growth through the S6kinase, Protein Kinase C (PKC), p21 and Glycogen Synthase Kinase 3β (GSK3β) activation [38]. These pathways change the cell cycle, ultimately promoting cell growth. Thus, increased dietary fat intake may potentially promote malignant cell growth through increased IGF-1 and decreased IGFBP-3, resulting in increased IGF-1 signaling through the IGF-1R, a receptor implicated in the transformation of healthy cells to cancerous cells and a mediator of cell growth through the IGF-1R/IRS-1 axis.

3.2. Increases in Androgen Signaling Due to Dietary Fat Intake

Along with IGF-1 signaling, androgen signaling is another pathway in which dietary fat intake can influence prostate cancer development. Some have demonstrated that decreased dietary fat intake is associated with decreased androgen [42,43] and testosterone levels [44–46], which subsequently improves signaling mediated through the IGF-1 signaling pathway. Androgens play a key role in the development of normal healthy prostate tissue; however, androgen signaling and, specifically, the androgen receptor, also known as nuclear receptor subfamily 3, group C, member 4, (NR3C4), is the principle stimulant of prostate cancer progression. In the early stages of development, malignant prostate cancer cells require androgen stimulation for growth [47]. However, increased androgen receptor growth is associated with the progression or switch of hormone sensitive cancers to hormone-resistant cancers, the more aggressive form of prostate cancer [47,48]. Androgens stimulate prostate cancer cell growth via the Erk-2 pathway, where Erk-2 activation increases the androgen receptor complex content in the prostate cells [49]. Androgens also increase IGF-1R expression [50], which is associated with prostate cancer development, as previously described, but IGF-1 can also have a more direct effect on the androgen receptor. Stimulation of the IGF-1 signaling cascade activates MAPK, which decreases the acetylation of heat shock protein (HSP) 90. HSP90 is a chaperone protein of the androgen receptor [51]. This decreased acetylation increases the association of the HSP90 with the androgen receptor, which further stimulates the signaling through the androgen receptor pathway. Ultimately, stimulation of this pathway results in upregulation of the androgen receptors, their associated proteins and androgen receptor regulated genes. High-fat diets have been shown to increase stimulation through the IGF-1 axis [33,34], as well as being associated with increased androgen and testosterone levels [42–46]. Diets low in total and saturated fat and high in *n*-3 fatty acids counter this pathway by inhibiting IGF-1 binding and decreasing HSP90 association with the androgen receptor [52]. Consequently, there is increased acetylation of androgen receptors resulting in their degradation, ultimately reducing androgen receptor proteins, as well as the number of androgen receptor-regulated genes.

3.3. Dietary Fat Mediation of Cell Proliferation and Angiogenesis

While total dietary fat and saturated fat intake have not been shown to have a direct effect in the cell cycle and angiogenesis, *n*-3 fatty acid intake has been shown to inhibit malignant cell proliferation and angiogenesis [53]. *n*-3 fatty acids work both intrinsically (mitochondrial pathway) and extrinsically (death receptor pathway) to induce apoptosis. Specifically, they can inhibit PI3K activity, which phosphorylates the Akt complex. Phosphorylated Akt regulates a number of downstream factors that can directly affect apoptosis and the cell cycle. Briefly, phosphorylated Akt inhibits caspase 9 and pro-apoptotic proteins Bad and BAK, leading to decreased apoptosis; inhabitation of these pathways via *n*-3 fatty acids ultimately results in increased cell death. Phosphorylated Akt also increases p27 and inactivates NFκB signaling, which can independently and directly halt the cell cycle. Thus, *n*-3 fatty acids may have an important role in inhibiting malignant cell proliferation and angiogenesis.

Total dietary fat and saturated fat may work indirectly to enhance cell proliferation and angiogenesis through the creation of reactive oxygen species (ROS) [54]. ROS generated endogenously and externally are associated with cancer progression by inducing a number of neoplastic transformations. ROS alter the conformational structure of the p53 protein, resulting in changes in protein behaviour and causing a mutated phenotype. These types of p53 mutations are specifically important in prostate cancer progression. Total dietary fat, especially *n*-6 fatty acids, as well as androgens can all serve as oxidants directly increasing oxidative stress and altering a number of transcription factors. Oxidative stress has been shown to be higher in the benign epithelium of men with prostate cancer when compared to men without prostate cancer [54], while Lee *et al.* [55] demonstrated that inactivation of glutathione-s-transferase pi, a pro-oxidant scavenging enzyme, is critical in the development of prostate cancer carcinogenesis. Specifically, dietary fat consumption may contribute to the carcinogenesis of prostate tissue via lipid peroxidation [56], thus resulting in increased oxidative stress.

The relationship between dietary fat, cell proliferation and angiogenesis is less direct than some of the other relationships previously described in this review. There is little evidence to suggest that total and saturated fat intake play any part in malignant cell proliferation and angiogenesis. Dietary fat may be working though secondary pathways, such as ROS generation, to stimulate proliferation and angiogenesis. More research in these areas is needed to elucidate this complex relationship.

4. Fatty Acid Type and Its Relationship with Prostate Cancer

While there are many proposed mechanisms through which dietary fat may affect prostate cancer development and progression, much of the literature examining prostate cancer and dietary fat intake lacks a definite conclusion as to the negative impact of dietary fat in prostate cancer. This discrepancy may be, in part, attributed to the diverse physiological effects of different types and distributions of dietary fats; thus, an evaluation of total dietary fat intake may miss important relationships between specific types of dietary fat intake and prostate cancer development. The direct and indirect roles, as well as the interrelationships between saturated fatty acids (SFA), monounsaturated fatty acids (MUFA), polyunsaturated fatty acids (PUFA) and trans fatty acids (TFA) on prostate cancer development and progression need to be elucidated in future work.

There is diverse epidemiological evidence suggesting that SFA intake is a risk factor for prostate cancer. Some studies show increased risk of prostate cancer risk and progression, while others are inconclusive. Animal models suggest that the quality of dietary fat, and, specifically, the PUFA content of dietary fat intake, may be an important prognosticator [57,58]. Long-chain SFA may negatively affect prostate cancer, while short-chain fatty acids may be beneficial. Escobar *et al.* [59] fed rats two isocaloric low-fat diets, in which only 7% of total calorie content was derived from fat. In one diet, fat was derived from lard and the other from linseed oil, which Vereshagin and Novitskaya [60] identified as: 52%–55% α-linolenic acid, 18:3n-3; ~7% palmitic acid, 16:0; ~4% stearic acid, 18:0; ~18%–23% oleic acid, 18:1n-9; and ~14%–17% linoleic acid, 18:2n-6. The lard-derived diet, which was high in palmitic acid and oleic acid, increased prostate weight, testosterone, cell proliferation and androgen receptor expression, compared to the diet rich in α-linolenic acid. These data support the notion that long-chain SFA may have negative effects on various physiological factors in prostate cancer; however, this has yet to be investigated in humans.

The role of MUFA is less clear than the role of SFA in prostate cancer development and progression. The Mediterranean diet, which is rich in oleic acid (18:1n-9), was originally thought to reduce the risk of prostate cancer [61]; however, this early evidence remains inconclusive, as studies have demonstrated protective [62], no association [63,64] and negative effects of MUFA on prostate cancer [65,66]. As the Mediterranean diet contains a variety of potential protective agents, such as lycopene-rich tomatoes, fish that are high in n-3 fatty acids and low quantities of red meat, it is challenging to pinpoint the role of MUFA.

There is extensive research examining the role of PUFA in prostate cancer. It is reported that n-6 fatty acids increase prostate cancer risk, while n-3 fatty acids decrease prostate cancer risk [57,58]. Specifically, the anti-cancer benefits of a diet with low n-6-to-n-3 fatty acid ratios are supported in the literature [67]. This type of diet is in specific contrast to the Western style diet with a 30:1 ratio of n-6 to n-3 fatty acids [68–71]. The main mechanisms of action seem to converge on the IGF-1 signaling pathway, leading to prevention or inhibition of malignant growth in prostate cancer cells.

Conversely, a limited number of studies have examined the role of TFA in prostate cancer risk and development. Overall, they appear to suggest an increased risk of prostate cancer with increased serum TFA. Previously, Smith *et al.* [72] reviewed the role of TFA in a number of cancers and identified six studies that examined prostate cancer. Bakker *et al.* [73] conducted an ecological study examining the fatty acid component of adipose tissue in 690 participants across eight European countries and Israel and found no significant relationship between TFA levels and risk of prostate cancer. King *et al.* [74] and Chavarro *et al.* [75] used case-control and nested case-control methodologies, respectively, and demonstrated increased risk in prostate cancer with increased levels of the number of different TFA in both serum phospholipids [74] and whole blood [75]. Food frequency questionnaires have also been used to examine TFA intake and prostate cancer risk and have demonstrated the increased risk of advanced cancer [76] and no relationship [77,78]. More recently, Brasky *et al.* [79] demonstrated an inverse risk between serum TFA and high risk prostate cancer and suggested that the relationship between TFA and prostate cancer risk may be more complicated than earlier hypotheses. Interestingly, Laake *et al.* [80] demonstrated that the source of the TFAs may play a significant role in determining risk, as they demonstrated no association between dietary intake levels of TFA from vegetable sources, but increased risk of prostate cancer when the TFA source is a fish source. This evidence is in the very early stages, where data is associative; thus, more research is warranted to identify potential mechanisms in which prostate cancer is affected by TFA intake, as this relationship appears to be more complex than previously thought.

5. Dietary Fat in the Prostate Cancer Survivor

As it is the second most common malignancy diagnosed in men worldwide and because the survival rates are so high [1,2], the number of prostate cancer survivors is constantly increasing. Thus, understanding how manipulating dietary fat may positively influence quality of life in prostate cancer survivorship is important. Another important consideration for prostate cancer survivors is the use of aADT, a common treatment for aggressive prostate cancer, which causes significant loss of skeletal muscle and increases in adipose tissue and has been related to increased risk of cardiovascular disease and diabetes in prostate cancer survivors [7]. However, there is limited data examining dietary fat throughout this stage of the prostate cancer trajectory.

Early reports demonstrate that fat intake, specifically saturated fat intake, may decrease disease-specific survival. Fradet and colleagues [81] followed a group of men diagnosed with prostate cancer for an average of 5.2 years. After controlling for cancer grade, clinical stage, treatment age and total energy intake, men in the lowest tertile of saturated fat intake had a decreased risk of dying from prostate cancer as compared to those in the highest tertile of saturated fat intake (hazards ratio: 3.13; 95% CI: 1.28–7.67). These findings align with the idea that fat intake, specifically saturated fat intake, promotes an environment conducive to prostate cancer growth. While this observational evidence supports the hypothesis that high levels of dietary fat have negative effects on prostate cancer survival, well-designed intervention studies are needed to identify if manipulating dietary fat can have positive effects on survivorship. These interventions should also investigate different sources of dietary fat and their ability to improve quality of life for the prostate cancer survivor by mitigating cancer recurrence, as some literature suggests that plant-based fats may be less harmful than animal-based fats [31,32,59].

Davies and colleagues [82] reviewed the evidence of the effects of low-fat diets on prostate cancer progression and identified five studies that manipulated dietary fat intake in some way to examine the potentially protective effects of these interventions. Ornish *et al.* [83] used a randomized control trial (RCT) design to examine the effect of an entire lifestyle intervention, including low-fat vegan diet supplemented with fish oil and a number of other vitamins and minerals combined with physical activity and stress management techniques, in a group of prostate cancer survivors and examined the effects on the prostate specific antigen (PSA) levels and LNCaP (human prostatic adenocarcinoma) cell growth *in vitro*. This comprehensive lifestyle intervention demonstrated significant improvements for prostate cancer patients *versus* the control group; however, the combined nature of this intervention makes it difficult to discern the individual effects of the lifestyle components (*i.e.*, exercise *vs.* low-fat diet *vs.* stress management techniques). Perhaps the synergistic interactions between these components improve patient outcomes. Two studies have examined the effects of low-fat diets supplemented with flaxseed on prostate cancer outcomes. Demark-Wahnefried *et al.* [84] demonstrated decreased proliferation rates in the men supplemented with flaxseed and that the low-fat diet group had significantly reduced serum cholesterol levels following ~30 days of supplementation. Heymach *et al.* [85] demonstrated that, as compared to the control arm, a low-fat diet, a flaxseed-supplemented diet and a low-fat diet with a flaxseed supplementation for 30 days had each decreased a number of angiogenic factors, though the results were greatest in the low-fat diet alone group. They speculate that the NFκB pathway may be regulating this response. A review by Hori *et al.* [86] supports the hypothesis suggested by the flax-supplemented diet that *n*-3 fatty acid may be beneficial for prostate cancer patients. Like Ornish *et al.* [83], Aronson *et al.* [87] used an RCT design to look at the effects of a four-week low-fat diet intervention as compared to a traditional Western diet on the effects of LNCaP cell growth. Serum for the low-fat diet group decreased the growth of the LNCaP cells as compared to the serum from the men on the Westernized diet. While there appears to be some evidence as to the protective effect of a low-fat diet for prostate cancer survivors, more research is warranted to better elucidate the specific components of these lifestyle interventions that will be most effective for prostate cancer patients.

Androgen Deprivation Therapy and Dietary Fat

ADT is a common treatment for prostate cancer patients; however, its use can have negative consequences for prostate cancer survivors. Specifically, patients undergoing ADT lose skeletal muscle mass and gain fat mass [88]. These changes are associated with increased risk of cardiovascular disease and diabetes [7]. Because of the associated changes in body composition and risk of comorbidities in survivorship, dietary intervention may be useful for prostate cancer patients receiving ADT. However, these considerations are beyond the scope of this review. Saylor and Smith [89] suggest lifestyle intervention, including low-fat diet and increased physical activity and weight control, may be beneficial in the prevention of these comorbidities in men receiving ADT and that future investigations are justified.

6. Conclusions

The aim of this paper was to examine dietary fat throughout the prostate cancer trajectory, including risk, development and survivorship. In most cases, there is limited evidence linking dietary fat and prostate cancer; however, some trends do emerge. Dietary fat, and, in particular, high intake of animal and saturated fats, may be associated with prostate cancer risk. The IGF/Akt signaling pathway appears to be the key signaling pathway moderating malignant cell growth and changes in androgen receptor signaling. The type of fat consumed may mediate the relationship between dietary fat and prostate cancer. Saturated fat and TFA have been negatively associated with prostate cancer development, while PUFA may have a protective effect, though these relationships remain tenuous. For prostate cancer survivors, a diet low in fat and particularly low in saturated fat may be beneficial, as it may reduce tumor angiogenesis and cancer recurrence. Integrating research throughout the prostate cancer trajectory may provide new insights into the relationship between dietary fat intake and prostate cancer, as many of the same pathways are implicated throughout the trajectory. In conclusion, preliminary evidence suggests diets low in fat may be beneficial at any point in the prostate cancer trajectory; however, much more research is needed to elucidate the complex relationships that exist between dietary fat and prostate cancer biology.

Acknowledgments: Katie M. Di Sebastiano is supported by the Constantine Karayannopoulos Graduate Studentship from Prostate Cancer Canada, Grant No. GS2014-04. Support for this review was also provided through a Seed Grant from the Motorcycle Ride for Dad Foundation awarded to Marina Mourtzakis.

Author Contributions: Katie M. Di Sebastiano and Marina Mourtzakis were responsible for the conception, design, information collection, writing and revisions of the manuscript.

References

1. Ferlay, J.; Soerjomataram, I.; Ervik, M.; Dikshit, R.; Eser, S.; Mathers, C.; Rebelo, M.; Parkin, D.M.; Forman, D.; Bray, F. GLOBOVAN 2012 v1.0, Cancer Incidence and Mortality Worldwide: IARC CancerBase No. 11. Available online: http://globocan.iarc.fr/Pages/fact_sheets_cancer.aspx (accessed on 29 September 2014).

2. Bray, F.; Ren, J.S.; Masuyer, E.; Ferlay, J. Estimates of global cancer prevalence for 27 sites in the adult population in 2008. *Int. J. Cancer* **2013**, *132*, 1133–1145. [CrossRef] [PubMed]

3. Discacciati, A.; Orsini, N.; Wolk, A. Body mass index and incidence of localized and advanced prostate cancer—A dose-response meta-analysis of prospective studies. *Ann. Oncol.* **2012**, *23*, 1665–1671. [CrossRef] [PubMed]

4. Cao, Y.; Ma, J. Body mass index, prostate-cancer specific mortality, and biochemical recurrence: A systematic review and meta-analysis. *Cancer Prev. Res. (Phila)* **2011**, *4*, 486–501. [CrossRef]

5. Nguyen, P.L.; Alibhai, S.M.; Basaria, S.; D'Amico, A.V.; Kantoff, P.W.; Keating, N.L.; Penson, D.F.; Rosario, D.J.; Tombal, B.; Smith, M.R. Adverse effects of androgen deprivation therapy and strategies to mitigate them. *Eur. Urol.* **2014**, in press.

6. Bray, G.A.; Popkin, B.M. Dietary fat intake does affect obesity! *Am. J. Clin. Nutr.* **1998**, *68*, 1157–1173. [PubMed]

7. Keating, N.L.; O'Malley, A.J.; Freedland, S.J.; Smith, M.R. Diabetes and cardiovascular disease during androgen deprivation therapy: Observational study of veterans with prostate cancer. *J. Natl. Cancer Inst.* **2010**, *102*, 39–46. [CrossRef] [PubMed]

8. Resnick, M.J.; Koyama, T.; Fan, K.H.; Albertsen, P.C.; Goodman, M.; Hamilton, A.S.; Hoffman, R.M.; Potosky, A.L.; Stanford, J.L.; Stroup, A.M.; *et al.* Long-term functional outcomes after treatment for localized prostate cancer. *N. Engl. J. Med.* **2013**, *368*, 436–445. [CrossRef] [PubMed]

9. Andersson, S.O.; Wolk, A.; Bergstrom, R.; Adami, H.O.; Englholm, G.; Englund, A.; Nyrén, O. Body size and prostate cancer: A 20 year follow-up study among 135006 Swedish construction worker. *J. Natl. Cancer Inst.* **1997**, *5*, 385–389. [CrossRef]

10. Mandair, D.; Rossi, R.E.; Pericleous, M.; Whyand, T.; Caplin, M.E. Prostate cancer and the influence of dietary factors and supplements: A systematic review. *Nutr. Metab. (Lond.)* **2014**, *11*. [CrossRef]

11. Pelser, C.; Mondul, A.M.; Hollenbeck, A.R.; Park, Y. Dietary fatty acids and risk of prostate cancer in the NIH-AARP diet and health study. *Cancer Epidemiol. Biomark. Prev.* **2013**, *22*, 697–707. [CrossRef]

12. Hu, J.; la Vecchia, C.; de Groh, M.; Negri, E.; Morrison, H.; Mery, L. Dietary transfatty acids and cancer risk. *Eur. J. Cancer Prev.* **2011**, *20*, 530–538. [CrossRef] [PubMed]

13. Haenszel, W.; Kurihara, M. Studies of Japanese migrants. I. Mortality from cancer and other disease among Japanese in the United States. *J. Natl. Cancer Inst.* **1968**, *40*, 43–68. [PubMed]

14. Staszewski, W.; Haenszel, W. Cancer mortality among the Polish-born in the United States. *J. Natl. Cancer Inst.* **1965**, *35*, 291–297. [PubMed]

15. Armstrong, B.; Doll, R. Environmental factors and cancer incidence and mortality in different countries, with special reference to dietary practice. *Int. J. Cancer* **1975**, *15*, 617–631. [CrossRef] [PubMed]

16. Graham, S.; Haughey, B.; Marshall, J.; Priore, R.; Byers, T.; Rzepka, T.; Mettlin, C.; Pontes, J.E. Diet in the epidemiology of the carcinoma of the prostate gland. *J. Natl. Cancer Inst.* **1983**, *70*, 687–692. [PubMed]

17. Heshmat, M.Y.; Kaul, L.; Kovi, J.; Jackson, M.A.; Jackson, A.G.; Jones, G.W.; Edson, M.; Enterline, J.P.; Worrell, R.G.; Perry, S.L. Nutrition and prostate cancer: A case-control study. *Prostate* **1985**, *6*, 7–17. [CrossRef] [PubMed]

18. Kolonel, L.N.; Yoshizawa, C.N.; Hankin, J.H. Diet and prostatic cancer: A case-control study in Hawaii. *Am. J. Epidemiol.* **1988**, *127*, 999–1012. [PubMed]

19. West, D.W.; Slattery, M.L.; Robinson, L.M.; French, T.K.; Mahoney, A.W. Adult dietary intake and prostate cancer risk in Utah: A case-control study with special emphasis on aggressive tumors. *Cancer Causes Control* **1991**, *2*, 85–94. [CrossRef]

20. Ross, R.K.; Paganini-Hill, A.; Henderson, B.E. The etiology of prostate cancer: What does the epidemiology suggest? *Prostate* **1983**, *4*, 333–344. [CrossRef] [PubMed]

21. Kaul, L.; Heshmat, M.Y.; Kovi, J.; Jackson, M.A.; Jackson, A.G.; Jones, G.W.; Edson, M.; Enterline, J.P.; Worrell, R.G.; Perry, S.L. The role of diet in prostate cancer. *Nutr. Cancer* **1987**, *9*, 123–128. [CrossRef] [PubMed]

22. Mettlin, C.; Selenskas, S.; Natarajan, N.; Huben, R. Beta-carotene and animal fats an their relationship to prostate cancer risk. A case-control study. *Cancer* **1989**, *64*, 605–612. [CrossRef] [PubMed]

23. Ohno, Y.; Yoshida, O.; Oishi, K.; Okada, K.; Yamabe, H.; Schroeder, F.H. Dietary beta-carotene and cancer of the prostate: A case-control study is Kyoto, Japan. *Cancer Res.* **1988**, *48*, 1331–1336. [PubMed]

24. Hirayama, T. Epidemiology or prostate cancer with special reference to the role of diet. *Natl. Cancer Inst. Monogr.* **1979**, *53*, 149–155. [PubMed]

25. Hsing, A.W.; McLaughlin, J.K.; Schuman, L.M.; Bjelke, E.; Gridley, G.; Wacholder, S.; Chien, H.T.; Blot, W.J. Diet, tobacco use, and fatal prostate cancer: Results from the Lutheran Brotherhood Cohort Study. *Cancer Res.* **1990**, *50*, 6836–6840. [PubMed]

26. Severson, R.K.; Nomura, A.M.; Grove, J.S.; Stemmermann, G.N. A prospective study of demographics, diet, and prostate cancer among men of Japanese ancestry in Hawaii. *Cancer Res.* **1989**, *49*, 1857–1860. [PubMed]

27. Mills, P.K.; Beeson, W.L.; Phillips, R.L.; Fraser, G.E. Cohort study of diet, lifestyle, and prostate cancer in Adventist men. *Cancer* **1989**, *64*, 598–604. [CrossRef] [PubMed]

28. Snowdon, D.A.; Phillips, R.L.; Choi, W. Diet, obesity, and risk of fatal prostate cancer. *Am. J. Epidemiol.* **1984**, *120*, 244–250. [PubMed]

29. Giovannucci, E.; Rimm, E.B.; Colditz, G.A.; Stampfer, M.J.; Ascherio, A.; Chute, C.G.; Willett, W.C. A prospective study of dietary fat and risk of prostate cancer. *J. Natl. Cancer Inst.* **1993**, *85*, 1571–1579. [CrossRef] [PubMed]

30. Ma, R.W.L.; Chapman, K. A systematic review of the effect of diet in prostate cancer prevention and treatment. *J. Hum. Nutr. Diet* **2009**, *22*, 187–199. [CrossRef] [PubMed]

31. Bairati, I.; Meyer, F.; Fradet, Y.; Moore, L. Dietary fat and advanced prostate cancer. *J. Urol.* **1998**, *159*, 1271–1275. [CrossRef] [PubMed]

32. Gathirua-Mwangi, W.G.; Zhang, J. Dietary factors and risk for advanced prostate cancer. *Eur. J. Cancer Prev.* **2014**, *23*, 96–109. [CrossRef] [PubMed]

33. Kaklamani, V.G.; Linos, A.; Kaklamani, E.; Markaki, I.; Koumantaki, Y.; Mantzoros, C.S. Dietary fat and carbohydrates are independently associated with circulating insulin-like growth factor 1 and insulin-like growth factor-binging protein 3 concentrations in healthy adults. *J. Clin. Oncol.* **1999**, *17*, 3291–3298. [PubMed]

34. Holmes, M.D.; Pollack, M.N.; Willett, W.C.; Hankinson, S.E. Dietary correlates of plasma insulin-like growth factor 1 and insulin-like growth factor binding protein 3 concentrations. *Cancer Epidemiol. Biomark. Prev.* **2002**, *11*, 852–861.

35. Rowlands, M.A.; Gunnell, D.; Harris, R.; Vatten, L.J.; Holly, J.M.; Martin, R.M. Circulating insulin-like growth factor peptides and prostate cancer risk: A systematic review and meta-analysis. *Int. J. Cancer* **2009**, *124*, 2416–2429. [CrossRef] [PubMed]

36. Singh, P.; Alex, J.M.; Bast, F. Insulin receptor (IR) and insulin-like-growth factor receptor 1 (IGF-1R) signaling systems: Novel treatment strategies for cancer. *Med. Oncol.* **2014**, *31*, 1–14. [CrossRef]

37. Baserga, R.; Peruzzi, F.; Reiss, K. The IGF-1 receptor in cancer biology. *Int. J. Cancer* **2003**, *107*, 873–877. [CrossRef] [PubMed]

38. Vankateswaran, V.; Klotz, L.H. Diet and prostate cancer: Mechanisms of action and implications for chemoprevention. *Nat. Rev. Urol.* **2010**, *7*, 442–453. [CrossRef] [PubMed]

39. LeRoith, D.; Roberts, C.T., Jr. The insulin-like growth factor system and cancer. *Cancer Lett.* **2003**, *195*, 127–137. [CrossRef] [PubMed]

40. Rubin, R.; Baserga, R. Insulin-like growth factor-1 receptor. Its role in cell proliferation, apoptosis, and tumorigenicity. *Lab. Investig.* **1995**, *73*, 311–331. [PubMed]

41. Pollack, M. Insulin and insulin-like growth factor signaling in neoplasia. *Nat. Rev. Cancer* **2008**, *8*, 915–928. [CrossRef] [PubMed]

42. Hill, P.; Wynder, E.L.; Garbaczewski, L.; Garnes, H.; Walker, A.R. Diet and urinary steroids in black and white North American men and black South African men. *Cancer Res.* **1979**, *39*, 5101–5105. [PubMed]

43. Fleshner, N.; Zlotta, A.R. Prostate cancer prevention: Past present and future. *Cancer* **2007**, *110*, 1889–1899. [CrossRef] [PubMed]

44. Hamalainen, E.; Adlercreutz, H.; Puska, P.; Pietinen, P. Diet and serum sex hormones in healthy men. *J. Steroid Biochem.* **1984**, *20*, 459–464. [CrossRef] [PubMed]

45. Hamalainen, E.; Adlercreutz, H.; Puska, P.; Pietinen, P. Decrease of serum total and free testosterone during a low-fat high-fibre diet. *J. Steroid Biochem.* **1983**, *18*, 369–370. [CrossRef] [PubMed]

46. Rosenthal, M.B.; Barnard, R.J.; Rose, D.P.; Inkeles, S.; Hall, J.; Pritikin, N. Effects of a high-complex-carbohydrate, low-fat, low-cholesterol diet on levels of serum lipids and estradiol. *Am. J. Med.* **1985**, *78*, 23–27. [CrossRef] [PubMed]

47. Grossmann, M.; Cheung, A.S.; Zajac, J.D. Androgens and prostate cancer pathogenesis and deprivation therapy. *Best Pract. Res. Clin. Endocrinol. Metab.* **2013**, *27*, 603–616. [CrossRef] [PubMed]

48. Knudsen, K.E.; Scher, H.I. Starving the addiction: New opportunities for durable suppression of AR signaling in prostate cancer. *Clin. Cancer Res.* **2009**, *15*, 4792–4798. [CrossRef] [PubMed]

49. Chatterjee, B. The role of the androgen receptor in the development of prostatic hyperplasia and prostate cancer. *Mol. Cell. Biochem.* **2003**, *253*, 89–101. [CrossRef] [PubMed]

50. Wu, J.D.; Haugk, K.; Woodke, L.; Nelson, P.; Coleman, I.; Plymate, S.R. Interaction of IGF signaling and the androgen receptor in prostate cancer progression. *J. Cell. Biochem.* **2006**, *99*, 392–401. [CrossRef] [PubMed]

51. Chen, Y.; Sawyers, C.L.; Scher, H.I. Targeting the androgen receptor pathway in prostate cancer. *Curr. Opin. Pharmacol.* **2008**, *8*, 440–448. [CrossRef] [PubMed]

52. McCarty, M.F.; Hejazi, J.; Rastmanesh, R. Beyond androgen deprivation: Ancillary integrative strategies for targeting the androgen receptor addiction of prostate cancer. *Integr. Cancer Ther.* **2014**, *13*, 389–395. [CrossRef]

53. Spencer, L.; Mann, C.; Metcalfe, M.; Webb, M.; Pollard, C.; Spencer, D.; Berry, D.; Steward, W.; Dennison, A. The effects of omega-3 FAs on tumour angiogenesis and their therapeutic potential. *Eur. J. Cancer* **2009**, *45*, 2077–2086. [CrossRef] [PubMed]

54. Fleshner, N.E.; Klotz, L.H. Diet, androgens, oxidative stress and prostate cancer susceptibility. *Cancer Metastasis Rev.* **1999**, *17*, 325–330. [CrossRef]

55. Lee, W.H.; Morton, R.A.; Epstein, J.I.; Brooks, J.D.; Campbell, P.A.; Bova, G.S.; Hsieh, W.S.; Isaacs, W.B.; Nelson, W.G. Cytidine methylation of regulatory sequences near the pi-class glutathione S-transferase gene accompanies human prostatic carcinogenesis. *Proc. Natl. Acad. Sci. USA* **1994**, *91*, 11733–11737. [CrossRef] [PubMed]

56. Vaco, C.E.; Wilhelm, J.; Harms-Rigdahl, M. Interaction of lipid peroxidation products with DNA. A review. *Mutat. Res.* **1988**, *195*, 137–149. [CrossRef] [PubMed]

57. Berquin, I.M.; Edwards, I.J.; Kridel, S.J.; Chen, Y.Q. Polyunsaturated fatty acid metabolism in prostate cancer. *Cancer Metastasis Rev.* **2011**, *30*, 295–309. [CrossRef] [PubMed]

58. Chen, Y.Q.; Edwards, I.J.; Kridel, S.J.; Thornburg, T.; Berquin, I.M. Dietary fat-gene interactions in cancer. *Cancer Metastasis Rev.* **2007**, *26*, 535–551. [CrossRef] [PubMed]

59. Escobar, E.L.; Gomes-Marcondes, M.C.; Carvalho, H.F. Dietary fatty acid quality affects AR and PPARgamma levels and prostate growth. *Prostate* **2009**, *69*, 548–558. [CrossRef] [PubMed]

60. Vereshagin, A.G.; Novitskaya, G.V. The triglyceride composition of linseed oil. *J. Am. Oil Chem. Soc.* **1965**, *42*, 970–974. [CrossRef] [PubMed]

61. Trichopoulou, A.; Lagiou, P.; Kuper, H.; Trichopoulos, D. Cancer and Mediterranean dietary traditions. *Cancer Epidemiol. Biomark. Prev.* **2000**, *9*, 869–873.

62. Lopez-Miranda, J.; Perez-Jimenez, F.; Ros, E.; de Caterina, R.; Badimon, L.; Covas, M.I.; Escrich, E.; Ordovás, J.M.; Soriguer, F.; Abiá, R.; *et al.* Olive oil and health: Summary of the II international conference on olive oil and health consensus report, Jaen and Cordoba (Spain) 2008. *Nutr. Metab. Cardiovasc. Dis.* **2010**, *20*, 284–294. [CrossRef] [PubMed]

63. Park, S.Y.; Wilkens, L.R.; Henning, S.M.; le Marchand, L.; Gao, K.; Goodman, M.T.; Murphy, S.P.; Henderson, B.E.; Kolonel, L.N. Circulating fatty acids and prostate cancer risk in a nested case-control study: The Multiethnic Cohort. *Cancer Causes Control* **2009**, *20*, 211–223. [CrossRef] [PubMed]

64. Crowe, F.L.; Key, T.J.; Appleby, P.N.; Travis, R.C.; Overvad, K.; Jakobsen, M.U.; Johnsen, N.F.; Tjønneland, A.; Linseisen, J.; Rohrmann, S.; *et al.* Dietary fat intake and risk of prostate cancer in the European Prospective Investigation into Cancer and Nutrition. *Am. J. Clin. Nutr.* **2008**, *87*, 1405–1413. [PubMed]

65. Narita, S.; Tsuchiya, N.; Saito, M.; Inoue, T.; Kumazawa, T.; Yuasa, T.; Nakamura, A.; Habuchi, T. Candidate genes involved in enhanced growth of human prostate cancer under high fat feeding identified by microarray analysis. *Prostate* **2008**, *68*, 321–335. [CrossRef] [PubMed]

66. Bidoli, E.; Talamini, R.; Bosetti, C.; Negri, E.; Maruzzi, D.; Montella, M.; Franceschi, S.; la Vecchia, C. Macronutrients, fatty acids, cholesterol and prostate cancer risk. *Ann. Oncol.* **2005**, *16*, 152–157. [CrossRef] [PubMed]

67. Williams, C.D.; Whitley, B.M.; Hoyo, C.; Grant, D.J.; Iraggi, J.D.; Newman, K.A.; Gerber, L.; Taylor, L.A.; McKeever, M.G.; Freedland, S.J. A high ratio of dietary n-6/n-3 polyunsaturated fatty acids is associated with increased risk of prostate cancer. *Nutr. Res.* **2011**, *31*, 1–8. [CrossRef] [PubMed]

68. Kobayashi, N.; Barnard, R.J.; Said, J.; Hong-Gonzalez, J.; Corman, D.M.; Ku, M.; Doan, N.B.; Gui, D.; Elashoff, D.; Cohen, P.; *et al.* Effect of low-fat diet on development of prostate cancer and Akt phosphorylation in the Hi-Myc transgenic mouse model. *Cancer Res* **2008**, *68*, 3066–3073. [CrossRef] [PubMed]

69. Berquin, I.M.; Min, Y.; Wu, R.; Wu, J.; Perry, D.; Cline, J.M.; Thomas, M.J.; Thornburg, T.; Kulik, G.; Smith, A.; *et al.* Modulation of prostate cancer genetic risk by omega-3 and omega-6 fatty acids. *J. Clin. Investig.* **2007**, *117*, 1866–1875. [CrossRef] [PubMed]

70. Kobayashi, N.; Barnard, R.J.; Henning, S.M.; Elashoff, D.; Reddy, S.T.; Cohen, P.; Leung, P.; Hong-Gonzalez, J.; Freedland, S.J.; Said, J.; *et al.* Effect of altering dietary omega-6/omega-3 fatty acid ratios on prostate cancer membrane composition, cyclooxygenase-2, and prostaglandin E2. *Clin. Cancer Res.* **2006**, *12*, 4662–4670. [CrossRef] [PubMed]

71. Akinsete, J.A.; Ion, G.; Witte, T.R.; Hardman, W.E. Consumption of high omega-3 fatty acid diet suppressed prostate tumorigenesis in C3(1) Tag mice. *Carcinogenesis* **2012**, *33*, 140–148. [CrossRef] [PubMed]

72. Smith, B.K.; Robinson, L.E.; Nam, R.; Ma, D.W.L. Trans-fatty acids and cancer: A mini-review. *Br. J. Nutr.* **2009**, *102*, 1254–1266. [CrossRef] [PubMed]

73. Bakker, N.; Van't, V.P.; Zock, P.L. Adipose fatty acids and cancers of the breast, prostate and colon: An ecological study. *Int. J. Cancer* **1997**, *72*, 587–591. [CrossRef] [PubMed]

74. King, I.B.; Kristal, A.R.; Schaffer, S.; Thronquist, M.; Goodman, G.E. Serum trans-fatty acids are associated with risk of prostate cancer in b-Carotene and Retinol Efficacy Trial. *Cancer Epidemiol. Biomark. Prev.* **2005**, *14*, 988–992. [CrossRef]

75. Chavarro, J.E.; Stampfer, M.J.; Campos, H.; Kurth, T.; Willett, W.C.; Ma, J. A prospective study of trans-fatty acid levels in blood and risk of prostate cancer. *Cancer Epidemiol. Biomark. Prev.* **2008**, *17*, 95–101. [CrossRef]

76. Liu, X.; Schumacher, F.R.; Plummer, S.J.; Jorgenson, E.; Casey, G.; Witte, J.S. Trans-fatty acid intake and increased risk of advanced prostate cancer: Modification by RNASEL R462Q variant. *Carcinogenesis* **2007**, *28*, 1232–1236. [CrossRef] [PubMed]

77. Schuurman, A.G.; van den Brandt, P.A.; Dorant, E.; Brants, H.A.; Goldbohm, R.A. Association of energy and fat intake with prostate carcinoma risk: Results from The Netherlands Cohort Study. *Cancer* **1999**, *86*, 1019–1027. [CrossRef] [PubMed]

78. Hodge, A.M.; English, D.R.; McCredie, M.R.; Severi, G.; Boyle, P.; Hopper, J.L.; Giles, G.G. Foods, nutrients and prostate cancer. *Cancer Causes Control* **2004**, *15*, 11–20. [CrossRef] [PubMed]

79. Brasky, T.M.; Till, C.; White, E.; Neuhouser, M.L.; Song, X.; Goodman, P.; Thompson, I.M.; King, I.B.; Albanes, D.; Kristal, A.R. Serum phospholipid fatty acids and prostate cancer risk: Results from the prostate cancer prevention trial. *Am. J. Epidemiol.* **2011**, *173*, 1429–1439.

80. Laake, I.; Carlsen, M.H.; Pedersen, J.I.; Weiderpass, E.; Selmer, R.; Kirkhus, B.; Thune, I.; Veierød, M.B. Intake of trans fatty acids from partially hydrogenated vegetable and fish oil and ruminant fat in relation to cancer risk. *Int. J. Cancer* **2013**, *132*, 1389–1403. [CrossRef] [PubMed]

81. Fradet, Y.; Meyer, F.; Bairati, I.; Shadmani, R.; Moore, L. Dietary fat and prostate cancer progression and survival. *Eur. Urol.* **1999**, *35*, 388–391. [CrossRef] [PubMed]

82. Davies, N.J.; Batehup, L.; Thomas, R. The role of diet and physical Activity in breast, colorectal, and prostate cancer survivorship: A review of the literature. *Br. J. Cancer* **2011**, *105*, 52–73. [CrossRef]

83. Ornish, D.; Weidner, G.; Fair, W.R.; Marlin, R.; Pettengill, E.B.; Raisin, C.J.; Dunn-Emke, S.; Crutchfield, L.; Jacobs, F.N.; Barnard, R.J.; et al. Intensive lifestyle changes may affect the progression of prostate cancer. *J. Urol.* **2005**, *174*, 1065–1070.

84. Demark-Wahnefried, W.; Polascik, T.J.; George, S.L.; Switzer, B.R.; Madden, J.F.; Ruffin, M.T.; Snyder, D.C.; Owzar, K.; Hars, V.; Albala, D.M.; et al. Flaxseed supplementation (not dietary fat restriction) reduces prostate cancer proliferation rates in men pre surgery. *Cancer Epidemiol. Biomarkers Prev.* **2008**, *17*, 3577–3587. [CrossRef] [PubMed]

85. Heymach, J.V.; Schackleford, T.J.; Tran, H.T.; Yoo, S.Y.; Do, K.A.; Wergin, M.; Saintigny, P.; Vollmer, R.T.; Polascik, T.J.; Snyder, D.; et al. Effects of low-fat diets on plasma levels of NF-kB-regulated inflammatory cytokine and angiogenic factors in men with prostate cancer. *Cancer Prev. Res. (Phila)* **2011**, *4*, 1590–1598. [CrossRef]

86. Hori, S.; Butler, E.; McLoughlin, J. Prostate cancer and diet: Food for thought? *BJUI Int.* **2011**, *107*, 1348–1359. [CrossRef]

87. Aronson, W.J.; Barnard, R.J.; Freedland, S.J.; Henning, S.; Elashoff, D.; Jardack, P.M.; Cohen, P.; Heber, D.; Kobayashi, N. Growth inhibitory effect of low fat diet on prostate cancer cells: Results of a prospective, randomized dietary intervention trial in men with prostate cancer. *J. Urol.* **2010**, *183*, 345–350. [CrossRef] [PubMed]

88. Haseen, F.; Murray, L.J.; Cardwell, C.R.; O'Sullivan, J.M.; Cantwell, M.M. The effects of androgen deprivation therapy on body composition in men with prostate cancer: Systematic review and meta-analysis. *J. Cancer Surviv.* **2010**, *4*, 128–139. [CrossRef] [PubMed]

89. Saylor, P.J.; Smith, M.R. Prostate cancer: How can we improve the health of men who receive ADT? *Nat. Rev. Urol.* **2009**, *6*, 529–531. [CrossRef] [PubMed]

10

Effects of Perioperative Supplementation with Omega-3 Fatty Acids on Leukotriene B$_4$ and Leukotriene B$_5$ Production by Stimulated Neutrophils in Patients with Colorectal Cancer

Lone S. Sorensen [1,*], Ole Thorlacius-Ussing [1,2], Henrik H. Rasmussen [3], Søren Lundbye-Christensen [4], Philip. C. Calder [5], Karen Lindorff-Larsen [6] and Erik B. Schmidt [4]

[1] Department of Surgical Gastroenterology, Aalborg University Hospital, 9000 Aalborg, Denmark; otu@rn.dk
[2] Institute of Clinical Medicine, Aarhus University Hospital, Aarhus 8000, Denmark
[3] Center for Nutrition and Bowel Disease, Aalborg University Hospital, 9000 Aalborg, Denmark; hhr@rn.dk
[4] Department of Cardiology, Center for Cardiovascular Research, Aalborg University Hospital, 9000 Aalborg, Denmark; solc@rn.dk (S.L.); ebs@rn.dk (E.B.S.)
[5] National Institute for Health Research Southampton Biomedical Research Center, University Hospital Southampton NHS Foundation Trust and University of Southampton, Southampton SO16 6YD, UK; p.c.calder@soton.ac.uk
[6] NordSim, Center for Simulation, Skills Training, Science and Innovation, Aalborg University Hospital, 9000 Aalborg, Denmark; kgll@rn.dk
* Author to whom correspondence should be addressed; lss@rn.dk

Abstract: Omega-3 fatty acids (*n*-3 FA) may have beneficial clinical and immune-modulating effects in surgical patients. In a randomized, double-blind, prospective, placebo-controlled trial, 148 patients referred for elective colorectal cancer surgery received an *n*-3 FA-enriched oral nutritional supplement (ONS) providing 2.0 g of eicosapentaenoic acid (EPA) and 1.0 g of docosahexaenoic acid (DHA) per day or a standard ONS for seven days before surgery. On the day of operation, there was a significant increase in the production of leukotriene B$_5$ (LTB$_5$) ($p < 0.01$) and 5-hydroxyeicosapentaenoic acid (5-HEPE) ($p < 0.01$), a significant decrease in the production of leukotriene B$_4$ (LTB$_4$) ($p < 0.01$) and a trend for a decrease in the production of 5-hydroxyeicosatetraenoic acid (5-HETE) ($p < 0.1$) from stimulated neutrophils in the active group compared with controls. There was no association between LTB$_4$ values and postoperative complications. In conclusion, oral *n*-3 FA exerts anti-inflammatory effects in surgical patients, without reducing the risk of postoperative complications.

Keywords: colorectal cancer; omega-3 fatty acids; immunomodulation; fish oil; leukotrienes

1. Introduction

Patients undergoing surgery are at risk of developing complications in the postoperative period [1–3]. This is believed to be partly caused by changes in the immune response following surgery [4]. Thus, initially, a hyper-inflammatory response followed by a phase of relative immune incompetence occurs in relation to major surgery [5].

The pathophysiological changes are complex, but may be driven by excessive production of various lipid mediators, including the very potent pro-inflammatory leukotriene B$_4$ (LTB$_4$) produced from the omega-6 fatty acid (*n*-6 FA) arachidonic acid (AA) present in cell membranes.

Among factors known to influence the clinical course of patients after surgery are nutritional status and specific biologically active nutrients [2,6–10] that might include the marine omega-3 fatty acids (*n*-3 FA) with the main biologically active *n*-3 FAs being eicosapentaenoic acid (EPA) and docosahexaenoic acid (DHA). Consumption of fish and fish oils oil increases the concentration of EPA and DHA in blood, cells and tissues [11,12] and alters the physical properties of cell membranes and the function of membrane proteins, including receptors, transporters and signalling proteins [13,14]. *n*-3 FA are incorporated into cell membranes in competition with the more abundant *n*-6 FA, AA, at the expense of the latter. AA may be liberated by phospholipases from cell membranes and induces leucocytes to produce the pro-inflammatory LTB_4 and the side product, 5-hydroxyeicosatetraenoic acid (5-HETE). In contrast, leukotriene B_5 (LTB_5) and the side product, 5-hydroxyeicosapentaenoic acid (5-HEPE), derived from EPA [15], have considerably less potent biological activities in comparison to LTB_4 [15,16]. Replacement of *n*-6 FA with *n*-3 FA in membranes of immune active cells may therefore lead to reduced formation of pro-inflammatory compounds, and by this, and other [5,12] mechanisms, *n*-3 FA may decrease infectious complications after surgery [7,17–20]. The influence of enteral feeds, including *n*-3 FA on AA-derived eicosanoids (e.g., LTB_4), has been the subject of much attention [5,21–23]. Several studies have indicated that *n*-3 FAs modulate the generation of inflammatory eicosanoids in gastrointestinal surgical patients [24–26] and may help to counteract the surgery-induced decline in antigen-presenting cell activity [20] and T-cell cytokine production [27].

The aim of the present study was to evaluate the production of LTB_4, 5-HETE, LTB_5 and 5-HEPE from stimulated neutrophils after seven days of preoperative treatment with an *n*-3 FA-enriched oral nutritional supplement (ONS) in patients undergoing colorectal cancer surgery and to study the possible impact on clinical outcome. Furthermore, the correlation between LTB_4 values and postoperative complications was investigated.

2. Materials and Methods

2.1. Study Design

This was a sub-study of a randomized, double-blind, prospective, placebo-controlled single-centre interventional trial involving 148 participants (Figure 1) awaiting colorectal cancer surgery [28]. Participants were recruited consecutively from the outpatient clinic of the Department of Surgical Gastroenterology, Aalborg University Hospital. All eligible participants were asked to participate.

Exclusion criteria were diabetes mellitus, consumption of >5 alcoholic drinks per day, emergency surgery, inability to understand the spoken and written information in Danish, untreated psychiatric conditions, pregnancy or breast-feeding, reduced kidney function (plasma creatinine > 130 µmol/L), use of *n*-3 FA supplements, anticipated poor compliance, immunosuppressive diseases and participation in another clinical trial.

After providing oral and written informed consent, participants were randomly assigned to treatment with *n*-3 FA (active treatment) or control (a standard ONS without marine *n*-3 FA), 200 mL twice per day (morning and afternoon) for 7 days before surgery. Randomization was performed using sealed non-transparent envelopes containing the randomization number and kept at the investigation site according to CONSORT (Consolidated Standards of Reporting Trials) guidelines [29]. The active and the control ONS cartons looked identical and had identical taste and scent (coffee). The main investigator and a study nurse enrolled the participants at the outpatient clinic and randomly assigned them to active treatment or control. The participants, carers, investigators and other researchers were blinded to treatment allocation throughout the study. The investigators had no access to the code until after completion of the study. Statistical analyses were completed before the code was broken.

Information collected included demographic data, tumour location and American Society of Anaesthesiologists (ASA) risk score [30]. All patients underwent standard Nutritional Risk Screening (NRS 2002) [31]. A food questionnaire focusing on consumption of seafood on a monthly basis was completed at baseline.

The study was approved by the regional ethics committee (N-VN-20050035) and conducted according to the Hong Kong amendment to the Declaration of Helsinki. The trial was registered at ClinicalTrials.gov: ID NCT00488904 [32].

2.2. Intervention

Participants in the active or control group received the ONS as a sip feed (200 mL twice a day morning and afternoon) for 7 days before surgery. The feeds (Supportan®) were isocaloric (1.5 kcal/mL) and isonitrogenous (Table 1) and were provided by Fresenius Kabi (Bad Homburg, Germany). Both feeds contained the same amounts of carbohydrate, protein, total fat and n-6 FA (Table 1).

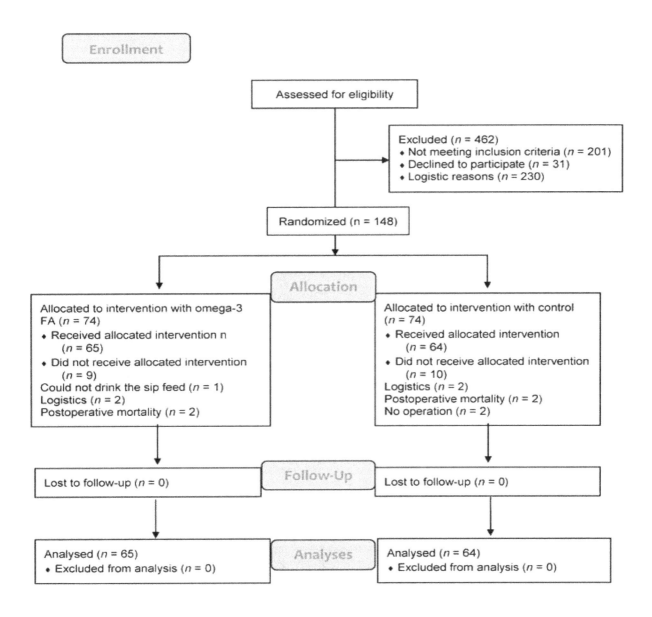

Figure 1. Patient flow through the study.

Table 1. Daily intake of energy and nutrients from the *n*-3 FA-enriched and the control oral nutritional supplement.

Daily dose	Control	*n*-3 FA (Active)
Energy (kcal)	600	600
Protein (g)	40	40
Carbohydrate (g)	49.6	49.6
Fat (g)	26.8	26.8
EPA (g)	0	2
DHA (g)	0	1
Total *n*-6 FA (g)	3.3	3.3

Fat content of the supplement was comprised of medium chain triglycerides, sunflower oil and safflower oil. The active supplement also contained additional fish oil at a level to achieve 2 g EPA and 1 g DHA per day (Table 1). Participants were provided with the sip feeds at inclusion, to consume twice a day for 7 days at home before hospitalization. A questionnaire regarding compliance preoperatively was completed, and good compliance was defined as self-reported consumption of at least 12 of the 14 ONS cartons before surgery.

2.3. Isolation of Blood Neutrophils

Blood was drawn in the fasting state on the day of the surgery. Neutrophils were separated from anticoagulated (K-EDTA 1.6 mg/mL) blood layered on top of PolymorphprepTM (AXIS-SHIELD PoC AS, Rodeloekka, Norway) and separated by a one-step centrifugation technique at 450 g for 40 min. Neutrophils were harvested and washed twice in tissue culture medium (RPMI 1640, Sigma-Aldrich, Ayrshire, UK), at ambient temperature and centrifuged for 10 min at $520 \times g$. Subsequently, neutrophils were counted and red cells eliminated by the addition of ice-cold 0.2% saline for 35 s. Next, 1.6% ice-cold saline was added in order to obtain an isotonic 0.9% concentration, followed by centrifugation at $300 \times g$ at 5 °C for 5 min, which was repeated once. Neutrophils were then washed in a phosphate buffer containing glucose and human albumin (PBS) and resuspended in PBS adjusting the concentration to 1×10^7 neutrophils/mL PBS. Isolated neutrophils were stored at -80 °C until analysis.

2.4. Analysis of Leukotrienes, 5-HEPE and 5-HETE

The neutrophil suspension (0.9 mL of 1×10^7 granulocytes/mL PBS) was prewarmed to 37 °C, and $CaCl_2$, $MgCl_2$ and calcium ionophore (A23187) at a final concentration of 10 μM were added to initiate stimulation. After 10 min, the reaction was terminated by the addition of 100% ice-cold ethanol, and the mixtures were centrifuged at 4 °C at $700 \times g$. The supernatant was stored at -80 °C for later analysis. C18 cartridges (Sep-Pak VAC RC, Waters Co., Milford, MA, USA) were used for the extraction of leukotrienes (LT), 5-HEPE and 5-HETE. The ethanol mixture was thawed and centrifuged, and international standard prostaglandin B_2 (PGB_2) and trifluoroacetic acid were added. The cartridges were conditioned and equilibrated using methyl formate, 100% ethanol and water. The acidified sample was loaded onto the cartridge, washed with 15% ethanol, water and hexane and eluted with methyl formate. The solvent was evaporated to dryness under nitrogen, and the sediment was dissolved in the mobile phase (31% H_2O, 27% methanol, 42% acetonitrile and 0.025% trifluoroacetic acid).

Analysis was performed by high pressure liquid chromatography (Dionex Ultimate LPG-3400A) on an Acclaim RSLC 2.1 mm × 100 mm C18 column (Dionex Corporation, Sunnyvale, CA, USA).

Concentrations were calculated using the internal standard and response factors. The response factors were calculated by analysis of a non-stimulated neutrophil suspension after the addition of known amounts of standards of LTB_4, LTB_5, 5-HETE and 5-HEPE, as well as an internal standard (PGB_2). Samples were extracted and analysed using high performance liquid chromatography, and eventually, the recovery factors were calculated.

2.5. Granulocyte Fatty Acid Analysis

Blood was drawn in the fasting state on the day of surgery. Granulocytes were prepared as described previously [33]. FA profiles were determined by gas chromatography using a Varian 3900 gas chromatograph, CP-8400 autosampler and CP 8414 autoinjector (Varian, Middelburg, The Netherlands), as well as a flame ionization detector. In split injection mode, a CP-sil 88.60-m $\times$ 0.25-mm capillary column (Varian, Middelburg, The Netherlands), temperature programming from 90 to 205 °C, a constant flow rate of 1.0 mL/min and helium carrier gas were used. Results for individual FAs are expressed as a percentage of the total FA content.

2.6. Statistical Analysis

The basic characteristics of the trial population were analysed with Fisher's exact test for categorical variables and unpaired t-tests for continuous variables. Differences between treatment groups were analysed using unpaired t-tests. If variances differed between groups, Welch's approximation was used. The distribution of continuous data was analysed for normality. As the values for 5-HEPE, 5-HETE and LTs were right skewed distributed, log transformed observations were analysed, and these were normally distributed. Distributions of 5-HEPE, 5-HETE and LT were described with median and inter-quartile range (IQR). Relative differences between groups in medians were calculated by exponentiation of the differences between log-transformed means. Associations between LTB_4 values and postoperative complications were analysed using logistic regression. The associations between log-transformed LT values 5-HEPE and AA, EPA and AA/EPA were analysed using linear regression. Analyses were performed blinded to treatment groups. The active and control groups were not identified until after the statistical analyses had been conducted. All p-values were two-tailed, and differences were reported with 95% confidence intervals (CI). p-values below 0.05 were considered significant. All analyses were performed using Stata version 11.2 (StataCorp, 2009; Texas City, TX, USA).

3. Results

3.1. Participants Characteristics

All eligible participants (n = 610) were asked to participate, but 230 participants were not included. This was due to a change in clinical practice during the study, such that many patients were offered surgery within a five-day period, which did not allow for participants to complete the seven-day intervention. Furthermore, some participants did not meet the inclusion criteria (201), and 31 participants declined to participate. Baseline characteristics of the included *vs.* the non-included participants did not differ.

A total of 148 consecutive patients (68 females, 80 males; mean age 71 (range 41–89) years) were included in the study. The majority of participants had open surgery; laparoscopic resection was only performed in nine patients in the control group and nine in the *n*-3 FA group. Participant characteristics did not differ between treatment groups (Table 2).

Table 2. Characteristics of patients in the control and active groups.

Variable	Control ($n = 74$)	Active ($n = 74$)	p
Demographic data			
Age, years, mean (SD)	71 (10)	69 (11)	0.164
Sex (male/female)	36/38	44/30	0.248
Body weight, kg, mean (SD)	76 (19)	77(17)	0.570
Height, cm, mean (SD)	169 (11)	171 (9)	0.301
BMI, kg/m^2, mean (SD)	26 (5)	26 (5)	0.651
Weight loss * (n)	19	11	0.068
Clinical characteristics			
Smoking/non-smoking (n)	11/60	17/54	0.292
Unknown smoking status	3	3	
Cancer location			
Colon/rectum (n)	40/34	38/36	0.869
Surgical procedure			0.977
Right hemicolectomy + transverse colon (n)	16	17	
Left hemicolectomy + sigmoid colon (n)	10	12	
Laparoscopic resection of sigmoid colon (n)	9	9	
Low anterior resection of rectum or abdominoperineal resection	28	30	
Colectomy (n)	4	3	
Other rectum resection (n)	7	3	
Nutritional status **			0.089
No risk (NRS score <3) (n)	23	34	
At risk (NRS score ≥3) (n)	50	39	
Unknown (n)	1	1	

Notes: There were no significant differences between groups ($p > 0.068$); BMI, body mass index; * defined as loss of more than 5% of body weight; ** defined according to NRS 2002 [31].

3.2. Fatty Acid Composition of Neutrophils

Neutrophil EPA and DHA were significantly higher, and AA and linoleic acid was significantly lower in the group receiving n-3 FA than in the control group (Table 3) [28].

The food questionnaire indicated an average dietary intake of n-3 FA of 0.6 g per day, with no difference in preoperative intake between groups ($p = 0.770$). None of the included participants received more than 150 mg of anti-inflammatory drugs daily. Both supplements were well tolerated with no adverse effects reported. Nine participants randomized to active treatment and 10 participants in the control group did not receive the allocated intervention for reasons listed in Figure 1.

Preoperatively, 63 of 65 participants in the active group were compliant compared with 56 of 64 participants in the control group ($p = 0.266$). Two participants died in each group. In the active group, death was caused by pneumonia and a myocardial infarction, whereas the participants in the control group died from septicaemia and sudden cardiac death.

Conversely, in the active group, neutrophils showed a significantly lower (by 12%) production of LTB$_4$ ($p < 0.001$) and a trend towards lower (by 7%) production of 5-HETE ($p = 0.059$). LTB$_4$/LTB$_5$ was significantly different between groups (by 68%) ($p < 0.001$) (Table 4). There was no statistically significant difference in clinical outcomes (total number of complications, infectious complications, non-infectious complications, intensive care unit stay, mortality, readmissions and hospital stay) between groups, as reported previously [28].

Table 3. Granulocyte fatty acids on day of operation in the control and active groups.

	Weight% of Total FA Content	
	Control	Active
EPA	0.54 (0.42–0.74)	2.10 (1.83–2.55) *
DPA	0.54 (0.42–0.74)	2.11 (1.83–2.55) *
DHA	1.31 (1.10–1.57)	1.61 (1.34–1.84) *
Total n-3 FA	2.44 (1.98–2.97)	5.95 (5.20–6.75) *
Arachidonic acid	12.51 (11.65–13.19)	11.61 (10.67–12.48) *
Linoleic acid	8.94 (8.24–9.49)	9.42 (8.72–10.19) **

Notes: Values are the median (IQR); FA, fatty acid; ONS, oral nutritional supplement; EPA, eicosapentaenoic acid; DPA, docosapentaenoic acid; DHA, docosahexaenoic acid; * $p < 0.001$; ** $p < 0.05$ *versus* the control group.

3.3. Production of Mediators from Neutrophils

Furthermore, compared to neutrophils from controls, those from participants in the n-3 FA group showed a significantly higher (by 176% and 306%, respectively) production of LTB$_5$ ($p < 0.001$) and 5-HEPE ($p < 0.001$) (Table 4).

Table 4. Formation of leukotrienes (LT) and side products (5-HEPE; 5-HETE) from activated neutrophils according to treatment group.

Eicosanoids	Control	Active	% Difference
LTB$_5$	5.8 (4.9–7.6)	17.5 (13.5–22.8)	176 *** (143–215)
LTB$_4$	186.8 (156.8–230.7)	163.5 (136.6–199.9)	−12 *** (−21−−3)
5-HETE	293.1 (246.5–357.8)	273.7 (221.8–320.7)	−7 * (−14−−0)
5-HEPE	34.2 (25.7–55.3)	154.7 (122.4–190.4)	306 *** (255–364)
LTB$_4$/LTB$_5$	31.8 (25.0–40.1)	9.6 (7.8–11.4)	−68*** (−72−−65)

Notes: Data are the median (IQR) ng/10^7 neutrophils and the percentage of difference between estimated medians; *** indicates $p < 0.01$; * indicates $p < 0.1$; ng/10^7 = nanogram/10^7 neutrophils.

There was no statistically significant association between the values of the proinflammatory LTB$_4$ production and any clinical outcome, including total number of complications ($p = 0.524$), infectious complications ($p = 0.660$) and non-infectious complications ($p = 0.307$) (Table 5). The ratio LTB$_4$/LTB$_5$ did not have a statistically significant association with the total number of complications ($p = 0.707$), infectious complications ($p = 0.711$) and non-infectious complications ($p = 0.143$) (Table 4).

However, There were strong associations between the content of AA and EPA in neutrophils and production of LTB$_4$ and LTB$_5$ (Figure 2) (all $p < 0.01$).

These graphs illustrate that the higher the content of EPA in the cell membranes, the higher the production of LTB$_5$. Furthermore, it can be seen that the higher the content of AA in cell membranes, the lower the production of LTB$_5$. Furthermore, there were strong associations between AA/EPA in neutrophils and LTB$_4$ and LTB$_5$ production (both $p < 0.01$) (results not shown) and between AA, EPA, AA/EPA and 5-HEPE production (all $p < 0.001$) (results not shown).

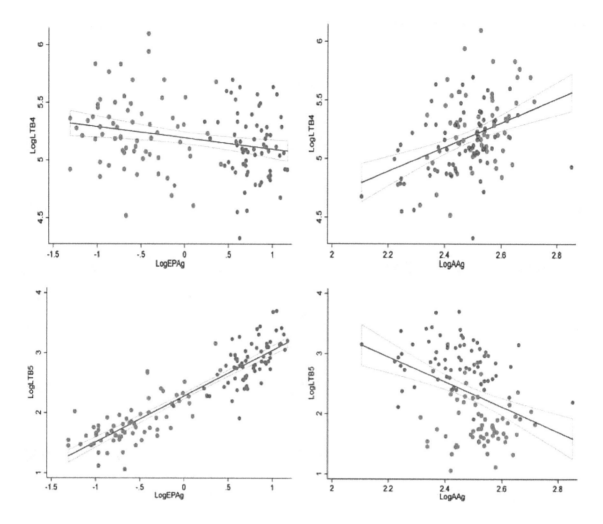

Figure 2. Associations between log-transformed AAg (AA content in the cell membranes of the granulocytes) and EPAg (EPA content in the cell membranes of the granulocytes) in the neutrophils, as well as the formation of LTs (LTB$_4$ and LTB$_5$ (ng/10^7)) by neutrophils, illustrated using scatter plots with regression lines and confidence bands added. Control group, red dots; active group, blue dots.

Table 5. Associations between LTs production by neutrophils and clinical outcome described by odds ratio (OR), CI and p-values for a unit change in LTB$_4$ and LTB$_4$/LTB$_5$, respectively.

	LTB$_4$			LTB$_4$/LTB$_5$		
	OR	**CI**	**p**	**OR**	**CI**	**p**
Infectious complications	1.00	1.00–1.01	0.660	1.00	0.97–1.03	0.711
Non-infectious complications	1.00	0.99–1.00	0.307	0.98	0.94–1.00	0.143
Total number of complications	1.00	0.99–1.00	0.524	1.00	0.98–1.03	0.707

4. Discussion

In this prospective randomized, double-blind, single-centre, placebo controlled study, it was demonstrated that seven days of enteral supplementation with 3 g of EPA + DHA daily resulted in a higher neutrophil production of LTB$_5$ and a lower production of LTB$_4$ compared to the control group. In addition, there was a higher neutrophil 5-HEPE production and a trend to lower production of 5-HETE in the active group compared to the control. While the differences in LTB$_4$ and LTB$_5$ production indicate an anti-inflammatory action of the supplement, it is unknown whether the difference in formation of 5-HETE and 5-HEPE between groups is of clinical relevance. However, 5-HETE enhances lymphocyte proliferation, whereas 5-HEPE only has one-tenth the potency of 5-HETE regarding this [34]. Thus, the current study demonstrates that preoperative supplementation with n-3 FA for one week can modulate immune function, assessed as the production of lipoxygenase mediators, in participants admitted for elective colorectal cancer surgery. However, this was not associated with a decrease in postoperative complication rates [28].

The strengths of the present study are that it was a randomized, prospective, relatively large clinical study, was double-blind, with an identical appearance for the sip feed cartons, the taste of n-3 FA was undetectable and that compliance was acceptable. Furthermore, the study population was relatively homogenous.

One limitation of the present study is that we only had data on eicosanoid formation from the day of surgery, whereas postoperative changes would also have been of interest. The short duration of the intervention (seven days) may have limited the incorporation of n-3 FA and the decrease of AA in neutrophils and, thereby, limited the impact on LTB_4 production, but a longer period of supplementation was not possible, as participants were operated on soon after cancer diagnosis. However, we showed in earlier publications that 3 g of n-3 FA for seven days before surgery was sufficient to assure significant incorporation of n-3 FA into neutrophils and into colonic tissue [28,35]. The required sample size was based on a reduction in postoperative infection rates from 30% to 10% and was calculated to be 148 participants in all, but we were only able to analyse data from 129 of these. A final limitation is the discrepancy between the number of eligible (610) and analysed participants (129) due to a change in clinical practice during the study, such that many patients were offered surgery within a five-day period, which did not allow for participants to complete the seven-day intervention.

Our findings are consistent with the results from three recent studies in humans [24,36,37]. In a prospective double-blind study, Wang et al. [37] randomized 64 participants with a need for postoperative parenteral nutrition after surgery into two groups. The study population was a mix of surgical patients (22 gastric cancers; 29 colonic cancers; 13 with other digestive diseases). They received either fish oil containing lipid emulsion (a mixture of soybean oil, MCT and fish oil) as part of the intravenous regimen, or a mix of soybean oil and MCT for 5 days after surgery. There was a significant increase in the neutrophil LTB_5/LTB_4 ratio but no effect on clinical outcome, infectious complications and bleeding events. Grimm et al. [36] randomized 33 participants undergoing major abdominal surgery into two groups in a prospective double-blind study to receive parenteral nutrition providing either a fish oil containing lipid emulsion (a mixture of soybean oil, MCT, olive oil and fish oil) or soybean oil for five days after surgery. The study population was again a mix of surgical patients. The initial production of LTB_4 and LTB_5 by neutrophils was similar in both groups. The production of LTB_5 from neutrophils was significantly increased, and the release of LTB_4 was decreased, though not significantly, in the participants receiving fish oil. The length of hospital stay was significantly shorter in the intervention group. Finally, Köller et al. [24] conducted a prospective double-blind randomized study with 30 participants undergoing colorectal surgery. Participants received parenteral nutrition, providing either a fish oil containing lipid emulsion (a mixture of soybean oil, MCT and fish oil) or soybean oil for five days post-surgery. This study also found a significant increase in LTB_5 production by leukocytes in the fish oil group, but without a concomitant decrease in LTB_4 production. These three studies all made use of intravenous (IV) nutrition given postoperatively. The present study, which used enteral nutrition given preoperatively, agrees with these earlier findings of increased LTB_5 production and decreased LTB_4 production after fish oil provision, but with limited clinical impact.

Some earlier studies have reported beneficial effects of oral n-3 FA supplementation in gastrointestinal surgery patients. Wachtler et al. [26] analysed leukocyte function in 40 participants undergoing major upper gastrointestinal surgery in a placebo-controlled double-blind study. One group received an n-3 FA-enriched (0.33 g/100 mL) oral supplement, also containing arginine and ribonucleic acid, and the other group received a standard control supplement for five days preoperatively. There was a significantly higher production of LTB_5 from neutrophils in the intervention group when compared to controls. However, no changes in LTB_4 were evident in the intervention group. The authors reported a low number of postoperative complications. In another study, Shimizu *et al.* [38] gave 12 children with ulcerative colitis 1.8 g EPA orally per day for two months. LTB_4 production by leucocytes and colonic mucosa were assessed before and after the intervention. Biopsies were taken from the rectal mucosa during sigmoidoscopy before and after initiation of EPA supplementation. After two months of supplementation, there was a decrease in LTB_4 production by leucocytes and colonic mucosa, while no information regarding LTB_5 production was given.

IV administration of *n*-3 FA ensures a quicker incorporation of the presumed active substances (*n*-3 FA) into the membranes of immune cells [39,40]. However, this format is not feasible in the pre-operative setting. ONSs are less expensive and enable the use of the gut prior to surgery. Two studies providing IV *n*-3 FA for five days post-operatively did not show any decrease in the production of LTB_4 [24,36]. Importantly many of these studies did not provide explicit information about the amount of *n*-3 FA given.

In the present study, seven days of oral supplementation with 3 g of *n*-3 FA daily ensured significant incorporation of EPA into neutrophils and a significant decrease in the formation of LTB_4. However, to achieve an anti-inflammatory response meditated by *n*-3 FA, it is probably more important that the formation of the AA-derived LTB_4 is suppressed than an increase in LTB_5. Despite this, there was no effect on clinical outcome in the current study. One explanation for this may be that *n*-3 FA incorporation was not sufficiently high. A higher *n*-3 FA dose or a longer duration of intervention could have had an impact on clinical outcome. The ratio LTB_4/LTB_5 was 68% lower in the active group, which is a considerable decrease, but still did not have any effect on clinical outcome.

One other important factor may be that the nutritional status of the patients, evaluated by NRS 2002, was generally good for most participants. A weight loss of more than 5% of body weight was only detected in 23% of participants entering the study. This could account for the lack of clinical improvement with the *n*-3 FA-enriched ONS, since it is likely that malnourished participants might benefit the most from ONS and from oral *n*-3 FA.

5. Conclusions

In summary, the current study shows that an ONS providing 3 g of *n*-3 FA daily for seven days before surgery was able to induce a significant decrease in the formation of the pro-inflammatory LTB_4 from neutrophils with a simultaneous increased production of LTB_5. A decrease in the formation of 5-HETE, though not significant, and a significant rise in 5-HEPE was also seen. However, the clinical consequences of these changes are unknown. Associations between values of LTB_4 or LTB_4/LTB_5 and postoperative complication rates were not seen. This indicates either that the changes observed were too small or that the formation of LTs from activated neutrophils is not an important determinant of surgical complications. Whether a longer period (months) of *n*-3 FA intake could be of a benefit for patients operated on for colorectal cancer regarding shorter stay in hospital or longer survival needs to be investigated in larger trials.

Abbreviations

AA	arachidonic acid
ASA	American Society of Anaesthesiologists
BMI	body mass index
CI	confidence intervals
DHA	docosahexaenoic acid
EPA	eicosapentaenoic acid
5-HEPE	5-hydroxyeicosapentaenoic acid
5-HETE	5-hydroxyeicosatetraenoic acid
IV	intravenous;
IQR	inter-quartile range
LT	leukotrienes
LTB_4	leukotriene B_4
LTB_5	leukotriene B_5

n-3 FA	*n*-3 fatty acids
n-6 FA	*n*-6 fatty acids
MCT	medium-chain triglycerides
ng	nanograms
NRS 2002	Nutritional Risk Screening
ONS	oral nutritional supplement
OR	odds ratio
PBS	phosphate-buffered saline
PGB$_2$	prostaglandin B$_2$

Acknowledgments: This work was kindly supported by Fresenius Kabi (Bad Homburg, Germany), The Obelske Family Foundation, the Hoejmosegaard Grant, the Aase and Ejnar Danielsens Foundation and the North Jutland Medical Association.

We thank study nurse Anne Madsen and the staff at the Lipid Research Clinic at Aalborg University Hospital for invaluable assistance in connection with completion of the study. We also thank Hanne Madsen for proofreading.

Author Contributions: Lone Schmidt Sorensen: study concept and design; acquisitions of data; analysis and interpretations of data; drafting of the manuscript; statistical analysis; obtained funding; study supervision; approval of the final version of the manuscript.

Henrik Hojgaard Rasmussen: study concept and design; critical revision of the manuscript; study supervision; approval of the final version of the manuscript.

Søren Lundbye-Christensen: statistical support; critical revision of the manuscript; approval of the final version of the manuscript.

Ole Thorlacius-Ussing: study concept and design; critical revision of the manuscript; study supervision; approval of the final version of the manuscript.

Karen Lindorff-Larsen: study concept and design; acquisitions of data; critical revision of the manuscript; study supervision; approval of the final version of the manuscript.

Erik Berg Schmidt: study concept and design; critical revision of the manuscript; study supervision; approval of the final version of the manuscript.

Philip C. Calder: study concept and design; critical revision of the manuscript; approval of the final version of the manuscript.

References

1. Platt, J.J.; Ramanathan, M.L.; Crosbie, R.A.; Anderson, J.H.; McKee, R.F.; Horgan, P.G.; McMillan, D.C. C-reactive protein as a predictor of postoperative infective complications after curative resection in patients with colorectal cancer. *Ann. Surg. Oncol.* **2012**, *19*, 4168–4177. [CrossRef]

2. Zhu, M.W.; Tang, D.N.; Hou, J.; Wei, J.M.; Hua, B.; Sun, J.H.; Cui, H.Y. Impact of fish oil enriched total parenteral nutrition on elderly patients after colorectal cancer surgery. *Chin. Med. J. (Engl.)* **2012**, *125*, 178–181.

3. The Danish Colorectal Cancer Database, The Danish Colorectal Cancer Group. Annual review. Available online: http://www.dccg.dk/03_Publikation/02_arsraport_pdf/aarsrapport_2011.png (accessed on 3 April 2013).

4. Kehlet, H.; Dahl, J.B. Anaesthesia, surgery, and challenges in postoperative recovery. *Lancet* **2003**, *362*, 1921–1928. [CrossRef]

5. Calder, P.C. *n*-3 fatty acids, inflammation, and immunity—Relevance to postsurgical and critically ill patients. *Lipids* **2004**, *39*, 1147–1161. [CrossRef]

6. Bozzetti, F.; Braga, M.; Gianotti, L.; Gavazzi, C.; Mariani, L. Postoperative enteral *versus* parenteral nutrition in malnourished patients with gastrointestinal cancer: A randomised multicentre trial. *Lancet* **2001**, *358*, 1487–1492. [CrossRef]

7. Braga, M.; Gianotti, L.; Vignali, A.; Carlo, V.D. Preoperative oral arginine and *n*-3 fatty acid supplementation improves the immunometabolic host response and outcome after colorectal resection for cancer. *Surgery* **2002**, *132*, 805–814. [CrossRef]

8. Gustafsson, U.O.; Ljungqvist, O. Perioperative nutritional management in digestive tract surgery. *Curr. Opin. Clin. Nutr. Metab. Care* **2011**, *14*, 504–509. [CrossRef]

9. Jie, B.; Jiang, Z.M.; Nolan, M.T.; Zhu, S.N.; Yu, K.; Kondrup, J. Impact of preoperative nutritional support on clinical outcome in abdominal surgical patients at nutritional risk. *Nutrition* **2012**, *28*, 1022–1027. [CrossRef]

10. Ryan, A.M.; Reynolds, J.V.; Healy, L.; Byrne, M.; Moore, J.; Brannelly, N.; McHugh, A.; McCormack, D.; Flood, P. Enteral nutrition enriched with eicosapentaenoic acid (EPA) preserves lean body mass following esophageal cancer surgery: Results of a double-blinded randomized controlled trial. *Ann. Surg.* **2009**, *249*, 355–363. [CrossRef]

11. Senkal, M.; Haaker, R.; Linseisen, J.; Wolfram, G.; Homann, H.H.; Stehle, P. Preoperative oral supplementation with long-chain Omega-3 fatty acids beneficially alters phospholipid fatty acid patterns in liver, gut mucosa, and tumor tissue. *J. Parenter. Enter. Nutr.* **2005**, *29*, 236–240. [CrossRef]

12. Senkal, M.; Geier, B.; Hannemann, M.; Deska, T.; Linseisen, J.; Wolfram, G.; Adolph, M. Supplementation of omega-3 fatty acids in parenteral nutrition beneficially alters phospholipid fatty acid pattern. *J. Parenter. Enter. Nutr.* **2007**, *31*, 12–17. [CrossRef]

13. Calder, P.C. Mechanisms of action of (*n*-3) fatty acids. *J. Nutr.* **2012**, *142*, 592S–599S. [CrossRef]

14. Stubbs, C.D.; Smith, A.D. The modification of mammalian membrane polyunsaturated fatty acid composition in relation to membrane fluidity and function. *Biochim. Biophys. Acta* **1984**, *779*, 89–137. [CrossRef]

15. Calder, P.C. The relationship between the fatty acid composition of immune cells and their function. *Prostaglandins Leukot. Essent. Fatty Acids* **2008**, *79*, 101–108. [CrossRef]

16. Terano, T.; Salmon, J.A.; Moncada, S. Biosynthesis and biological activity of leukotriene B5. *Prostaglandins* **1984**, *27*, 217–232. [CrossRef]

17. Jiang, Z.M.; Wilmore, D.W.; Wang, X.R.; Wei, J.M.; Zhang, Z.T.; Gu, Z.Y.; Wang, S.; Han, S.M.; Jiang, H.; Yu, K. Randomized clinical trial of intravenous soybean oil alone versus soybean oil plus fish oil emulsion after gastrointestinal cancer surgery. *Br. J. Surg.* **2010**, *97*, 804–809. [CrossRef]

18. Senkal, M.; Mumme, A.; Eickhoff, U.; Geier, B.; Spath, G.; Wulfert, D.; Joosten, U.; Frei, A.; Kemen, M. Early postoperative enteral immunonutrition: Clinical outcome and cost-comparison analysis in surgical patients. *Crit. Care Med.* **1997**, *25*, 1489–1496. [CrossRef]

19. Tsekos, E.; Reuter, C.; Stehle, P.; Boeden, G. Perioperative administration of parenteral fish oil supplements in a routine clinical setting improves patient outcome after major abdominal surgery. *Clin. Nutr.* **2004**, *23*, 325–330.

20. Weiss, G.; Meyer, F.; Matthies, B.; Pross, M.; Koenig, W.; Lippert, H. Immunomodulation by perioperative administration of *n*-3 fatty acids. *Br. J. Nutr.* **2002**, *87* (Suppl. 1), S89–S94. [CrossRef]

21. Furst, P.; Kuhn, K.S. Fish oil emulsions: What benefits can they bring? *Clin. Nutr.* **2000**, *19*, 7–14.

22. Grimm, H.; Mayer, K.; Mayser, P.; Eigenbrodt, E. Regulatory potential of *n*-3 fatty acids in immunological and inflammatory processes. *Br. J. Nutr.* **2002**, *87* (Suppl. 1), S59–S67. [CrossRef]

23. Mayer, K.; Grimm, H.; Grimminger, F.; Seeger, W. Parenteral nutrition with *n*-3 lipids in sepsis. *Br. J. Nutr.* **2002**, *87* (Suppl. 1), S69–S75. [CrossRef]

24. Koller, M.; Senkal, M.; Kemen, M.; Konig, W.; Zumtobel, V.; Muhr, G. Impact of omega-3 fatty acid enriched TPN on leukotriene synthesis by leukocytes after major surgery. *Clin. Nutr.* **2003**, *22*, 59–64. [CrossRef]

25. Morlion, B.J.; Torwesten, E.; Lessire, H.; Sturm, G.; Peskar, B.M.; Furst, P.; Puchstein, C. The effect of parenteral fish oil on leukocyte membrane fatty acid composition and leukotriene-synthesizing capacity in patients with postoperative trauma. *Metabolism* **1996**, *45*, 1208–1213. [CrossRef]

26. Wachtler, P.; Axel, H.R.; Konig, W.; Bauer, K.H.; Kemen, M.; Koller, M. Influence of a pre-operative enteral supplement on functional activities of peripheral leukocytes from patients with major surgery. *Clin. Nutr.* **1995**, *14*, 275–282. [CrossRef]

27. Schauder, P.; Rohn, U.; Schafer, G.; Korff, G.; Schenk, H.D. Impact of fish oil enriched total parenteral nutrition on DNA synthesis, cytokine release and receptor expression by lymphocytes in the postoperative period. *Br. J. Nutr.* **2002**, *87* (Suppl. 1), S103–S110. [CrossRef]

28. Sorensen, L.S.; Thorlacius-Ussing, O.; Schmidt, E.B.; Rasmussen, H.H.; Lundbye-Christensen, S.; Calder, P.C.; Lindorff-Larsen, K. Randomized clinical trial of perioperative omega-3 fatty acid supplements in elective colorectal cancer surgery. *Br. J. Surg.* **2014**, *101*, 33–42. [CrossRef]

29. Moher, D.; Hopewell, S.; Schulz, K.F.; Montori, V.; Gotzsche, P.C.; Devereaux, P.J.; Elbourne, D.; Egger, M.; Altman, D.G. CONSORT 2010 Explanation and Elaboration: Updated guidelines for reporting parallel group randomised trials. *J. Clin. Epidemiol.* **2010**, *63*, e1–e37. [CrossRef]

30. Wolters, U.; Wolf, T.; Stutzer, H.; Schroder, T. ASA classification and perioperative variables as predictors of postoperative outcome. *Br. J. Anaesth.* **1996**, *77*, 217–222. [CrossRef]

31. Kondrup, J.; Rasmussen, H.H.; Hamberg, O.; Stanga, Z. Nutritional risk screening (NRS 2002): A new method based on an analysis of controlled clinical trials. *Clin. Nutr.* **2003**, *22*, 321–336. [CrossRef]

32. A Service of the U.S. National Institutes of Health. Available online: http://clinicaltrials.gov/ct2/show/ NCT00488904?term=NCT00488904&rank=1 (accessed on 4 September 2010).

33. Nielsen, M.S.; Gammelmark, A.; Madsen, T.; Obel, T.; Aardestrup, I.; Schmidt, E.B. The effect of low-dose marine *n*-3 fatty acids on the biosynthesis of pro-inflammatory 5-lipoxygenase pathway metabolites in overweight subjects: A randomized controlled trial. *Prostaglandins Leukot. Essent. Fatty Acids* **2012**, *87*, 43–48. [CrossRef]

34. Powell, W.S.; Gravel, S.; Gravelle, F. Formation of a 5-oxo metabolite of 5,8,11,14,17-eicosapentaenoic acid and its effects on human neutrophils and eosinophils. *J. Lipid Res.* **1995**, *36*, 2590–2598.

35. Sorensen, L.S.; Rasmussen, H.H.; Aardestrup, I.V.; Thorlacius-Ussing, O.; Lindorff-Larsen, K.; Schmidt, E.B.; Calder, P.C. Rapid Incorporation of omega-3 Fatty Acids Into Colonic Tissue After Oral Supplementation in Patients With Colorectal Cancer: A Randomized, Placebo-Controlled Intervention Trial. *J. Parenter. Enter. Nutr.* **2013**, *38*, 617–624. [CrossRef]

36. Grimm, H.; Mertes, N.; Goeters, C.; Schlotzer, E.; Mayer, K.; Grimminger, F.; Furst, P. Improved fatty acid and leukotriene pattern with a novel lipid emulsion in surgical patients. *Eur. J. Nutr.* **2006**, *45*, 55–60.

37. Wang, J.; Yu, J.C.; Kang, W.M.; Ma, Z.Q. Superiority of a fish oil-enriched emulsion to medium-chain triacylglycerols/long-chain triacylglycerols in gastrointestinal surgery patients: A randomized clinical trial. *Nutrition* **2012**, *28*, 623–629. [CrossRef]

38. Shimizu, T.; Fujii, T.; Suzuki, R.; Igarashi, J.; Ohtsuka, Y.; Nagata, S.; Yamashiro, Y. Effects of highly purified eicosapentaenoic acid on erythrocyte fatty acid composition and leukocyte and colonic mucosa leukotriene B4 production in children with ulcerative colitis. *J. Pediatr. Gastroenterol. Nutr.* **2003**, *37*, 581–585. [CrossRef]

39. Carpentier, Y.A.; Simoens, C.; Siderova, V.; Vanweyenberg, V.; Eggerickx, D.; Deckelbaum, R.J. Recent developments in lipid emulsions: Relevance to intensive care. *Nutrition* **1997**, *13*, 73S–78S. [CrossRef]

40. Barros, K.V.; Carvalho, P.O.; Cassulino, A.P.; Andrade, I.; West, A.L.; Miles, E.A.; Calder, P.C.; Silveira, V.L. Fatty acids in plasma, white and red blood cells, and tissues after oral or intravenous administration of fish oil in rats. *Clin. Nutr.* **2013**, *32*, 993–998. [CrossRef]

11

The Anti-Proliferative Effects of Enterolactone in Prostate Cancer Cells: Evidence for the Role of DNA Licencing Genes, mi-R106b Cluster Expression, and PTEN Dosage

Mark J. McCann [1,2,*], Ian R. Rowland [3] and Nicole C. Roy [1,2,4]

[1] Food Nutrition & Health, Food and Bio-based Products, AgResearch Grasslands Research Centre, Palmerston North 4442, New Zealand; nicole.roy@agresearch.co.nz

[2] Gravida: National Centre for Growth and Development, The University of Auckland, Auckland 1142, New Zealand

[3] Department of Food and Nutritional Sciences, P.O. Box 226, Whiteknights, Reading RG6 6AP, UK; i.rowland@reading.ac.uk

[4] The Riddet Institute, Massey University, Palmerston North 4442, New Zealand

[*] Author to whom correspondence should be addressed; mark.mccann@agresearch.co.nz

Abstract: The mammalian lignan, enterolactone, has been shown to reduce the proliferation of the earlier stages of prostate cancer at physiological concentrations *in vitro*. However, efficacy in the later stages of the disease occurs at concentrations difficult to achieve through dietary modification. We have therefore investigated what concentration(s) of enterolactone can restrict proliferation in multiple stages of prostate cancer using an *in vitro* model system of prostate disease. We determined that enterolactone at 20 µM significantly restricted the proliferation of mid and late stage models of prostate disease. These effects were strongly associated with changes in the expression of the DNA licencing genes (GMNN, CDT1, MCM2 and 7), in reduced expression of the miR-106b cluster (miR-106b, miR-93, and miR-25), and in increased expression of the PTEN tumour suppressor gene. We have shown anti-proliferative effects of enterolactone in earlier stages of prostate disease than previously reported and that these effects are mediated, in part, by microRNA-mediated regulation.

Keywords: enterolactone; lignan; prostate; proliferation; PTEN; miR-106b cluster

1. Introduction

Prostate cancer is the second most common cancer in men worldwide with seventy percent of annual diagnoses occurring in Westernised societies [1]. The incidence of the disease is considerably higher in the EU, North America and New Zealand than in China (14, 22 and 25-fold, respectively) [2–5] Whilst risk factors for prostate cancer such as age, ethnic origin and heredity are important, geographical and economic differences in diet and lifestyle appear to influence prostate disease risk to a greater extent [6–8]. A clear link between diet and prostate cancer is yet to be shown, due in part to a lack of understanding of the effects, or absence of effect of dietary components on the mechanisms of prostate tumourigenesis.

Enterolactone (ENL) is a weakly-oestrogenic (100 to 1000-fold less compared to natural oestradiol) mammalian metabolite that is produced by the metabolism of plant lignans by intestinal bacteria, but may also be present in low amounts in dairy foods and meat as a consequence of ruminant intestinal metabolism (reviewed [9–11]), [12–16]. ENL has been reported to have anti-cancer, anti-oxidant, anti-inflammatory and anti-angiogenic properties [10,11,17–21], but ecological studies examining ENL exposure and disease risk, especially with regard to prostate cancer, have been inconclusive [9–11]. This is due, in part, to a lack of understanding of how the inter-individual response to ENL may be affected by diet and lifestyle, genetic and/or epigenetic factors and intestinal microbiota composition.

Serum or urinary ENL levels, a biomarker of exposure, vary considerably by population and dietary preference, and typically ranges from 0.1 to 10 µM [9–11]. There is, however, some evidence that ENL can accumulate to higher levels (up to 25-fold higher) in prostate tissue and fluid, suggesting a biological function for ENL in the prostate [22]. Although there are human, animal and *in vitro* studies showing that purified ENL, or foods rich in ENL, can inhibit the development and progression of prostate cancer for example by reducing proliferation [18–21] or affecting steroid metabolism and activity [23], it is not yet clear if these effects occur at concentrations achievable through dietary intake alone [9–11]. There is a distinct lack of data available on the concentration of ENL in prostate tissue pre and post-intervention with ENL precursors, which restricts our understanding of how bio-available ENL is in the prostate. We have recently shown that physiologically-relevant concentrations of ENL can reduce the proliferation of early-stage prostate disease *in vitro* and that these effects are associated with alterations in the expression of DNA replication licencing genes [19].

The correct initiation of DNA replication requires the licencing of origin of replications by the minichromosome maintenance complex (MCM) [24]. The loading of this MCM complex is facilitated, in part, by chromatin licensing and DNA replication factor 1 (CDT1), which is itself negatively regulated by geminin (GMMN). Abnormal expression of GMNN, CDT1, and MCM2 and 7 have been linked with the malignant progression of prostate cancer [25–31]. Another key signalling pathway disrupted in prostate cancer is the phosphoinositide-3-kinase (PI3K)-AKT signalling pathway. The phosphatase and tensin homolog (PTEN) tumour suppressor gene negatively regulates the PI3K/AKT pathway and PTEN is one of the most common tumour suppressor genes whose appropriate function is compromised in prostate cancer (~70% of cases) [32–34], which leads to abnormal proliferation and cell death. Initiation of DNA replication and PTEN tumour suppression are transcriptionally-linked as one of the MCMs (MCM7) has a microRNA cluster (miR-106b, -93, and 25) in one of its introns that suppresses PTEN translation and dysregulation of the cluster is also linked to cancer [35].

Cancer is not composed of abnormal cells at the same stage of disease; rather it is a series of abnormal cells at differing stages of disease that collectively compromise the appropriate function of the tissue. Previous research has shown anti-proliferative effects of ENL in one or in limited stages of disease, rather than efficacy in a range of disease states [18–21]. Therefore, we hypothesised that ENL could restrict the proliferation of more than just the later stages of prostate disease. To investigate our hypothesis we used an *in vitro* model system of six prostate cell lines representing the early (RWPE-1 and WPE1-NA22), mid (WPE1-NB14 and WPE1-NB11) and later (WPE1-NB26 and LNCaP) stages of prostate tumourigenesis [36,37]. The LNCaP cell line is a model of the switch between androgen sensitivity and insensitivity during prostate disease that occurs in the later stages of carcinogenesis [37]. This *in vitro* model system was used to assess how the metabolic activity, growth rate, cell cycle progression changes with ENL exposure over 24 and 48 h. Based on these data we explored potential mechanisms for the anti-proliferative activity by measuring the expression of the GMMN, CDT1, MCM2 and MCM7, miR-106b cluster, and PTEN genes.

2. Experimental Section

2.1. Cell Culture and Enterolactone Preparation

Authenticated RWPE-1 (P52), WPE1-NA22 (P20), WPE1-NB14 (P16), WPE1-NB11 (P24), WPE1-NB26 (P15), and LNCaP (P22) cell lines were purchased from the American Type Culture Collection (Manassas, VA, USA) to test the effects of ENL. All cell culture reagents were obtained from Life Technologies (Auckland, New Zealand) unless otherwise stated. The cell lines were cultured and maintained as described previously [19], with all experiments were completed within ten sub-cultures from the original ATCC stock.

A stock solution of ENL (45199, Sigma-Aldrich, Auckland, New Zealand) at 16.76 mM (100% DMSO) was prepared and used to prepare test concentrations of ENL in cell-line specific medium. Etoposide (Sigma-Aldrich, Auckland New Zealand) was used as a positive control for proliferation as it blocks DNA synthesis resulting in apoptosis. The negative control for all experiments was cell-line specific medium adjusted to contain 0.36% v/v of DMSO.

2.2. Cell Viability—Mitochondrial Activity Assay

The effect of 10 to 100 μM ENL on the metabolic activity of the six cell lines over 48 h was measured using the water soluble tetrazolium cytotoxicity assay (WST-1, Clontech, Mountain View, CA, USA) as described previously [19]. The negative control and each concentration of ENL were tested on twenty-four biological replicates for both time points. The absorbance of the formazan dye produced was measured at 450 and 650 nm using a SpectraMax 250 spectrophotometer (Molecular Devices, Sunnyvale, CA, USA). For all measurements (including the blank), the background absorbance (650 nm) was subtracted from the detection wavelength (450 nm) and these corrected values were used for analysis.

2.3. Cell Viability—Growth Kinetics Assay

The effect of 10 to 60 μM ENL on the viability of each cell line over 48 h was measured using trypan blue staining and the number of non-blue (viable) cells counted as described previously [19]. For each of three separate assays for each time point, each concentration was tested on two technical replicates with an initial seeding density of 5×10^5 cells. From these data the effect of ENL on the doubling time of the cell lines was calculated.

2.4. Cell Viability—Cell Cycle Profile Assay

The effect of 20 μM ENL on the cell cycle profile of six cell lines over 48 h was measured with the Dead Cell Apoptosis Kit with Annexin V Alexa Fluor® 488 & Propidium Iodide from Life Technologies (Auckland, New Zealand). This kit is a flow cytometry kit used to measure early apoptosis by detecting phosphatidyl serine expression and membrane permeability [18,38].

Each assay was completed according to the manufacturer's instructions. For each of three separate assays for each time point, each concentration was tested on three technical replicates with an initial seeding density of 5×10^5 cells. The fluorescence intensities of Alexa Fluor 488 and Propidium Iodide in each sample, at 585 nm, were measured using a FACSCalibur flow cytometer with CELLQuest Pro Software (BD Biosciences, Auckland, New Zealand), and analysed using FlowJo V7.6.3 (TreeStar, Ashland, OR, USA).

2.5. Quantification of Gene Expression—mRNA and miRNA Genes

The expression of GMNN, CDT1, MCMs 2 and 7, PTEN, hsa-miR-106b, hsa-miR-93, and hsa-miR-25 by the six cell lines treated with 20 μM ENL over 48 h was quantified using probe-based real-time PCR. All reagents were obtained from Life Technologies (Auckland, New Zealand) unless otherwise stated. For each gene and time point, two biological replicates (with triplicate qPCR measurements) of 5×10^5 cells were used.

The NucleoSpin® miRNA kit (Macherey-Nagel, Düren, Germany) was used to extract large and small RNA in separate fractions from each of the samples according to the manufacturer's instructions. RNA quantity and integrity was determined based on A260:280 and A260:230 nm ratios using a NanoDrop 1000 spectrophotometer (Thermo Fisher Scientific, Melbourne, Australia) and a Agilent 2100 bioanalyser (Agilent, Santa Clara, CA, USA). Only RNA with both absorbance ratios of 1.8 to 2.1 and with a RIN value of 9 or greater were considered to be of sufficient quality and integrity.

For the large RNA fractions, 500 ng was reverse transcribed into cDNA using a high capacity RNA-to-cDNA kit according to the manufacturer's instructions. The expression levels of the mRNA transcripts of the GMNN, CDT1, MCMs 2 and 7, and PTEN genes were quantified using pre-validated PrimeTime Nuclease assays (Hs.PT.51.14706721.g, Hs.PT.53.27448129.gs, Hs.PT.53.25820936, Hs.PT.53.23112694.g, and Hs.PT.51.14706721.g) (Integrated DNA Technologies, Singapore, Singapore). The HPRT1 (Hs.PT.39a.22214821) reference gene was used to normalise for RNA content.

For the small RNA fractions, 10 ng was reverse transcribed into cDNA with gene specific primers using the TaqMan microRNA RT kit according to the manufacturer's instructions. The expression levels of the mature hsa-miR-106, hsa-miR-93, and hsa-miR-25 genes were quantified using pre-validated TaqMan assays (000442, 002139, and 002442). The RNU6B reference gene (001093) was used to normalise for RNA content.

All real-time PCR assays were prepared as triplicate 10 µL reactions comprising a 9.0 µL aliquot of master mix (5.0 µL of 2x Kapa Fast Probe mix (Kapa Biosystems, Wilmington, DE, USA), 0.5 µL of 20x mRNA or miRNA gene assay, 3.5 µL of nuclease-free water, and 1 µL of cDNA (10-fold dilution in nuclease-free water). The thermal profile used was: 95 °C for 20 s, followed by 40 cycles of 95 °C for 3 s and 60 °C for 30 s. The experiment was completed using a RotorGene 6000 qPCR instrument (Qiagen, Hilden, Germany). Data were normalised to the appropriate reference gene and analysed for expression level changes (ratio compared to untreated) using the ΔCq method with efficiency correction. The efficiencies for all PCRs ranged between 1.91 and 2.03, where 2.0 represents 100% efficiency.

2.6. Statistical Analyses

All data were analysed for statistical significance using a one-way ANOVA with SigmaStat 12.3 (Systat Software Inc., San Jose, CA, USA). The normality of the data was tested using the Shapiro-Wilk method and the equality of variance using the Leven Median test. Non-normally distributed data was ranked and analysed using the Kruskal-Wallis ANOVA method. Following ANOVA, significantly different means were identified using the Dunnett's post-hoc test. A probability (p) value of less than 0.05 was considered to show a significant difference.

3. Results

3.1. ENL Reduces the Viability of Mid to Later Stage Prostate Disease Cell Lines

ENL exerted differential effects on the mitochondrial metabolic activity and growth kinetics of the prostate cell lines at 24 and 48 h of exposure (Figures 1 and 2).

At 24 h, 20 µM ENL or greater significantly reduced the metabolic activity of the WPE1-NB14, WPE1-NB11, WPE1-NB26, and LNCaP cell lines. At 48 h, 40 µM ENL or greater reduced the activity of all cell lines. However, the activity of the WPE1-NA22 (10 and 20 µM), WPE1-NB14 (10 and 20 µM), WPE1-NB11 (10 and 20 µM), WPE1-NB26 (10 and 20 µM), and LNCaP (20 µM) cell lines was reduced at this time point. The RWPE-1 cell line tolerated up 40 µM ENL without significant alterations in metabolic activity. The metabolic activity of the WPE1-NB44, WPE1-NB11, WPE1-NB26, and LNCaP cell lines were significantly reduced in a dose dependent manner at concentrations of 20 µM of greater at both time points. The WPE1-NB14 and WPE1-NB11 cells were particularly sensitive to ENL at 24 and 48 h.

These data indicate that the lowest concentration of ENL that affects the metabolic activity in the "diseased" cell lines, but does not affect the "normal" cell line is 20 µM. As 40 to 100 µM ENL clearly affected all cell lines, these concentrations were excluded from further analysis. As changes in metabolic activity may result in altered growth rates, *i.e.*, a change in the time taken for a population of cells to double in number, we measured the doubling times of the cell lines in response to 10 and 20 µM ENL over 48 h.

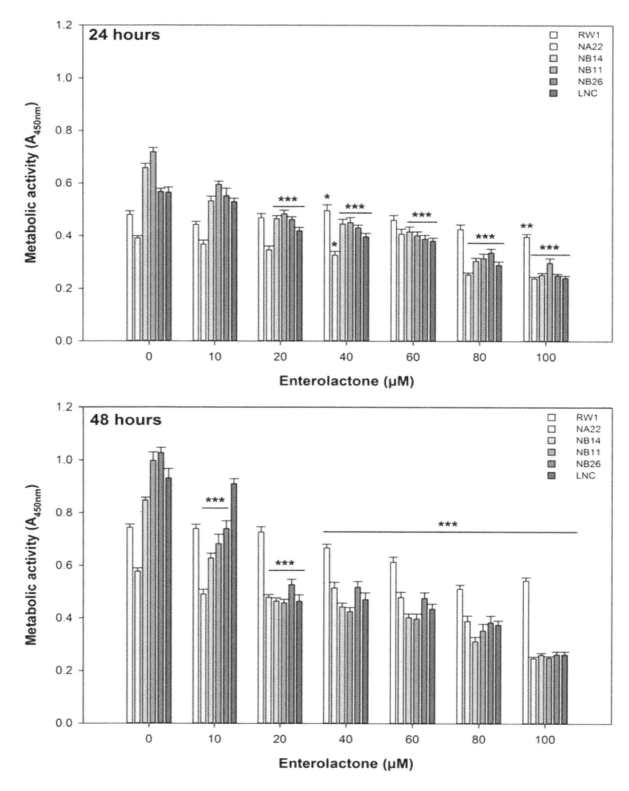

Figure 1. The effect of ENL on the metabolic activity of prostate cell lines over 48 h. The data are expressed as the mean absorbance ±SEM (n = 24). A statistical difference between untreated and treated samples is indicated by * ($p < 0.05$), ** ($p < 0.01$), or *** ($p < 0.002$).

The growth kinetics, based on the time for the population to double in number, of the RWPE-1 and WPE1-NA22 cell lines were unaltered by ENL. The positive control, 20 μM etoposide, significantly ($p < 0.018$) decreased the metabolic activity and increased in the doubling time of the cell lines over 48 h. The WPE1-NB14, WPE1-NB11, and WPE1-NB26 cell lines were the most sensitive to the ENL-induced increased doubling time (*i.e.*, slower growth) of these cell lines. The doubling time of the LNCaP cell line was only affected by 20 μM ENL.

As 20 μM ENL was the lowest concentration that affected both the metabolic activity and doubling times of the WPE1 and LNCaP cell lines, but not the RWPE-1 cell line (the least diseased cell line in our model and an approximation of a "normal" cell line) this concentration was selected for further study.

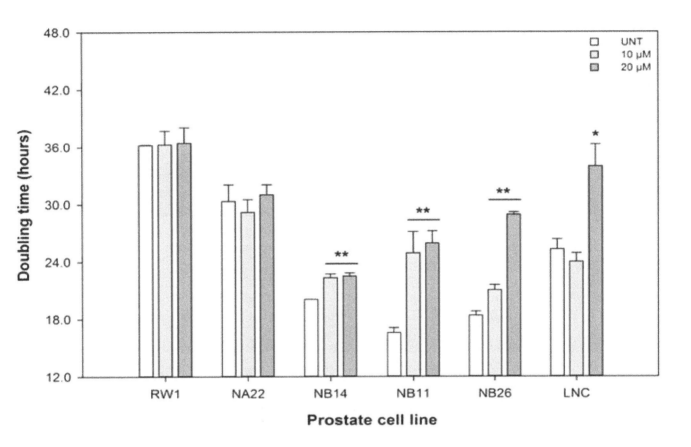

Figure 2. The effect of ENL on the doubling times of prostate cell lines over 48 h. The data are expressed as the mean doubling time ±SEM (*n* = 3). A statistical difference between untreated (UNT) and treated samples is indicated by * ($p < 0.05$), or ** ($p < 0.01$).

3.2. ENL Restricts the Cell Cycle of and Induces Apoptosis in Mid to Later Stage Prostate Disease Cell Lines

The restriction of cell cycle progression in the cell lines with 20 μM ENL over 48 h is shown in Figure 3 to Figure 4. The positive control, 20 μM etoposide, significantly increased the S-phase and level of apoptosis of the cell lines over 48 h ($p < 0.014$).

At 24 h, there was an increase in the percentage of cells in the G_0/G_1 phase of the cell cycle for the RWPE-1, WPE1-NB14, WPE1-NB11, WPE1-NB26, and LNCaP cell lines in response to 20 μM ENL. For the LNCaP cell line there was also decrease in the percentage of cells in the G_2/M phase. At 48 h, the cell cycle of the WPE1-NB14 and WPE1-NB11 cell lines remained altered (NB14: increased G_0/G_1, decreased S, and NB11: decreased G_0/G_1, increased S, decreased G_2/M) by ENL. The G_0/G_1 and G_2/M phases of the LNCaP cell line were also restricted, both reduced, after 48 h.

The data in Figures 3 and 4 also show that 20 μM ENL induces apoptosis in the WPE1-NB14, WPE1-NB11, and WPE1-NB26 after 24 and 48 h. At 48 h, the WPE1-NA22 and LNCaP cell lines also had increased levels of apoptosis in response to ENL.

These data indicate that the disrupted viability (metabolic activity and doubling times), shown in Figures 1 and 2, of the cell lines is due, in part, to alterations in cell cycling and cell death. Given the alterations shown Figures 3 and 4, the effect of 20 μM ENL on the expression of genes involved in two key pathways during abnormal growth and carcinogenesis was quantified to explore potential mechanisms of action.

3.3. ENL Alters the Expression of DNA Licencing Genes in Mid to Later Stage Prostate Disease Cell Lines

The expression of the DNA licencing genes in response to 20 μM ENL by the six cell lines are shown in Figure 5. The co-efficient of variation for the HPRT1 reference gene amongst the untreated cell lines was 9% and 5%, at 24 and 48 h respectively. These data show that the expression of GMNN (CDT1 inhibitor) is increased approximately 2 to 3 fold in the WPE1-NB14 and WPE1-NB11 cell lines after 24 and 48 h. The expression of CDT1 was reduced in these cell lines by approximately 2 fold. The expression of the MCM2 and 7 genes was reduced in the majority of cell lines at 24 h, but only in the WPE1-NA2, WPE1-NB14, and WPE1-NB11 cell lines at 48 h. These changes in expression imply that the licencing of DNA for replication is reduced and would results in cell cycle restrictions (particularly in the G_0/G_1 and S phases), reduced proliferation, and/or increased cell death.

The reduced expression of MCM7 suggests that the miR-106b cluster (located in one of the introns of MCM7) may also be influenced by ENL and if so this may affect the expression of the PTEN gene.

3.4. ENL Alters the Expression of the miR-106b Cluster Leading to Increased PTEN Expression

The expression of the miR-106b cluster and PTEN genes in response to 20 μM ENL by the six cell lines are shown in Figure 6. The co-efficient of variation for the rnu6b reference gene in the untreated cell lines was 2.3% and 2%, at 24 and 48 h respectively. These data show that the expression of miR-106b, miR-93, and miR-25 are decreased in the WPE1-NB14, WPE1-NB11, WPE1-NB26, and LNCaP cell lines after 24 and 48 h. The expression of PTEN is substantially increased in the WPE1 and LNCaP cell lines.

These data suggest that the repression of the miR-106b cluster leads, in part, to increased PTEN expression. However, the expression of PTEN was increased by ENL in the WPE1-NA22 cell line despite no substantial change in the expression of the miR-106b cluster.

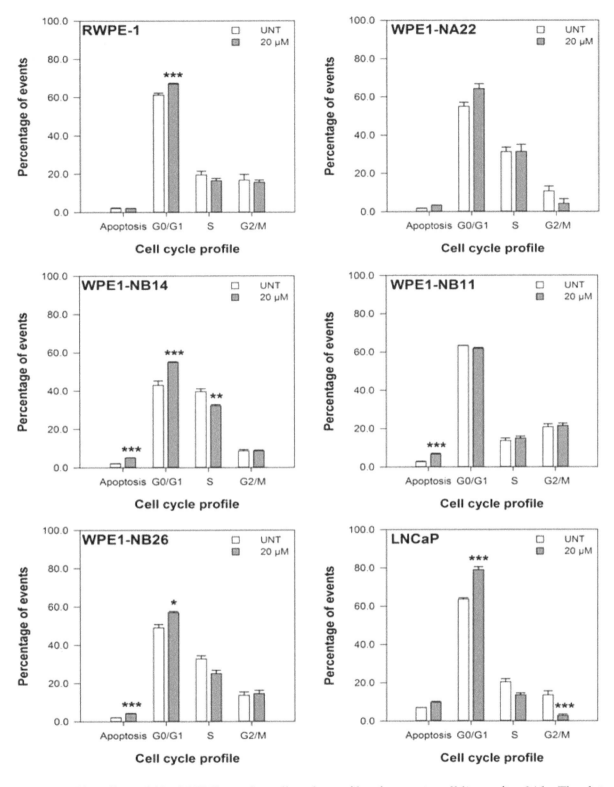

Figure 3. The effect of 20 μM ENL on the cell cycle profile of prostate cell lines after 24 h. The data are expressed as the mean percentage of events in each phase ±SEM ($n = 3$). A statistical difference between untreated and treated samples is indicated by * ($p < 0.05$), ** ($p < 0.01$), or *** ($p < 0.002$).

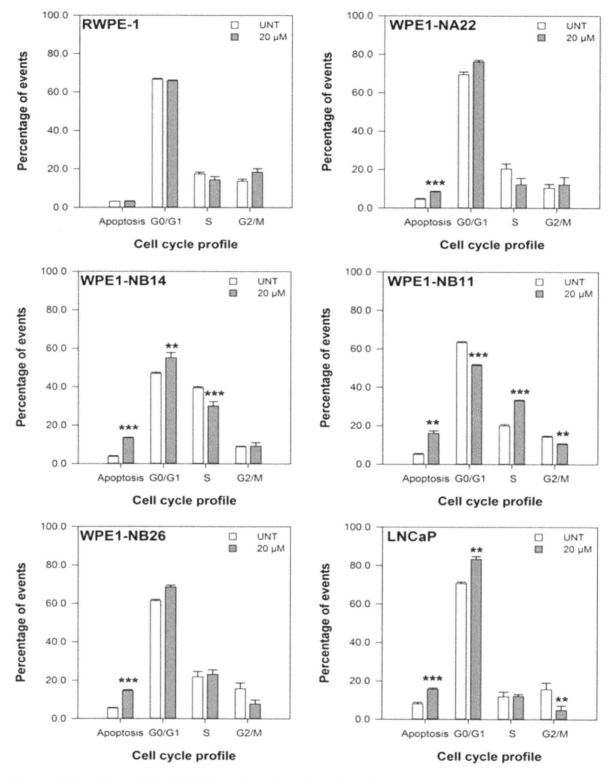

Figure 4. The effect of 20 µM ENL on the cell cycle profile of prostate cell lines after 48 h. The data are expressed as the mean percentage of events in each phase ±SEM ($n = 3$). A statistical difference between untreated and treated samples is indicated by * ($p < 0.05$), ** ($p < 0.01$), or *** ($p < 0.002$).

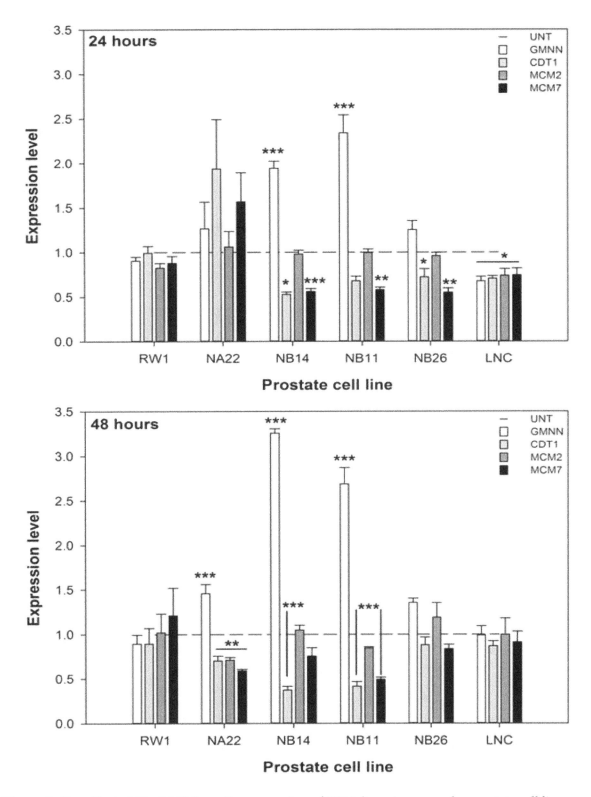

Figure 5. The effect of 20 μM ENL on the expression of DNA licencing genes by prostate cell lines over 48 h. The data are expressed as the mean expression level ±SEM ($n = 3$). For each cell line, a difference between untreated and treated samples is indicated by * ($p < 0.05$), ** ($p < 0.01$), or *** ($p < 0.002$).

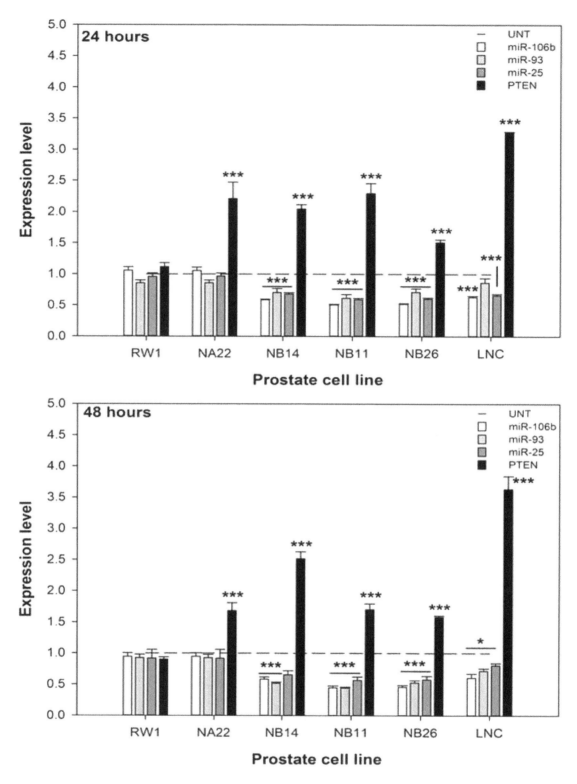

Figure 6. The effect of ENL on the expression of the PTEN gene and miR-106b cluster genes by prostate cell lines over 48 h. The data are expressed as the mean expression level ±SEM (*n* = 3). For each cell line, a difference between untreated and treated samples is indicated by * (*p* < 0.05), or *** (*p* < 0.002).

4. Discussion

The present study provides further evidence that a pure mammalian lignan inhibits the *in vitro* proliferation of prostate cell lines. To our knowledge, this is the first study to examine the correlation between the expression of genes associated with DNA licencing and miR-106b cluster mediated PTEN and biological end-points of proliferation *in vitro*.

Previous *in vitro* studies examining how the prostate cell lines respond to ENL have reported anti-proliferative effects for concentrations ranging from 25 to 100 μM and our data are in agreement with these findings [18,20]. In contrast to the previous studies we have studied the effects of ENL on the proliferation of a range of prostate cell models, rather than the late-stage models generally used, and explored potential mechanisms of action. We have shown that ENL at 20 μM over 48 h is sufficient to restrict the proliferation of primarily mid to later stage prostate cancer cells without any effects on the approximately "normal" RWPE-1 cell line. However, this cell line is immortalised and is not truly normal. Additionally we have shown that the anti-proliferative effects of ENL are strongly associated with: (1) improved negative regulation of abnormal DNA licencing (increased GMNN expression and decreased CDT1 expression); and (2) inhibition of miR-106b cluster expression leading to increased expression of the tumour suppressive gene PTEN.

The ENL-induced changes in genes required for DNA replication initiation may explain the effects of ENL on cell cycle control and consequently proliferation in the prostate cell lines. However, the effect of altering the GMNN/CDT1 balance in tumourigenic cells (which express higher levels of these genes compared to normal cells [31]) is unclear as there is debate about how the GMNN/CDT1 balance influences the development and progression of cancer [26–28,39,40]. Additionally we have also shown that the expression of MCM2 and MCM7 is reduced by ENL in the prostate cell lines used, and this may be linked altered CDT1 expression as CDT1 is required for the loading of the MCM complex during the initiation of DNA replication [24]. MCM7, in particular, is known to be oncogenic [25,29,41] not only for its role in DNA licencing, but also due to other interactions such as: (1) MCM7 overexpression can inhibit the retinoblastoma-controlled cell G_1/S cell cycle block [42,43]; (2) MCM7 interacts with the androgen receptor [44], appropriate androgen signalling and the consequences of androgen insensitivity are key factors in prostate carcinogenesis and relapse [45,46]; and (3) one of the introns of MCM7 contains the mir-106b cluster [35] which targets two key tumour suppressor genes implicated in the prostate cancer, PTEN and CDKN1A (p21) [47–49].

Reduced PTEN expression can contribute to cancer development due to decreased negative regulation of the PI3K/AKT pathway (known as quasi-sufficiency) [50]. Unlike the classic "two-hit" model of tumour suppression, it is the amount of functional PTEN (which can be affected by several factors not just transcription) that determines its tumour suppressive capacity. We have shown that ENL can increase PTEN expression, which may restore the appropriate regulation by PTEN of the PI3K/AKT pathway. However, the LNCaP cell line has a mutated and non-functional PTEN gene [32] and therefore the consequence of its increased expression by ENL is unclear.

The concentrations used in this study have yet to be shown to be achievable in the prostate *in vivo* either through dietary or pharmacological intervention. We also have only demonstrated a link between gene expression and proliferation markers—further work is needed to establish whether the expression changes result in functional changes at the post-transcriptional level. We have shown that there appears to be a relationship between ENL-mediated expression of the PTEN gene, perhaps via suppression of the miR-106b cluster, and proliferation in prostate cancer cell lines. If these are confirmed at the proteomic and functional level, it may represent a novel mechanism for the anti-proliferative activity of ENL.

5. Conclusions

In conclusion we have provided evidence for the anti-proliferative effects of ENL in mid and late prostate cell lines, and have shown that changes in the transcription of DNA licencing, miR-106b cluster, and PTEN genes may be involved in these effects. This is important as we have shown that ENL is effective in earlier stages of prostate cancer than previously reported and two important pathways in prostate tumourigenesis are linked through miRNA effects.

Acknowledgments: This work was supported by the Marsden Fund Council from NZ Government funding (administered by the Royal Society of New Zealand) and the Palmerston North Medical Research Foundation.

Author Contributions: Mark J. McCann wrote the manuscript and completed the experimental work. All of the authors reviewed the manuscript and contributed to the scientific content of this paper.

References

1.   Jemal, A.; Bray, F.; Center, M.M.; Ferlay, J.; Ward, E.; Forman, D. Global cancer statistics. *CA Cancer J. Clin.* **2011**, *61*, 69–90. [CrossRef]
2.   Center, M.M.; Jemal, A.; Lortet-Tieulent, J.; Ward, E.; Ferlay, J.; Brawley, O.; Bray, F. International variation in prostate cancer incidence and mortality rates. *Eur. Urol.* **2012**, *61*, 1079–1092. [CrossRef] [PubMed]
3.   Ferlay, J.; Shin, H.R.; Bray, F.; Forman, D.; Mathers, C.; Parkin, D.M. Estimates of worldwide burden of cancer in 2008: GLOBOCAN 2008. *Int. J. Cancer* **2010**, *127*, 2893–2917. [CrossRef] [PubMed]
4.   Baade, P.D.; Youlden, D.R.; Krnjacki, L.J. International epidemiology of prostate cancer: Geographical distribution and secular trends. *Mol. Nutr. Food Res.* **2009**, *53*, 171–184. [CrossRef] [PubMed]
5.   Cullen, J.; Elsamanoudi, S.; Brassell, S.A.; Chen, Y.; Colombo, M.; Srivastava, A.; McLeod, D.G. The burden of prostate cancer in Asian nations. *J. Carcinog.* **2012**, *11*, 7. [CrossRef] [PubMed]
6.   Venkateswaran, V.; Klotz, L.H. Diet and prostate cancer: Mechanisms of action and implications for chemoprevention. *Nat. Rev. Urol.* **2010**, *7*, 442–453. [CrossRef] [PubMed]
7.   Khan, N.; Afaq, F.; Mukhtar, H. Lifestyle as risk factor for cancer: Evidence from human studies. *Cancer Lett.* **2010**, *293*, 133–143. [CrossRef] [PubMed]
8.   Muller, D.C.; Severi, G.; Baglietto, L.; Krishnan, K.; English, D.R.; Hopper, J.L.; Giles, G.G. Dietary patterns and prostate cancer risk. *Cancer Epidemiol. Biomark. Prev.* **2009**, *18*, 3126–3129. [CrossRef]
9.   Saarinen, N.M.; Tuominen, J.; Pylkkanen, L.; Santti, R. Assessment of information to substantiate a health claim on the prevention of prostate cancer by lignans. *Nutrients* **2010**, *2*, 99–115. [CrossRef] [PubMed]
10.   Adlercreutz, H. Lignans and human health. *Crit. Rev. Clin. Lab. Sci.* **2007**, *44*, 483–525. [CrossRef] [PubMed]
11.   McCann, M.J.; Gill, C.I.; McGlynn, H.; Rowland, I.R. Role of mammalian lignans in the prevention and treatment of prostate cancer. *Nutr. Cancer* **2005**, *52*, 1–14. [CrossRef] [PubMed]
12.   Kuhnle, G.G.; Dell'Aquila, C.; Aspinall, S.M.; Runswick, S.A.; Mulligan, A.A.; Bingham, S.A. Phytoestrogen content of foods of animal origin: Dairy products, eggs, meat, fish, and seafood. *J. Agric. Food Chem.* **2008**, *56*, 10099–10104. [CrossRef] [PubMed]
13.   Setchell, K.D.; Lawson, A.M.; Mitchell, F.L.; Adlercreutz, H.; Kirk, D.N.; Axelson, M. Lignans in man and in animal species. *Nature* **1980**, *287*, 740–742. [CrossRef] [PubMed]
14.   Woting, A.; Clavel, T.; Loh, G.; Blaut, M. Bacterial transformation of dietary lignans in gnotobiotic rats. *FEMS Microbiol. Ecol.* **2010**, *72*, 507–514. [CrossRef] [PubMed]
15.   Clavel, T.; Borrmann, D.; Braune, A.; Dore, J.; Blaut, M. Occurrence and activity of human intestinal bacteria involved in the conversion of dietary lignans. *Anaerobe* **2006**, *12*, 140–147. [CrossRef] [PubMed]
16.   Clavel, T.; Henderson, G.; Engst, W.; Dore, J.; Blaut, M. Phylogeny of human intestinal bacteria that activate the dietary lignan secoisolariciresinol diglucoside. *FEMS Microbiol. Ecol.* **2006**, *55*, 471–478. [CrossRef] [PubMed]
17.   Saarinen, N.M.; Thompson, L.U. Prolonged administration of secoisolariciresinol diglycoside increases lignan excretion and alters lignan tissue distribution in adult male and female rats. *Br. J. Nutr.* **2010**, *104*, 833–841. [CrossRef] [PubMed]
18.   McCann, M.J.; Gill, C.I.; Linton, T.; Berrar, D.; McGlynn, H.; Rowland, I.R. Enterolactone restricts the proliferation of the LNCaP human prostate cancer cell line *in vitro*. *Mol. Nutr. Food Res.* **2008**, *52*, 567–580. [CrossRef] [PubMed]
19.   McCann, M.J.; Rowland, I.R.; Roy, N.C. Anti-proliferative effects of physiological concentrations of enterolactone in models of prostate tumourigenesis. *Mol. Nutr. Food Res.* **2013**, *57*, 212–224. [CrossRef] [PubMed]
20.   Chen, L.H.; Fang, J.; Li, H.; Demark-Wahnefried, W.; Lin, X. Enterolactone induces apoptosis in human prostate carcinoma LNCaP cells via a mitochondrial-mediated, caspase-dependent pathway. *Mol. Cancer Ther.* **2007**, *6*, 2581–2590. [CrossRef] [PubMed]

21. Lin, X.; Switzer, B.R.; Demark-Wahnefried, W. Effect of mammalian lignans on the growth of prostate cancer cell lines. *Anticancer Res.* **2001**, *21*, 3995–3999. [PubMed]

22. Morton, M.S.; Chan, P.S.; Cheng, C.; Blacklock, N.; Matos-Ferreira, A.; Abranches-Monteiro, L.; Correia, R.; Lloyd, S.; Griffiths, K. Lignans and isoflavonoids in plasma and prostatic fluid in men: Samples from Portugal, Hong Kong, and the United Kingdom. *Prostate* **1997**, *32*, 122–128. [CrossRef] [PubMed]

23. Adlercreutz, H.; Bannwart, C.; Wahala, K.; Makela, T.; Brunow, G.; Hase, T.; Arosemena, P.J.; Kellis, J.T., Jr.; Vickery, L.E. Inhibition of human aromatase by mammalian lignans and isoflavonoid phytoestrogens. *J. Steroid Biochem. Mol. Biol.* **1993**, *44*, 147–153. [CrossRef] [PubMed]

24. Masai, H.; Matsumoto, S.; You, Z.; Yoshizawa-Sugata, N.; Oda, M. Eukaryotic chromosome DNA replication: Where, when, and how? *Annu. Rev. Biochem.* **2010**, *79*, 89–130. [CrossRef]

25. Luo, J.H. Oncogenic activity of MCM7 transforming cluster. *World J. Clin. Oncol.* **2011**, *2*, 120–124. [CrossRef] [PubMed]

26. Hook, S.S.; Lin, J.J.; Dutta, A. Mechanisms to control rereplication and implications for cancer. *Curr. Opin. Cell Biol.* **2007**, *19*, 663–671. [CrossRef] [PubMed]

27. Lau, E.; Tsuji, T.; Guo, L.; Lu, S.H.; Jiang, W. The role of pre-replicative complex (pre-RC) components in oncogenesis. *FASEB J.* **2007**, *21*, 3786–3794. [CrossRef] [PubMed]

28. Montanari, M.; Macaluso, M.; Cittadini, A.; Giordano, A. Role of geminin: from normal control of DNA replication to cancer formation and progression? *Cell Death Differ.* **2006**, *13*, 1052–1056. [CrossRef] [PubMed]

29. Ren, B.; Yu, G.; Tseng, G.C.; Cieply, K.; Gavel, T.; Nelson, J.; Michalopoulos, G.; Yu, Y.P.; Luo, J.H. MCM7 amplification and overexpression are associated with prostate cancer progression. *Oncogene* **2006**, *25*, 1090–1098. [CrossRef] [PubMed]

30. Honeycutt, K.A.; Chen, Z.; Koster, M.I.; Miers, M.; Nuchtern, J.; Hicks, J.; Roop, D.R.; Shohet, J.M. Deregulated minichromosomal maintenance protein MCM7 contributes to oncogene driven tumorigenesis. *Oncogene* **2006**, *25*, 4027–4032. [CrossRef] [PubMed]

31. Xouri, G.; Lygerou, Z.; Nishitani, H.; Pachnis, V.; Nurse, P.; Taraviras, S. Cdt1 and geminin are down-regulated upon cell cycle exit and are over-expressed in cancer-derived cell lines. *Eur. J. Biochem.* **2004**, *271*, 3368–3378. [CrossRef] [PubMed]

32. Chen, Z.; Trotman, L.C.; Shaffer, D.; Lin, H.K.; Dotan, Z.A.; Niki, M.; Koutcher, J.A.; Scher, H.I.; Ludwig, T.; Gerald, W.; *et al.* Crucial role of p53-dependent cellular senescence in suppression of Pten-deficient tumorigenesis. *Nature* **2005**, *436*, 725–730. [CrossRef] [PubMed]

33. Pourmand, G.; Ziaee, A.A.; Abedi, A.R.; Mehrsai, A.; Alavi, H.A.; Ahmadi, A.; Saadati, H.R. Role of PTEN gene in progression of prostate cancer. *Urol. J.* **2007**, *4*, 95–100. [PubMed]

34. Vlietstra, R.J.; van Alewijk, D.C.; Hermans, K.G.; van Steenbrugge, G.J.; Trapman, J. Frequent inactivation of PTEN in prostate cancer cell lines and xenografts. *Cancer Res.* **1998**, *58*, 2720–2723. [PubMed]

35. Poliseno, L.; Salmena, L.; Riccardi, L.; Fornari, A.; Song, M.S.; Hobbs, R.M.; Sportoletti, P.; Varmeh, S.; Egia, A.; Fedele, G.; *et al.* Identification of the miR-106b~25 microRNA cluster as a proto-oncogenic PTEN-targeting intron that cooperates with its host gene MCM7 in transformation. *Sci. Signal.* **2010**, *3*, ra29. [CrossRef] [PubMed]

36. Webber, M.M.; Quader, S.T.; Kleinman, H.K.; Bello-DeOcampo, D.; Storto, P.D.; Bice, G.; DeMendonca-Calaca, W.; Williams, D.E. Human cell lines as an *in vitro/in vivo* model for prostate carcinogenesis and progression. *Prostate* **2001**, *47*, 1–13. [CrossRef] [PubMed]

37. Horoszewicz, J.S.; Leong, S.S.; Chu, T.M.; Wajsman, Z.L.; Friedman, M.; Papsidero, L.; Kim, U.; Chai, L.S.; Kakati, S.; Arya, S.K.; *et al.* The LNCaP cell line—A new model for studies on human prostatic carcinoma. *Prog. Clin. Biol. Res.* **1980**, *37*, 115–132. [PubMed]

38. Van Engeland, M.; Nieland, L.J.; Ramaekers, F.C.; Schutte, B.; Reutelingsperger, C.P. Annexin V-affinity assay: A review on an apoptosis detection system based on phosphatidylserine exposure. *Cytometry* **1998**, *31*, 1–9. [CrossRef] [PubMed]

39. Arentson, E.; Faloon, P.; Seo, J.; Moon, E.; Studts, J.M.; Fremont, D.H.; Choi, K. Oncogenic potential of the DNA replication licensing protein CDT1. *Oncogene* **2002**, *21*, 1150–1158. [CrossRef] [PubMed]

40. Blow, J.J.; Gillespie, P.J. Replication licensing and cancer—A fatal entanglement? *Nat. Rev. Cancer* **2008**, *8*, 799–806. [CrossRef]

41. Lei, M. The MCM complex: Its role in DNA replication and implications for cancer therapy. *Curr. Cancer Drug Targets* **2005**, *5*, 365–380. [CrossRef] [PubMed]

42. Sterner, J.M.; Dew-Knight, S.; Musahl, C.; Kornbluth, S.; Horowitz, J.M. Negative regulation of DNA replication by the retinoblastoma protein is mediated by its association with MCM7. *Mol. Cell. Biol.* **1998**, *18*, 2748–2757. [PubMed]

43. Mukherjee, P.; Winter, S.L.; Alexandrow, M.G. Cell cycle arrest by transforming growth factor beta1 near G1/S is mediated by acute abrogation of prereplication complex activation involving an Rb-MCM interaction. *Mol. Cell. Biol.* **2010**, *30*, 845–856. [CrossRef] [PubMed]

44. Shi, Y.K.; Yu, Y.P.; Zhu, Z.H.; Han, Y.C.; Ren, B.; Nelson, J.B.; Luo, J.H. MCM7 interacts with androgen receptor. *Am. J. Pathol.* **2008**, *173*, 1758–1767. [CrossRef] [PubMed]

45. Evans, C.P.; Lara, P.N., Jr. Prostate cancer: Predicting response to androgen receptor signalling inhibition. *Nat. Rev. Urol.* **2014**, *11*, 433–435. [CrossRef] [PubMed]

46. Balk, S.P. Androgen receptor functions in prostate cancer development and progression. *Asian J. Androl.* **2014**, *16*, 561–564. [CrossRef] [PubMed]

47. Song, M.S.; Salmena, L.; Pandolfi, P.P. The functions and regulation of the PTEN tumour suppressor. *Nat. Rev. Mol. Cell Biol.* **2012**, *13*, 283–296. [PubMed]

48. Sarker, D.; Reid, A.H.; Yap, T.A.; de Bono, J.S. Targeting the PI3K/AKT pathway for the treatment of prostate cancer. *Clin. Cancer Res.* **2009**, *15*, 4799–4805. [CrossRef] [PubMed]

49. Abbas, T.; Dutta, A. p21 in cancer: Intricate networks and multiple activities. *Nat. Rev. Cancer* **2009**, *9*, 400–414. [CrossRef] [PubMed]

50. Berger, A.H.; Knudson, A.G.; Pandolfi, P.P. A continuum model for tumour suppression. *Nature* **2011**, *476*, 163–169. [CrossRef] [PubMed]

12

An Investigation into the Association between DNA Damage and Dietary Fatty Acid in Men with Prostate Cancer

Karen S. Bishop [1,*], Sharon Erdrich [2], Nishi Karunasinghe [1], Dug Yeo Han [3], Shuotun Zhu [3], Amalini Jesuthasan [3] and Lynnette R. Ferguson [1,2,3]

[1]   Auckland Cancer Society Research Centre, FM & HS, University of Auckland, Private Bag 92019, Auckland 1142, New Zealand; n.karunasinghe@auckland.ac.nz (N.K.); l.ferguson@auckland.ac.nz (L.R.F.)

[2]   Discipline of Nutrition, FM & HS, University of Auckland, Private Bag 92019, Auckland 1142, New Zealand; sharon.erdrich@gmail.com

[3]   Nutrigenomics New Zealand, University of Auckland, Private Bag 92019, Auckland 1142, New Zealand; dy.han@auckland.ac.nz (D.Y.H.); st.zhu@auckland.ac.nz (S.Z.); amalini3@hotmail.com (A.J.)

*   Author to whom correspondence should be addressed; k.bishop@auckland.ac.nz;

Abstract: Prostate cancer is a growing problem in New Zealand and worldwide, as populations adopt a Western style dietary pattern. In particular, dietary fat is believed to be associated with oxidative stress, which in turn may be associated with cancer risk and development. In addition, DNA damage is associated with the risk of various cancers, and is regarded as an ideal biomarker for the assessment of the influence of foods on cancer. In the study presented here, 20 men with prostate cancer adhered to a modified Mediterranean style diet for three months. Dietary records, blood fatty acid levels, prostate specific antigen, C-reactive protein and DNA damage were assessed pre- and post-intervention. DNA damage was inversely correlated with dietary adherence ($p = 0.013$) and whole blood monounsaturated fatty acids ($p = 0.009$) and oleic acid ($p = 0.020$). DNA damage was positively correlated with the intake of dairy products ($p = 0.043$), red meat ($p = 0.007$) and whole blood omega-6 polyunsaturated fatty acids ($p = 0.015$). Both the source and type of dietary fat changed significantly over the course of the dietary intervention. Levels of DNA damage were correlated with various dietary fat sources and types of dietary fat.

Keywords: DNA damage; Mediterranean style diet; fatty acids; prostate cancer

1. Introduction

Prostate cancer in New Zealand and worldwide is an increasing problem with respect to prevalence and receipt of appropriate, and in some countries, timely treatment. Prostate cancer is the most common cancer amongst men in New Zealand, accounting for 27% of all new male cancer cases [1]. In addition to older age, ethnicity and family history being risk factors for prostate cancer, lifestyle is also believed to play a role [2]. This belief is supported by evidence obtained from migrants who adopted the lifestyle of their new country to varying degrees [3]. Such migrants also adopted the risk levels associated with that country, rather than their country of origin, depending on the extent to which they changed their lifestyle [3]. It is widely accepted that diet plays an important role in the development of cancers and that a Mediterranean style diet, as opposed to a Western style diet, may ameliorate the risk and progression of prostate cancer due to the effect of various Mediterranean style dietary components on inflammation and oxidative stress, amongst other factors [4]. The source and components of dietary fat vary enormously between Mediterranean and Western dietary patterns. The former is higher in monounsaturated fatty acid (MUFA) rich-plant foods including oleic acid-rich olive oils, as well as the long chain omega 3 polyunsaturated fatty acids (PUFA) that are largely sourced from oily fish (which are high in the omega 3 fatty acids (n3PUFA), eicosapentanoiec acid (EPA) and docosahexaneoic acid (DHA)) [5]. A Western style dietary pattern on the other hand is higher in omega 6 fatty acids (n6PUFA) sourced largely from seed oils and animal fats [5].

Exogenous and endogenous factors can influence oxidative stress [6], which is caused by an imbalance between antioxidants and reactive oxygen species. Lifestyle and diet can be a source of antioxidants and can also promote oxidative stress. Examples of foods that promote oxidative stress include meat cooked at high temperature, as well as some processed and smoked meats [7,8]. Meat cooked at high heat can generate heterocyclic amines (HCA) and polycyclic aromatic hydrocarbons and these can induce DNA instability [7–10]. The susceptibility to prostate cancer risk as a result of consumption of such compounds may be modified by genotype [11]. The consumption of processed meats may also promote the formation of cancers as they contain potentially harmful nitrates and nitrites [9]. Other dietary sources of fat, such as dairy, contain calcium and angiotensin-converting enzyme inhibitors that may decrease oxidative stress, at least in people who are obese [12]. Despite such evidence, dairy intake has received mixed reviews with respect to association with prostate cancer risk [13–15].

There is some controversy regarding dietary fat intake and prostate cancer prevalence and progression [16–18]. Total and saturated fat intake has been positively associated with prostate specific antigen (PSA) levels [19], increased risk of prostate cancer, and aggressive prostate cancer [16,18], whilst saturated fat intake has been associated with fatal prostate cancer [18].

The dietary fatty acids that are discussed herein are shown in relation to one another in Figure 1. Both animal and plants consist of different types of fats in varying proportions. Animal fats consist predominantly of saturated fats (single carbon bonds in the hydrocarbon chains), and plant fats consist predominantly of unsaturated fats (with a varying number of double bonds). There are some exceptions, for example coconut oil contains predominantly saturated fat, and fish consists primarily of PUFA. Unsaturated trans fats are only found in trace amounts in meat and dairy, but they are often produced during the hydrogenation of vegetable oils to produce saturated fats, and therefore are common in processed foods [20].

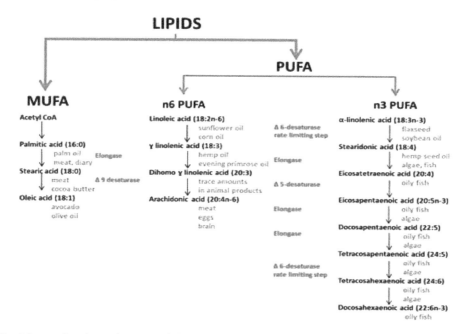

Figure 1. The biosynthesis pathways of the omega 3, 6 and 9 family of poly- and mono-unsaturated fatty acids (adapted from [21–23]).The main dietary sources are shown in blue text, and the enzymes in red text.

Linoleic and α-linolenic acid are essential fatty acids, whilst other fatty acids, to some degree, can be synthesised from precursors [22] (Figure 1). In the n3 PUFA and n6PUFA pathways there is competition for the Δ6-desaturase and Δ5-desaturase enzymes, although both enzymes preferentially catalyse the n3PUFA pathway [21]. In a Review by Plourde and Cunnane [24] the authors discuss the acceptance of the view that there is an "extremely limited efficiency" of the desaturase conversion of ALA to DHA. The controversy of the conversion of LA and ALA to the long chain PUFAs arose in part due to the early use of rat models and also due to using animals that were deficient in essential fatty acids [25]. These two approaches were misleading as rats have a more efficient conversion of LA and ALA to longer chain PUFA, and fatty acid deficiency stimulates the conversion of LA and ALA to longer chain PUFA [25]. Although EPA and DHA biosynthesis is generally regarded as being inefficient [22], the extent of this inefficiency is controversial as measurements of longer chain PUFA may be quite different in plasma *versus* levels measured in other tissues, and it is plasma levels that are more commonly measured and reported [24,26]. However, it seems that the most predictable means of achieving adequate levels of EPA and DHA in plasma and tissues is through consuming long chain PUFA from dietary sources.

The intake of animal, saturated and *trans*-unsaturated fats is associated with all-cause mortality [27] and death due to prostate cancer [18,27]. The consumption of MUFA, PUFA, and vegetable fats on the other hand are associated with a decreased risk of developing prostate cancer or death from prostate cancer [18,27].

Unrepaired DNA damage can result in mutations and some mutations can lead to the development of cancerous tumours. Polymorphisms, such as the single nucleotide polymorphism rs2853826 found in the mitochondrial gene *NADH dehydrogenase subunit*, can influence oxidative stress in women carrying the G allele (G10398), and who also consume alcohol [28]. In such an instance, genotype and alcohol consumption may therefore have an impact on the risk of breast cancer development. Unsurprisingly, cancers such as prostate cancer have been found to be associated with raised levels of DNA damage [29], and raised antioxidant levels can help activate the expression of the *glutathione S-transferase* gene and thereby help protect against this damage [30]. The measurement of DNA damage is regarded as an ideal biomarker for the assessment of the influence of foods or food components on cancer, and the alkaline comet assay (single cell gel electrophoresis) is regarded as a suitable technique for such an assessment [31,32].

The aim of this study was to determine the association between fat and oil intake, as part of a modified Mediterranean style dietary intervention study, and whole blood fatty acid profiles and their association with markers of inflammation and DNA damage in men with prostate cancer. It was hypothesised that the proposed diet would be associated with improvements in PSA, CRP, DNA damage and whole blood fatty acid levels. Evidence obtained could be used to support the prescribed diet as the basis for dietary guidelines that may benefit men with prostate cancer in the future.

2. Experimental Section

Ethical approval was obtained from the Northern B Health and Disability Ethics Committee, Auckland, New Zealand (Ethics number NTY/11/11/109) to perform this study. Study volunteers were selected from an existing cohort of men with prostate cancer based on their Gleason scores, such that those with a Gleason score of 6 (3 + 3) and 7 (3 + 4) were invited to participate in this dietary intervention. Neither a control group free from prostate cancer, nor a control group with prostate cancer and following a standard diet were included. The dietary intervention was explained in detail and a hardcopy of the guidelines and a lengthy compilation of recipes were provided [33]. From the point of view of fat intake, volunteers were asked to adhere to the following guidelines: to include 30–50 g of mixed, unsalted seeds and nuts daily; to include 15 mL or more of extra virgin olive oil and to avoid exposure of the oil to medium and high heat; to reduce dairy intake to one portion daily (information on alternative sources of dietary calcium was provided); to substitute butter and/or margarine with an olive oil based spread; to limit intake of red meat to less than 400 g a week and to substitute with oily fish and white meat; to avoid high temperature cooking of protein; to avoid processed meats; and to include oily fish in the diet at least once a week. The intention was not to change calorie intake, although there was a concern that this may increase due to nut and olive oil intake. Exercise was monitored at baseline and study end through the use of activity diaries. Light to moderate exercise was encouraged during the enrollment interview to encourage general well-being, but no support or resources were provided in this regard. Volunteers were provided with food samples due to the expense and novelty of some of the items, and blood samples were collected at baseline and at three months from volunteers in a non-fasting state. The blood samples were collected into vaccutainers and either kept on ice or at room temperature (plain, EDTA, Heparin and SST II Advance tubes were used). All blood tubes were processed within two hours of blood draw. The food samples supplied included 200 g of frozen vacuum packed salmon per week (Aoraki Smokehouse Salmon, Twizel, New Zealand) and 1 L of extra virgin olive oil (oleic acid content of 78.3%) per month (Seed Oil Extraction Ltd., Ashburton, New Zealand). Adherence to various aspects of the dietary intervention was assessed using a modified, validated questionnaire [34].

The fatty acid profiles were determined using the Holman Bloodspot fatty acid profile test (Lipid Technologies LLC (Austin, MN, USA) via Functional and Integrative Medicine Ltd. (Napier, New Zealand)). Frozen whole blood was thawed and approximately 75 μL was spotted onto the supplied filter cards. The composition of the fatty acids in the samples was derivatised to form fatty acid methyl esters and thereafter assessed using gas chromatography (Lipid Technologies LLC).

The comet assay can be used to detect lesions in DNA strands [35], and was used herein to assess change in DNA damage over time. Results were also obtained by additionally challenging DNA with hydrogen peroxide (H_2O_2) as described by Olive & Banáth [36]. This involved treating 20 μL of whole blood with 1 mL of a 200 μM solution of H_2O_2 in phosphate buffered saline solution, placing on ice for 30 min and discarding the supernatant after centrifugation. Thereafter the comet assay was performed on heparinised blood as outlined in Karunasinghe *et al.* [37,38]. DNA damage was quantitated using the Komet® version 6.0 digital imaging system (Andor Technology, Belfast, UK). The first 50 leucocytes suitable for capturing were scored. Leucocytes were visualised using an Axioskop 2 fluorescent microscope (Zeiss, Goettingen, Germany) and a CCD camera (Evolution VF, QI Imaging, Media Cybernetics, Warrendale, PA, USA). In this way DNA damage was induced wherever significant weakness was present in the DNA strands and hence H_2O_2-induced DNA damage was considered as an indicator of "DNA fragility". Data for percentage tail DNA were log-transformed as they were not normally distributed. The back-transformed mean of the log-transformed values was used for the statistical analysis.

Statistical analysis was carried out using SAS (V9.2 SAS Institute, Cary, NC, USA) as follows: the Students paired *t*-test was used for the comparison of variables at the baseline and three month time points and Spearman bivariate correlations were used to measure relationships between variables.

3. Results

The characteristics of the study participants are presented in Table 1 and summarised as follows: participants were aged between 52 and 74 years; 80% had a body mass index (BMI) of ≥ 25 kg/m^2 and over the course of the study mean body weight reduced by 2.3 kg ($p = 0.0007$); 60% had undergone prostatectomy, whilst 30% of participants were on watchful wait or active surveillance. All participants had a Gleason score of 6 (3 + 3) or 7 (3 + 4) at the time of prostatectomy or most recent biopsy.

Table 1. Baseline characteristics of the study participants.

Baseline Characteristics		n
Age (years) (range 52–74 years)	50–59	3
	60–69	12
	≥70	5
BMI (kg/m²) (range 23–33 kg/m²)	≤19.9	0
	20–24.9	4
	25–29.9	12
	≥30	4
Gleason score *	3 + 3	14
	3 + 4	6
Smoking status	Never	7
	Past	13
	Present	0
Supplements	Omega 3 (from fish oil)	3
	Vitamins	4
Treatment type	None	6
	Prostatectomy	10
	Prostatectomy + ADT + DxR	1
	Prostatectomy + DxR	1
	ADT + DxR	1
	Brachytherapy	1

BMI: Body mass index; ADT: Androgen deprivation therapy; DxR: Radiotherapy (other than Brachytherapy); * The Gleason score is based on tissue obtained from the prostatectomy. Where a prostatectomy was not performed, the Gleason score was based on a biopsy sample.

A modified Mediterranean adherence score was used to assess adherence to the study diet at baseline and at three months. The intake of olive oil, nuts, dairy, fish and red meat changed significantly over the course of the study (Table 2). Saturated fat intake, as a percentage of total fat intake at baseline and three months, decreased significantly ($p < 0.0001$). As expected, the source of dietary fat changed in response to the recommended dietary intervention. Figure 2 shows intake of MUFA increased and SFA and total fatty acid decreased significantly over the study period. However, the intake of total fat and PUFA, when measured in grams per day, did not change (Figure 2).

The source, type and amount of fatty acid intake influenced various physiological characteristics, as well as blood levels and ratios. At study end BMI was inversely and significantly correlated to blood n3PUFA ($r = -0.451$; $p = 0.046$). Decreases in BMI were associated with increased measurements of PUFA ($r = -0.484$; $p = 0.031$) and LA ($r = -0.463$; $p = 0.040$). In addition, increased whole blood arachidonic acid (AA) ($r = -0.455$; $p = 0.044$) levels were associated with weight loss but not a significant decrease in BMI.

Table 2. Changes in the sources of dietary fat from baseline to three months.

Dietary Component (Unit of Measure)	Mean (SE)		Mean Difference (95% CI)	p
	Baseline	Three Months		
Olive oil (mL/day)	14.5 (3.8)	28.8 (4.7)	14.2 (6.8–16.0)	**0.0008**
Nuts (Servings/week)	2.3 (0.5)	5.1 (0.6)	2.9 (1.5–4.2)	**0.0003**
Butter/cream/margarine (Servings/day)	2.1 (0.3)	1.0 (0.3)	−1.1 (−0.6−−1.6)	**0.0002**
Dairy products (Servings/week)	7.4 (0.9)	4.4 (0.7)	−2.9 (−1.2−−4.7)	**0.0025**
Fish (Servings/week)	1.7 (0.2)	3.5 (0.5)	1.8 (0.9–2.7)	**0.0005**
Red and processed meat (Servings/week)	3.9 (0.5)	1.9 (0.4)	−2.0 (−2.6−−1.3)	**0.0005**

SE: standard error; CI: confidence interval.

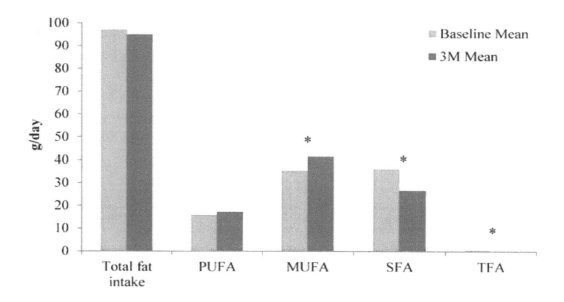

Figure 2. Changes in types of dietary fat intake from baseline to three months.* Statistically significant p values; PUFA: polyunsaturated fatty acids; MUFA: monounsaturated fatty acids; SFA: saturated fatty acids; TFA: trans fatty acids.

Total SFA significantly decreased at study end, partly due to a significant decrease in stearic acid intake (Table 3). Total MUFA, PUFA or any individual fatty acid within those synthesis pathways, showed no change, with the exception of DHA and DHA + EPA which showed a statistically significant increase in blood levels (Table 3). In addition, the ratios of n6PUFA:n3PUFA and AA:EPA had both decreased by study end (Table 3).

No significant correlations were noted between fatty acid measurements obtained from the blood fatty acid profile and food intake assessed via FoodWorks®7 (Xyris software Pty Ltd. 2012, Kenmore Hills, Australia). However, some statistically significant correlations were evident between various fatty acids reported from the blood fatty acid profile and food items as assessed in an adherence questionnaire (Table 4). Dairy intake in particular was inversely correlated with total n3PUFA, EPA and EPA + DHA, and positively correlated with the ratio of AA to EPA (Table 4).

C-reactive protein, PSA and DNA damage were measured at baseline and at three months. Neither C-reactive protein nor PSA changed significantly over the course of the study period. However, a significant, inverse relationship between adherence to the modified Mediterranean diet and basal DNA damage emerged. Spearman correlation was used to identify relationships between intake of individual food items that were recommended as part of the dietary intervention and DNA damage at three months. Foods high in animal fat were significantly positively associated with basal DNA damage (Table 5). In addition, association of DNA fragility with various fat related dietary components was assessed and the DNA fragility was inversely correlated with fish intake ($r = -0.452$; $p = 0.045$) whilst dairy intake was found to be positively associated with DNA fragility ($r = 0.571$; $p = 0.008$).

Significant correlations were observed between basal DNA damage and dietary fat sources, as measured by an adherence questionnaire, as well as various fatty acids reported from the blood fatty acids profile at three months (Table 5). No associations were evident when analysing fatty acid intake, as measured by the diet diaries and analysed via FoodWorks®7 (Xyris software Pty Ltd. 2012), and basal DNA damage. A representative example of various levels of DNA damage is evident in Figure 3.

Results show that total MUFA and n9MUFA (particularly oleic acid), were inversely associated with DNA damage while total n6PUFA, and a higher ratio of n6PUFA to n3PUFA, were associated with increased DNA damage.

Table 3. Whole blood fatty acid profile expressed as mean percent, at baseline and three months.

Blood Fatty Acids	Mean (SE)		Mean Difference (95% CI)	p
	Baseline	Three Months		
Total SFA	34.7 (0.3)	33.7 (0.4)	−1.0 (0.4–1.5)	**0.002**
16:0 Palmitic acid	22.6 (0.3)	22.3 (0.4)	−0.3 (−0.1–0.7)	0.161
18:0 Stearic acid	10.5 (0.2)	10.0 (0.2)	−0.5 (0.2–0.9)	**0.002**
Total MUFA	23.4 (0.4)	23.7 (0.4)	0.3 (0.4–1.0)	0.366
Total n9MUFA	23.1 (0.4)	23.4 (0.4)	0.3 (−0.4–1.0)	0.380
18:1ω9 Oleic acid	22.7 (0.4)	23.2 (0.4)	0.5 (−0.2–1.1)	0.162
Total PUFA	39.5 (0.5)	40.3 (0.5)	0.9 (−0.1–1.8)	0.079
Total n6PUFA	32.8 (0.4)	33.0 (0.5)	0.2 (−0.7–1.2)	0.636
18:2ω6 LA	19.6 (0.7)	19.4 (0.9)	−0.2 (−1.7–1.4)	0.832
20:4ω6 AA	9.1 (0.3)	8.9 (0.3)	−0.2 (−0.7–0.3)	0.379
Total n3PUFA	6.6 (0.4)	7.3 (0.3)	0.6 (−0.0–1.3)	0.057
18:3ω3 LNA	0.5 (0.0)	0.6 (0.1)	0.0 (−0.1–0.2)	0.689
20:5ω3 EPA	1.4 (0.9)	1.5 (0.7)	0.1 (−0.2–0.5)	0.463
22:6ω3 DHA	3.0 (0.9)	3.5 (0.1)	0.5 (0.2–0.8)	**0.001**
EPA + DHA	4.4 (0.4)	5.0 (0.2)	0.6 (0.3–1.2)	**0.042**
Modified WBS n3 Index	6.1 (0.5)	7.0 (0.3)	0.9 (0.0–1.7)	**0.043**
n6PUFA:n3PUFA	5.2 (0.3)	4.7 (0.2)	−0.6 (−1.0−−0.1)	**0.019**
AA:EPA	8.58 (0.9)	6.9 (0.6)	−1.6 (−3.1−−0.2)	**0.030**

Abbreviations: AA: Arachidonic acid; CI: confidence interval; DHA: docosahexaneoic acid; DPA: docosapentaenoic acid; EPA: eicosapentaenoic acid; LA: linoleic acid; LNA: linolenic acid; MUFA: monounsaturated fatty acids; n9MUFA: omega 9 monounsaturated fatty acids; n3PUFA: omega 3 polyunsaturated fatty acids; n6PUFA: omega 6 polyunsaturated fatty acids; p: probability value; PUFA: polyunsaturated fatty acids; SE: standard error; SFA: saturated fatty acids; WBS: whole blood spot.

Table 4. Correlation between various whole blood fatty acid levels and intake of selected food items at three months.

Blood Fatty Acids	Dietary Fat Source	Correlation	p
	Fish intake	0.210	0.374
Total n3PUFA	Nut intake	0.341	0.141
	Dairy intake	−0.433	0.057
	Red meat intake	0.082	0.732
	Fish intake	0.172	0.468
EPA	Nut intake	0.147	0.535
	Dairy intake	−0.580	**0.007**
	Red meat intake	−0.475	**0.034**
	Fish intake	0.123	0.605
EPA + DHA	Nut intake	0.222	0.347
	Dairy intake	−0.609	**0.004**
	Red meat intake	0.055	0.817
	Fish intake	0.192	0.418
n6PUFA:n3PUFA	Nut intake	−0.349	0.132
	Dairy intake	−0.147	0.537
	Red meat intake	0.486	**0.029**
	Fish intake	0.233	0.323
AA:EPA	Nut intake	0.084	0.725
	Dairy intake	0.409	0.073
	Red meat intake	−0.029	0.904

Abbreviations: EPA: eicosapentanoiec acid; DHA: docosahexaneoic; n3PUFA: omega 3 polyunsaturated fatty acid, n6PUFA: omega 6 polyunsaturated fatty acid; AA: arachidonic acid.

Table 5. Correlation between DNA damage and dietary fatty acid intake and blood fatty acids.

Outcome of Interest	Dietary Fat Sources	Baseline		Three Months	
		Correlation	p	Correlation	p
	Olive oil	0.002	0.995	−0.370	0.109
DNA damage	Servings of butter, cream, margarine	0.278	0.235	0.456	**0.043**
	Servings of fish	0.202	0.393	0.510	0.829
	Servings of red meat	0.066	0.783	0.576	**0.007**
	Total MUFA	0.200	0.3988	−0.565	**0.009**
	Total n9MUFA	0.211	0.371	−0.561	**0.010**
Blood Fatty Acid	Oleic acid	0.220	0.352	−0.514	**0.020**
	Total n6PUFA	−0.116	0.627	0.536	**0.015**
	Total n3PUFA	−0.314	0.178	−0.224	0.342
	n6PUFA:n3PUFA ratio	0.330	0.155	0.507	**0.023**

Abbreviations: MUFA: mono-unsaturated fatty acids; n9MUFA: omega 9 polyunsaturated fatty acids; n6PUFA: omega 6 polyunsaturated fatty acids; n3PUFA: omega 3 polyunsaturated fatty acids.

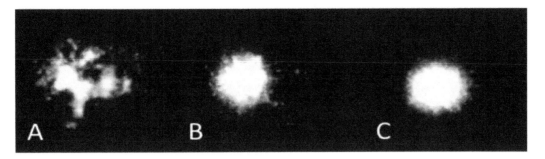

Figure 3. Representative images of different levels of DNA damage as measured by the Comet assay. **A**: extensive damage; **B**: moderate damage; **C**: minor damage.

4. Discussion

Dietary fat intake was measured by assessing whole blood fatty acid levels, as well as by using four-day food diaries and assessing intake via FoodWorks®7 software (Xyris software Pty Ltd. 2012). A modified Mediterranean diet adherence questionnaire was used to evaluate conformity to a Mediterranean style dietary pattern, which is generally high in both $n3$ and $n6$PUFA, and to measure intake and change in intake of specific high fat foods in response to the dietary intervention.

The Holman Bloodspot fatty acid profile test (Lipid Technologies LLC), requiring whole blood samples, was used to assess fatty acid profiles at baseline and study end. Although other fatty acid profile tests can be used to measure fatty acid levels from other components of blood samples, whole blood was regarded as preferable as it can be used to assess fatty acid intake over the previous two months. Both Rise *et al.* [39] and Sun *et al.* [40] state that erythrocyte fatty acid profiles provide a better reflection of long term PUFA intake than plasma fatty acid profiles, and this view is supported by work carried out by Katan *et al.* [41]. In their study, Katan *et al.* concluded that erythrocyte fatty acid profiles reflected intake over the past one to two months [41]. It is clear that plasma and serum fatty acid profiles reflect more recent fatty acid intake than erythrocyte, whole blood or adipose tissue fatty acid profiles [39,40,42]. Based on this evidence it is likely that the Holman Bloodspot test captures fatty acid intake over the two months prior to blood collection.

A number of statistically significant changes in fatty acid profiles (Table 3) were noted such as the increase in DHA whole blood levels from 3.0% to 3.5% ($p = 0.001$). However, although the changes in EPA levels were not statistically significant, they did increase from 1.36% to 1.5% over the three month study period. Together, these changes contributed to a statistically significant increase in the modified WBS $n3$ index ($p = 0.043$) (Table 3).

Fatty acid profiles were measured from whole blood spots (WBS) and this presents challenges with regards to calculating a red blood cell (RBC) $n3$ index. A RBC $n3$ index is typically calculated from the sum of EPA and DHA (from RBC membranes) as a percentage of total RBC fatty acids [43]. Bailey-Hall *et al.* compared DHA and EPA levels from whole blood obtained from a finger prick with values obtained from RBCs (venipuncture) [44]. Although the mean percentage for DHA was approximately 150% lower from capillary whole blood than in RBCs, the DHA and EPA values from the two sample types were highly correlated [44]. As mentioned in the "Experimental" section, the fatty acid profiles were determined by Lipid Technologies LLC (Austin Minnesota) using Holman Bloodspot fatty acid profile tests. Results were presented as a percentage of total lipid content from WBS. An RBC $n3$ index was reported and as this percentage was calculated from WBS, it was therefore necessary to apply a conversion factor wherein the relationship between DHA from whole blood *versus* DHA from red blood cells, was taken into account [44]. The actual algorithm used is proprietary information [45]. Rather than refer to this value as the RBC $n3$ index, which could be viewed as misleading, the authors have used the term "modified WBS $n3$ index" (Table 3). Due to the relationship between blood fatty acids in whole blood *vs.* RBC from venipuncture established by Bailey-Hall [44] upon which the algorithm developed by Lipid Technologies is based [45], the authors have considered the modified WBS $n3$

index as equivalent to the widely used RBC $n3$ index. The RBC $n3$ index is negatively associated with death, particularly sudden death, from coronary heart disease [43]. Although the most desirable levels might be influenced by cultural background, maximal cardioprotection and slowest rate of telomere loss takes place at an RBC $n3$ index $\geq 8\%$ and 8.7% respectively [43]. The increase in the modified WBS $n3$ index found in this study (from 6.10% to 6.98%) was significant, yet it remained below the target value for the reduction of coronary heart disease risk. However, it is believed that any increase in the modified WBS $n3$ index would be beneficial as $n3$ fatty acids can alter membrane biophysical properties and in addition to lipid metabolism, this may impact on inflammatory responses [46]. In addition, the dietary intervention continued for only three months and it is possible that the modified WBS $n3$ index may have continued to increase until target levels were reached.

Fatty acid profiles have predominantly been analysed from either plasma [47–49] or serum [50] and therefore results from these studies are not comparable with our own due to the different substrates used. However, in a recent Australian study data were collected on fasting whole blood fatty acids, but only intake in grams of SFA, MUFA and PUFA were shown, as well as a limited number of blood fatty acid ratios [51]. Total fat, as well as SFA, MUFA and PUFA intake (all measured in grams per day) were all comparatively higher in our study, relative to the study carried out by Alhazmi *et al.* [51].

An association between a change in dietary pattern over a three month time period, and whole blood fatty acids was investigated. Importantly, overall fat intake did not change despite a Mediterranean dietary pattern being traditionally high in fat. This lack of change is due to a substitution in source of fats, such that meats high in saturated fat were replaced by oily fish, and although dairy intake decreased significantly, olive oil and nut intake also increased significantly (Table 2). These changes are consistent with the adoption of a Mediterranean style dietary pattern. The change in fat source is supported by the statistically significant decrease in total SFA (Figure 2), particularly stearic acid (Table 3). Changes in blood fatty acid profiles, although physiologically small, were statistically significant (Table 3). This is largely due to the fact that the percentage values are small and therefore a large physiological change is unlikely.

In this dietary intervention study the intake of olive oil, oily fish, seeds and nuts was promoted, and therefore the dietary intake of MUFA and PUFA increased (Table 2). This increase is partly reflected in the change in blood fatty acid levels (Table 3). The intake of dietary sources of MUFA increased significantly ($p = 0.0243$) (Figure 2), as did the whole blood levels of $n3$PUFAs DHA ($p = 0.001$) and EPA + DHA ($p = 0.042$) (Table 3).

The increase in the modified WBS $n3$ index was consistent with the reported intake of dietary items containing $n3$PUFAs. Increased intake of $n3$PUFA is often associated with a reduction in $n6$PUFA blood levels partially due to competitive inhibition of rate limiting desaturase enzymes [23] (Figure 1), although there is some debate regarding this perhaps overly simplistic view [24,26]. However, there were no correlating significant changes in percentage $n6$PUFA in our study. While we expected that intake of some sources of $n6$PUFA, such as the cheaper vegetable oils that are often found in processed foods (e.g., soybean, sunflower, rice-bran, cottonseed and corn oils) would decrease due to substitution with olive oil, which is much lower in $n6$PUFA, there is no evidence that this occurred. Although we assessed for olive oil intake, we did not question the intake of other oils. An alternative explanation could lie in the fatty acid composition of nuts. We recommended and observed an increased consumption of nuts. Nut consumption increased from a mean of 2.2 to 5.2 servings per week. Many nuts are high in $n6$PUFA, thus off-setting the decrease of $n6$PUFA from other sources. In spite of this, the increase in $n3$PUFA contributed to a statistically significant decrease in the $n6$:$n3$ ratio, indicating a shift towards a less inflammatory profile. Correlations between intake of dietary fatty acids and blood fatty acids were not evident (values not reported). The levels of blood fatty acids are not only affected by intake [48,49], but also by the rate at which fatty acids are transformed (Figure 1). This transformation is often inefficient and influenced by rate limiting enzymes such as the delta-6-desaturase enzymes [52].

It is also important to consider whether *n*3PUFAs from plant sources decreased as this might counter-balance the increase in fish intake. However, one would expect this to be evident from the blood fatty acid profiles, as sources of EPA and DHA would largely be from oily fish and the limited conversion of alpha linolenic acid via elongation and desaturation reactions to stearidonic acid, EPA and finally DHA [23]. EPA and DHA can also be obtained from certain algal species [23], but only one of the study participants took algae-based supplements. The output from FoodWorks®7 software (Xyris software Pty Ltd. 2012) is in the form of food components and therefore we are comparing measurements of whole foods, such as fish, from the adherence tool, with measurement of food components such as *n*3PUFA, which can be sourced from a number of different foods including fish, refined vegetable oils and nuts for example.

What is of particular interest and relevance is that EPA intake was inversely associated with intake of dairy products ($p = 0.007$) and red meat ($p = 0.034$); and blood percentage EPA + DHA was significantly inversely associated with dairy intake. Due to the study design, the effect of dietary intake on prostate cancer risk could not be assessed. However, it is interesting to note that the above mentioned association between increased EPA and DHA intake with decreased dairy was also reported in a study where the influence of various dietary components on prostate cancer risk was assessed [53]. These results support evidence obtained from the adherence questionnaires that fish, as the primary dietary source of EPA, partially replaced the intake of meat, and some dairy products.

The Comet assay is a standard method for measuring DNA damage in eukaryotic cells, regardless of how that damage has been caused [54]. Leucocytes, as in this study, are usually used for the analysis of comets, but one of the drawbacks is that these cells are not usually a target tissue for cancer [54]. However, DNA damage in leucocytes, as measured in a Comet assay, may still present as a reliable marker for increased cancer risk as genomic instability is a common and widely accepted characteristic amongst cancers. A number of studies have been reported wherein DNA damage has been used to assess response to genotoxic stress in terms of cancer risk or effect on cancer related pathways [55–57]. Machowetz *et al.* and Colomer *et al.* both reported a reduction in DNA damage in response to olive oil consumption [58,59]. For this reason it was anticipated that a similar reduction in DNA damage would be observed in our own study participants as their consumption of extra virgin olive oil had increased significantly from 14.83 mL/day to 28.75 mL/day (Table 2). While an inverse association was seen between olive oil consumption and DNA damage, this was not significant ($p = 0.109$) (Table 5). However, the percentage of oleic acid in the blood (along with total MUFA and total omega 9), was inversely associated with basal DNA damage at the end of the study, which is consistent with published results [60]. As this association occurred in spite of only a minor increase in the blood oleic acid ratio, the relationship may serve as a marker for an unmeasured, associated factor, such as olive oil polyphenols.

When investigating food sources of fatty acids, it was clear that DNA damage was associated with a higher intake of dairy products and red meat (Table 5). Increased MUFA intake (Figure 2), supported by statistically significant MUFA blood levels (Table 3) were inversely correlated with basal DNA damage at three months (Table 5). Total *n*6PUFA and *n*6PUFA:*n*3PUFA on the other hand were positively correlated with DNA damage (Table 5) and this was not unexpected as *n*6PUFA is believed to be pro-inflammatory and low *n*6PUFA:*n*3PUFA ratios are believed to be anti-inflammatory.

While we did not question participants to obtain detailed information about culinary fats at baseline, we predicted that most participants would have been consuming olive oil with a lower level of polyphenols than that provided by the extra virgin olive oil supplied for this study (Oil Seed Extractions Ltd., Ashburton, New Zealand). Furthermore, our requirement of just one or more tablespoons of olive oil daily was perhaps too low to boost oleic acid levels sufficiently. In a study by Mitjavila *et al.* [61] olive oil was supplemented at a rate of a litre per week (equivalent to just over 140 mL/day), the usual Mediterranean diet includes 60 mL/day of extra virgin olive oil [34]. However, this was thought to be too high an expectation for a New Zealand population that does not have a tradition of olive oil consumption.

The inclusion of oily fish was an important component of the modified Mediterranean diet. The diet was modified to promote the inclusion of oily fish due to the $n3$PUFA content in fish being a good source of the anti-inflammatory fatty acids, EPA and DHA. From the adherence questionnaire the reported intake of fish doubled (Table 2), and this increase was statistically significant ($p = 0.0005$). No significant correlation was seen between any of the blood fatty acids and fish intake (correlations ranged from $r = 0.017$ to 0.21 (Table 4)). These results are not entirely inconsistent with those reported by Norrish *et al.*, in which fish intake was "moderately correlated" to EPA and DHA when measured from red blood cells obtained from New Zealand men ($r = 0.26$ and 0.32 respectively, the p values were not reported) [62]. The whole blood fatty acid profile is a reflection of oily fish intake over the preceding two months, whilst the diet diaries are a measure of intake the week prior to the blood draw. Some of the volunteers indicated that they had consumed all their salmon donations by this stage and may have been unwilling to purchase additional oily fish. This highlights the advantage of blood biomarkers that reflect both short and longer-term intake over diet diaries or food frequency questionnaires to assess dietary intake.

In addition to changes in the consumption of fish, it can be seen that intake from other sources of dietary fat also changed. Statistically significant changes were seen in the consumption of olive oil and nuts, where consumption increased, and dairy products, where consumption decreased (Table 2). This could result in the increased intake of $n3$PUFA and the decreased intake of $n6$PUFA, depending on the type and quantity of nuts consumed. The type of nuts consumed was not recorded.

Although the authors cannot speculate as to whether the modified Mediterranean diet detailed herein would increase longevity, it is clear that indicators of general health were enhanced. This view is supported by the fact that many of the men who were carrying excess weight, decreased their body weight during the study period; that whole blood fatty acid profiles improved, specifically DHA levels and the modified WBS $n3$ index (a marker of heart health); and that DNA damage levels decreased. In addition, anecdotal reports show that one of the study volunteers reported improved sleep patterns, thought to be due to decreased nocturia (nocturia being a common side-effect of prostate cancer treatment and prostatic disease); one volunteer experienced reduced arthritic pain; another experienced a reduced need for anti-inflammatory medication, whilst a number of volunteers commented on an improved feeling of well-being.

5. Conclusions

Dietary change to promote the intake of oily fish and olive oil as part of a Mediterranean style diet can be achieved in men with prostate cancer. Both the source and type of dietary fat intake changed significantly over the course of the dietary intervention. The intake of olive oil, nuts and fish increased significantly, whilst the intake of dairy and red meat decreased significantly from baseline to three months. The whole blood levels of the SFA, stearic acid decreased significantly, whilst the levels of DHA increased significantly. Although the whole blood levels of total $n6$PUFAs did not change significantly over the course of the intervention, care should be taken to provide advice regarding the increased intake of nuts to ensure that the type and quantity of nuts consumed maintains $n6$PUFA within levels associated with reduced health risks. Whilst dietary fat intake significantly changed over the course of the study, this change was not statistically associated with the significant changes in blood fatty acid profiles. However, total MUFA and oleic acid levels in the volunteers adhering to this dietary intervention were associated with a significant reduction in DNA damage. DNA damage was positively correlated with the ratio of $n6$PUFA to $n3$PUFA, as well as to the intake of red and processed meats, and dairy products.

Acknowledgments: Fatty acid tests were sponsored by Lipid Technologies LLC via Functional and Integrative Medicine Ltd.; Salmon was donated by Aoraki Smokehouse Salmon, Twizel, New Zealand; Olive oil was donated by Oil Seed Extraction Ltd., Ashburton, New Zealand.
The Volunteers and their partners are acknowledged for their commitment to this study.

Author Contributions: K.S.B. planned and initiated the study; planned and wrote the manuscript; S.E. and K.S.B. carried out the study; N.K. and S.E. carried out the Comet assays and interpreted the results; planned and edited drafts of the manuscript; D.Y.H. carried out the statistical analysis and edited drafts of the manuscript; A.J. processed and stored the samples; S.Z. performed the phlebotomy; L.R.F. helped plan the study and edited drafts of the manuscript.

References

1. Cancer: New Registrations and Deaths 2010. Available online: http://www.health.govt.nz/publication/cancer-new-registrations-and-deaths-2010 (accessed on 22 August 2014).

2. Bishop, K.S.; Chi, H.-J.K.; Han, D.Y.; Ferguson, L.R. Prostate cancer prevention in the developing world—What are we waiting for? *Curr. Pharmacogenomics Pers. Med.* **2012**, *10*, 70–86. [CrossRef]

3. Itsiopoulos, C.; Hodge, A.; Kaimakamis, M. Can the Mediterranean diet prevent prostate cancer? *Mol. Nutr. Food Res.* **2009**, *53*, 227–239. [CrossRef] [PubMed]

4. Melnik, B.C.; John, S.M.; Schmitz, G. Over-stimulation of insulin/IGF-1 signaling by western diet may promote diseases of civilization: Lessons learnt from Laron syndrome. *Nutr. Metab.* **2011**, *8*, 41. [CrossRef]

5. Serra-Majem, L.; de la Cruz, J.N.; Ribas, L.; Salleras, L. Mediterranean diet and health: Is all the secret in olive oil? *Pathophysiol. Haemost. Thromb.* **2003**, *33*, 461–465. [CrossRef] [PubMed]

6. Breen, A.P.; Murphy, J.A. Reactions of oxyl radicals with DNA. *Free Radic. Biol. Med.* **1995**, *18*, 1033–1077. [CrossRef] [PubMed]

7. Sugimura, T.; Wakabayashi, K.; Nakagama, H.; Nagao, M. Heterocyclic amines: Mutagens/carcinogens produced during cooking of meat and fish. *Cancer Sci.* **2004**, *95*, 290–299. [CrossRef] [PubMed]

8. Norrish, A.E.; Ferguson, L.R.; Knize, M.G.; Felton, J.S.; Sharpe, S.J.; Jackson, R.T. Heterocyclic amine content of cooked meat and risk of prostate cancer. *J. Natl. Cancer Inst.* **1999**, *91*, 2038–2044. [CrossRef] [PubMed]

9. John, E.M.; Stern, M.C.; Sinha, R.; Koo, J. Meat consumption, cooking practices, meat mutagens, and risk of prostate cancer. *Nutr. Cancer* **2011**, *63*, 525–537. [CrossRef] [PubMed]

10. Joshi, A.D.; Corral, R.; Catsburg, C.; Lewinger, J.-P.; Koo, J.; John, E.M.; Ingles, S.; Stern, M.C. Red meat and poultry, cooking practices, genetic susceptibility and risk of prostate cancer: Results from the California Collaborative Prostate Cancer Study. *Carcinogenesis* **2012**, *33*, 2108–2118. [CrossRef]

11. Van Hemelrijck, M.; Rohrmann, S.; Steinbrecher, A.; Kaaks, R.; Teucher, B.; Linseisen, J. Heterocyclic aromatic amine (HCA) intake and prostate cancer risk: Effect modification by genetic variants. *Nutr. Cancer* **2012**, *64*, 704–713.

12. Zemel, M.B.; Sun, X. Dietary calcium and dairy products modulate oxidative and inflammatory stress in mice and humans. *J. Nutr.* **2008**, *138*, 1047–1052. [PubMed]

13. Ganmaa, D.; Li, X.M.; Wang, J.; Qin, L.Q.; Wang, P.Y.; Sato, A. Incidence and mortality of testicular and prostatic cancers in relation to world dietary practices. *Int. J. Cancer* **2002**, *98*, 262–267. [CrossRef] [PubMed]

14. Torfadottir, J.E.; Steingrimsdottir, L.; Mucci, L.; Aspelund, T.; Kasperzyk, J.L.; Olafsson, O.; Fall, K.; Tryggvadottir, L.; Harris, T.B.; Launer, L.; *et al.* Milk intake in early life and risk of advanced prostate cancer. *Am. J. Epidemiol.* **2012**, *175*, 144–153. [CrossRef] [PubMed]

15. Pettersson, A.; Kasperzyk, J.L.; Kenfield, S.A.; Richman, E.L.; Chan, J.M.; Willett, W.C.; Stampfer, M.J.; Mucci, L.A.; Giovannucci, E.L. Milk and dairy consumption among men with prostate cancer and risk of metastases and prostate cancer death. *Cancer Epidemiol. Biomark. Prev.* **2012**, *21*, 428–436. [CrossRef]

16. Giovannucci, E.; Rimm, E.B.; Colditz, G.A.; Stampfer, M.J.; Ascherio, A.; Chute, C.G.; Willett, W.C. A prospective study of dietary fat and risk of prostate cancer. *J. Natl. Cancer Inst.* **1993**, *85*, 1571–1579. [CrossRef] [PubMed]

17. Salem, S.; Salahi, M.; Mohseni, M.; Ahmadi, H.; Mehrsai, A.; Jahani, Y.; Pourmand, G. Major dietary factors and prostate cancer risk: A prospective multicenter case-control study. *Nutr. Cancer* **2011**, *63*, 21–27. [PubMed]

18. Pelser, C.; Mondul, A.M.; Hollenbeck, A.R.; Park, Y. Dietary fat, fatty acids, and risk of prostate cancer in the NIH-AARP diet and health study. *Cancer Epidemiol. Biomark. Prev.* **2013**, *22*, 697–707. [CrossRef]

19. Ohwaki, K.; Endo, F.; Kachi, Y.; Hattori, K.; Muraishi, O.; Nishikitani, M.; Yano, E. Relationship between dietary factors and prostate-specific antigen in healthy men. *Urol. Int.* **2012**, *89*, 270–274. [CrossRef] [PubMed]

20. Erkkilä, A.; de Mello, V.D.F.; Risérus, U.; Laaksonen, D.E. Dietary fatty acids and cardiovascular disease: An epidemiological approach. *Prog. Lipid Res.* **2008**, *47*, 172–187. [CrossRef] [PubMed]

21. White, H.M.; Richert, B.T.; Latour, M.A. Impacts of Nutrition and Environmental Stressors on Lipid Metabolism. In *Lipid Metabolism*; Baeze, R.V., Ed.; InTech: Rijeka, Croatia, 2013; Chapter 10. [CrossRef]

22. Fatty Acids: Methylene-Interrupted Double Bonds. Available online: http://lipidlibrary.aocs.org/Lipids/fa_poly/index.htm (accessed on 22 August 2014).

23. Lenihan-Geels, G.; Bishop, K.S.; Ferguson, L.R. Alternative sources of omega-3 fats: Can we find a sustainable substitute for fish? *Nutrients* **2013**, *5*, 1301–1315. [CrossRef] [PubMed]

24. Plourde, M.; Cunnane, S.C. Extremely limited synthesis of long chain polyunsaturates in adults: Implications for their dietary essentiality and use as supplements. *Appl. Physiol. Nutr. Metab.* **2007**, *32*, 619–634. [CrossRef] [PubMed]

25. Plourde, M.; Fortier, M.; Vandal, M.; Tremblay-Mercier, J.; Freemantle, E.; Begin, M.; Pifferi, F.; Cunnane, S.C. Unresolved issues in the link between docosahexaenoic acid and Alzheimer's disease. *Prostaglandins Leukot. Essent. Fat. Acids* **2007**, *77*, 301–308. [CrossRef]

26. Barcelo-Coblijn, G.; Murphy, E.J. Alpha-linolenic acid and its conversion to longer chain *n*-3 fatty acids: Benefits for human health and a role in maintaining tissue *n*-3 fatty acid levels. *Prog. Lipid Res.* **2009**, *48*, 355–374. [CrossRef] [PubMed]

27. Richman, E.; Kenfield, S.A.; Chavarro, J.E.; Stampfer, M.J.; Giovannucci, E.L.; Willett, W.C.; Chan, J.M. Fat intake after diagnosis and risk of lethal prostate cancer and all-cause mortality. *JAMA* **2013**, *173*, 1–8.

28. Blein, S.; Berndt, S.; Joshi, A.D.; Campa, D.; Ziegler, R.G.; Riboli, E.; Cox, D.G.; Gaudet, M.M.; Stevens, V.L.; Diver, W.R.; *et al.* Factors associated with oxidative stress and cancer risk in the breast and prostate cancer cohort consortium. *Free Radic. Res.* **2014**, *48*, 380–386. [CrossRef]

29. Lockett, K.L.; Hall, M.C.; Clark, P.E.; Chuang, S.C.; Robinson, B.; Lin, H.Y.; Su, L.J.; Hu, J.J. DNA damage levels in prostate cancer cases and controls. *Carcinogenesis* **2006**, *27*, 1187–1193. [CrossRef] [PubMed]

30. Kanwal, R.; Pandey, M.; Bhaskaran, N.; Maclennan, G.T.; Fu, P.; Ponsky, L.E.; Gupta, S. Protection against oxidative DNA damage and stress in human prostate by glutathione *S*-transferase P1. *Mol. Carcinog.* **2014**, *53*, 8–18. [CrossRef] [PubMed]

31. Wasson, G.R.; McKelvey-Martin, V.J.; Downes, C.S. The use of the comet assay in the study of human nutrition and cancer. *Mutagenesis* **2008**, *23*, 153–162. [CrossRef] [PubMed]

32. Liao, W.; McNutt, M.A.; Zhu, W.G. The comet assay: A sensitive method for detecting DNA damage in individual cells. *Methods* **2009**, *48*, 46–53. [CrossRef] [PubMed]

33. Erdrich, S.; Bishop, K. The Modified Mediterranean Diet for Men: Recipe Collection. Available online: https://cdn.auckland.ac.nz/assets/fmhs/sms/nutrition/pcd/docs/recipes.png (accessed on 16 June 2014).

34. Martinez-Gonzalez, M.A.; Garcia-Arellano, A.; Toledo, E.; Salas-Salvado, J.; Buil-Cosiales, P.; Corella, D.; Covas, M.I.; Schroder, H.; Aros, F.; Gomez-Gracia, E.; *et al.* A 14-item Mediterranean diet assessment tool and obesity indexes among high-risk subjects: The PREDIMED trial. *PLoS One* **2012**. [CrossRef]

35. Dhillon, V.S.; Thomas, P.; Fenech, M. Comparison of DNA damage and repair following radiation challenge in buccal cells and lymphocytes using single-cell gel electrophoresis. *Int. J. Radiat. Biol.* **2004**, *80*, 517–528. [CrossRef] [PubMed]

36. Olive, P.L.; Banath, J.P. The comet assay: A method to measure DNA damage in individual cells. *Nat. Protoc.* **2006**, *1*, 23–29. [CrossRef] [PubMed]

37. Karunasinghe, N.; Ryan, J.; Tuckey, J.; Masters, J.; Jamieson, M.; Clarke, L.C.; Marshall, J.R.; Ferguson, L.R. DNA stability and serum selenium levels in a high-risk group for prostate cancer. *Cancer Epidemiol. Biomark. Prev.* **2004**, *13*, 391–397.

38. Ferguson, L.R.; Han, D.Y.; Fraser, A.G.; Huebner, C.; Lam, W.J.; Morgan, A.R.; Duan, H.; Karunasinghe, N. Genetic factors in chronic inflammation: Single nucleotide polymorphisms in the STAT-JAK pathway, susceptibility to DNA damage and Crohn's disease in a New Zealand population. *Mutat. Res.* **2010**, *690*, 108–115. [CrossRef]

39. Rise, P.; Eligini, S.; Ghezzi, S.; Colli, S.; Galli, C. Fatty acid composition of plasma, blood cells and whole blood: Relevance for the assessment of the fatty acid status in humans. *Prostaglandins Leukot. Essent. Fat. Acids* **2007** *76*, 363–369. [CrossRef]

40. Sun, Q.; Ma, J.; Campos, H.; Hankinson, S.E.; Hu, F.B. Comparison between plasma and erythrocyte fatty acid content as biomarkers of fatty acid intake in US women. *Am. J. Clin. Nutr.* **2007**, *86*, 74–81. [PubMed]

41. Katan, M.B.; Deslypere, J.P.; van Birgelen, A.P.; Penders, M.; Zegwaard, M. Kinetics of the incorporation of dietary fatty acids into serum cholesteryl esters, erythrocyte membranes, and adipose tissue: An 18-month controlled study. *J. Lipid Res.* **1997**, *38*, 2012–2022. [PubMed]

42. Katan, M.B.; Grundy, S.M.; Willett, W.C. Should a low-fat, high-carbohydrate diet be recommended for everyone? Beyond low-fat diets. *N. Engl. J. Med.* **1997**, *337*, 563–566; discussion 566–567. [PubMed]

43. Harris, W.S. The omega-3 index: Clinical utility for therapeutic intervention. *Curr. Cardiol. Rep.* **2010**, *12*, 503–508. [CrossRef] [PubMed]

44. Bailey-Hall, E.; Nelson, E.B.; Ryan, A.S. Validation of a rapid measure of blood PUFA levels in humans. *Lipids* **2008**, *43*, 181–186. [CrossRef] [PubMed]

45. Bibus, D.M.; Lipid Technologies, LLC, Austin, MN, USA. Personal communication, 2014.

46. Harris, W.S. The omega-3 index as a risk factor for coronary heart disease. *Am. J. Clin. Nutr.* **2008**, *87*, 1997S–2002S. [PubMed]

47. Gann, P.H.; Hennekens, C.H.; Sacks, F.M.; Grodstein, F.; Giovannucci, E.L.; Stampfer, M.J. Prospective study of plasma fatty acids and risk of prostate cancer. *J. Natl. Cancer Inst.* **1994**, *86*, 281–286. [CrossRef] [PubMed]

48. Ma, J.; Folsom, A.R.; Shahar, E.; Eckfeldt, J.H. Plasma fatty acid composition as an indicator of habitual dietary fat intake in middle-aged adults. The Atherosclerosis Risk in Communities (ARIC) Study Investigators. *Am. J. Clin. Nutr.* **1995**, *62*, 564–571. [PubMed]

49. Saadatian-Elahi, M.; Slimani, N.; Chajes, V.; Jenab, M.; Goudable, J.; Biessy, C.; Ferrari, P.; Byrnes, G.; Autier, P.; Peeters, P.H.; *et al.* Plasma phospholipid fatty acid profiles and their association with food intakes: Results from a cross-sectional study within the European Prospective Investigation into Cancer and Nutrition. *Am. J. Clin. Nutr.* **2009**, *89*, 331–346. [CrossRef] [PubMed]

50. Holub, B.J.; Wlodek, M.; Rowe, W.; Piekarski, J. Correlation of omega-3 levels in serum phospholipid from 2053 human blood samples with key fatty acid ratios. *Nutr. J.* **2009**, *8*, 58. [CrossRef] [PubMed]

51. Alhazmi, A.; Stojanovski, E.; Garg, M.L.; McEvoy, M. Fasting whole blood fatty acid profile and risk of type 2 diabetes in adults: A nested case control study. *PLoS One* **2014**. [CrossRef]

52. Surette, M.E. Dietary omega-3 PUFA and health: Stearidonic acid-containing seed oils as effective and sustainable alternatives to traditional marine oils. *Mol. Nutr. Food Res.* **2013**, *57*, 748–759. [CrossRef] [PubMed]

53. Leitzmann, M.F.; Stampfer, M.J.; Michaud, D.S.; Augustsson, K.; Colditz, G.C.; Willett, W.C.; Giovannucci, E.L. Dietary intake of *n*-3 and *n*-6 fatty acids and the risk of prostate cancer. *Am. J. Clin. Nutr.* **2004**, *80*, 204–216. [PubMed]

54. Collins, A. The comet assay for DNA damage and repair. *Mol. Biotechnol.* **2004**, *26*, 249–261. [CrossRef] [PubMed]

55. Waters, D.J.; Shen, S.; Glickman, L.T.; Cooley, D.M.; Bostwick, D.G.; Qian, J.; Combs, G.F.; Morris, J.S. Prostate cancer risk and DNA damage: Translational significance of selenium supplementation in a canine model. *Carcinogenesis* **2005**, *26*, 1256–1262. [CrossRef] [PubMed]

56. Mroz, R.M.; Schins, R.P.F.; Li, H.; Jimenez, L.A.; Drost, E.M.; Holownia, A.; MacNee, W.; Donaldson, K. Nanoparticle-driven DNA damage mimics irradiation-related carcinogenesis pathways. *Eur. Respir. J.* **2008**, *31*, 241–251. [CrossRef] [PubMed]

57. Karanika, S.; Karantanos, T.; Li, L.; Corn, P.G.; Thompson, T.C. DNA damage response and prostate cancer: Defects, regulation and therapeutic implications. *Oncogene* **2014**. [CrossRef]

58. Machowetz, A.; Poulsen, H.E.; Gruendel, S.; Weimann, A.; Fito, M.; Marrugat, J.; de la Torre, R.; Salonen, J.T.; Nyyssonen, K.; Mursu, J.; *et al.* Effect of olive oils on biomarkers of oxidative DNA stress in Northern and Southern Europeans. *FASEB J.* **2007**, *21*, 45–52. [CrossRef] [PubMed]

59. Colomer, R.; Menendez, J.A. Mediterranean diet, olive oil and cancer. *Clin. Transl. Oncol.* **2006**, *8*, 15–21. [CrossRef] [PubMed]

60. Weinbrenner, T.; Fito, M.; de la Torre, R.; Saez, G.T.; Rijken, P.; Tormos, C.; Coolen, S.; Albaladejo, M.F.; Abanades, S.; Schroder, H.; *et al.* Olive oils high in phenolic compounds modulate oxidative/antioxidative status in men. *J. Nutr.* **2004**, *134*, 2314–2321. [PubMed]

61. Mitjavila, M.T.; Fandos, M.; Salas-Salvado, J.; Covas, M.I.; Borrego, S.; Estruch, R.; Lamuela-Raventos, R.; Corella, D.; Martinez-Gonzalez, M.A.; Sanchez, J.M.; *et al.* The Mediterranean diet improves the systemic lipid and DNA oxidative damage in metabolic syndrome individuals. A randomized, controlled, trial. *Clin. Nutr.* **2013**, *32*, 172–178. [CrossRef] [PubMed]

62. Norrish, A.E.; Skeaff, C.M.; Arribas, G.L.; Sharpe, S.J.; Jackson, R.T. Prostate cancer risk and consumption of fish oils: A dietary biomarker-based case-control study. *Br. J. Cancer* **1999**, *81*, 1238–1242. [CrossRef] [PubMed]

Permissions

The contributors of this book come from diverse backgrounds, making this book a truly international effort. This book will bring forth new frontiers with its revolutionizing research information and detailed analysis of the nascent developments around the world.

We would like to thank all the contributing authors for lending their expertise to make the book truly unique. They have played a crucial role in the development of this book. Without their invaluable contributions this book wouldn't have been possible. They have made vital efforts to compile up to date information on the varied aspects of this subject to make this book a valuable addition to the collection of many professionals and students.

This book was conceptualized with the vision of imparting up-to-date information and advanced data in this field. To ensure the same, a matchless editorial board was set up. Every individual on the board went through rigorous rounds of assessment to prove their worth. After which they invested a large part of their time researching and compiling the most relevant data for our readers.

The editorial board has been involved in producing this book since its inception. They have spent rigorous hours researching and exploring the diverse topics which have resulted in the successful publishing of this book. They have passed on their knowledge of decades through this book. To expedite this challenging task, the publisher supported the team at every step. A small team of assistant editors was also appointed to further simplify the editing procedure and attain best results for the readers.

Apart from the editorial board, the designing team has also invested a significant amount of their time in understanding the subject and creating the most relevant covers. They scrutinized every image to scout for the most suitable representation of the subject and create an appropriate cover for the book.

The publishing team has been an ardent support to the editorial, designing and production team. Their endless efforts to recruit the best for this project, has resulted in the accomplishment of this book. They are a veteran in the field of academics and their pool of knowledge is as vast as their experience in printing. Their expertise and guidance has proved useful at every step. Their uncompromising quality standards have made this book an exceptional effort. Their encouragement from time to time has been an inspiration for everyone.

The publisher and the editorial board hope that this book will prove to be a valuable piece of knowledge for researchers, students, practitioners and scholars across the globe.

List of Contributors

Laura Keaver
Department of Health and Nutritional Science, Institute of Technology Sligo, FP1 YW50 Sligo, Ireland
Friedman School of Nutrition Science and Policy, Tufts University, Boston, MA 02111, USA

Fang Fang Zhang
Friedman School of Nutrition Science and Policy, Tufts University, Boston, MA 02111, USA

Ioanna Yiannakou
Department of Medicine, Boston University, Boston, MA 02215, USA

Julie Richards
Abbott Nutrition, Bob Evans Farms, Columbus, OH 43212, USA

Mary Beth Arensberg, Sara Thomas, Kirk W. Kerr and Refaat Hegazi
Abbott Nutrition Division of Abbott, Columbus, OH 43219, USA

Michael Bastasch
Department of Medicine and Division of Radiation Oncology, University of Texas East Health, Athens, TX 75751, USA

Vassiliki Diakatou
Children's & Adolescents' Oncology Radiotherapy Department, Athens General Children's Hospital "Pan. & Aglaia Kyriakou", GR-11527 Athens, Greece
Department of Public Health Policy, School of Public Health, University of West Attica, Athens University Campus, 196 Alexandras Avenue, GR-11521 Athens, Greece

Tonia Vassilakou
Department of Public Health Policy, School of Public Health, University of West Attica, Athens University Campus, 196 Alexandras Avenue, GR-11521 Athens, Greece

Maryam Ebadi and Vera C. Mazurak
Division of Human Nutrition, Department of Agricultural, Food and Nutritional Science, University of Alberta, 4-002 Li Ka Shing Centre for Health Research Innovation, Edmonton, AB T6G 2E1, Canada

Harmony F. Turk
Institut Curie, Paris 75248, France

Rita Ostan, Elisa Pini, Maria Scurti, Dario Vianello, Claudia Bertarelli, Cristina Fabbri, Morena Martucci and Aurelia Santoro
Department of Experimental, Diagnostic and Specialty Medicine (DIMES), University of Bologna, Via San Giacomo 12, 40126 Bologna, Italy

Catia Lanzarini, Elena Bellavista, Stefano Salvioli and Miriam Capri
Department of Experimental, Diagnostic and Specialty Medicine (DIMES), University of Bologna, Via San Giacomo 12, 40126 Bologna, Italy
Interdepartmental Centre "L. Galvani" (CIG) University of Bologna, Via San Giacomo 12, 40126 Bologna, Italy

Massimo Izzi, Giustina Palmas and Fiammetta Biondi
Interdepartmental Centre "L. Galvani" (CIG) University of Bologna, Via San Giacomo 12, 40126 Bologna, Italy

Claudio Franceschi
Department of Experimental, Diagnostic and Specialty Medicine (DIMES), University of Bologna, Via San Giacomo 12, 40126 Bologna, Italy
IRCCS, Institute of Neurological Sciences, Via Altura 3, 40139 Bologna, Italy
National Research Council of Italy, CNR, Institute for Organic Synthesis and Photoreactivity (ISOF), Via P. Gobetti 101, 40129 Bologna, Italy

Jennifer M. Monk and Krista A. Power
Department of Human Health and Nutritional Sciences, University of Guelph, Guelph, ON N1G 2W1, Canada
Guelph Food Research Centre, Agriculture and Agri-Food Canada, Guelph, ON N1G 5C9, Canada

Danyelle M. Liddle, Anna A. De Boer, David W.L. Ma and Lindsay E. Robinson
Department of Human Health and Nutritional Sciences, University of Guelph, Guelph, ON N1G 2W1, Canadat

Reema F. Tayyem, Suhad S. Abu-Mweis and Lana M. Agraib
Department of Clinical Nutrition & Dietetic, The Hashemite University, Zarqa 13115, Jordan

Hiba A. Bawadi
Department of Health Sciences, College of Arts and Sciences, Qatar University, Doha, Qatar

Ihab N. Shehadah
Chief Gastroenterology Division, King Hussein Cancer Center, Amman 11180, Jordan

Kamal E. Bani-Hani
Faculty of Medicine, The Hashemite University, Zarqa 13115, Jordan

Tareq Al-Jaberi
Department of General and Pediatric Surgery, Jordan University of Science and Technology, Irbid 22110, Jordan

Majed Al-Nusairr
Chief Gastroenterology Division, Prince Hamza Hospital, Amman 11118, Jordan

Dennis D. Heath
Cancer Prevention and Control Program, Moores Cancer Center, University of California, San Diego, La Jolla, CA 92093, USA

Andrea Dueregger, Isabel Heidegger, Philipp Ofer, Helmut Klocker and Iris E. Eder
Division of Experimental Urology, Department of Urology, Innsbruck Medical University, Innsbruck, A-6020 Austria

Bernhard Perktold and Reinhold Ramoner
Department of Dietetics, University of Applied Sciences Tyrol, Innsbruck A-6020, Austria

Katie M. Di Sebastiano and Marina Mourtzakis
Department of Kinesiology, University of Waterloo, 200 University Avenue W., Waterloo, ON N2L 3G1, Canada

Lone S. Sorensen
Department of Surgical Gastroenterology, Aalborg University Hospital, 9000 Aalborg, Denmark

Ole Thorlacius-Ussing
Department of Surgical Gastroenterology, Aalborg University Hospital, 9000 Aalborg, Denmark
Institute of Clinical Medicine, Aarhus University Hospital, Aarhus 8000, Denmark

Henrik H. Rasmussen
Center for Nutrition and Bowel Disease, Aalborg University Hospital, 9000 Aalborg, Denmark

Søren Lundbye-Christensen and Erik B. Schmidt
Department of Cardiology, Center for Cardiovascular Research, Aalborg University Hospital, 9000 Aalborg, Denmark

Philip. C. Calder
National Institute for Health Research Southampton Biomedical Research Center, University Hospital Southampton NHS Foundation Trust and University of Southampton, Southampton SO16 6YD, UK

Karen Lindorff-Larsen
NordSim, Center for Simulation, Skills Training, Science and Innovation, Aalborg University Hospital, 9000 Aalborg, Denmark

Mark J. McCann
Food Nutrition & Health, Food and Bio-based Products, AgResearch Grasslands Research Centre, Palmerston North 4442, New Zealand
Gravida: National Centre for Growth and Development, The University of Auckland, Auckland 1142, New Zealand

Ian R. Rowland
Department of Food and Nutritional Sciences, Whiteknights, Reading RG6 6AP, UK

Nicole C. Roy
Food Nutrition & Health, Food and Bio-based Products, AgResearch Grasslands Research Centre, Palmerston North 4442, New Zealand
Gravida: National Centre for Growth and Development, The University of Auckland, Auckland 1142, New Zealand
The Riddet Institute, Massey University, Palmerston North 4442, New Zealand

Karen S. Bishop and Nishi Karunasinghe
Auckland Cancer Society Research Centre, FM & HS, University of Auckland, Auckland 1142, New Zealand

Sharon Erdrich
Discipline of Nutrition, FM & HS, University of Auckland, Auckland 1142, New Zealand

Dug Yeo Han, Shuotun Zhu and Amalini Jesuthasan
Nutrigenomics New Zealand, University of Auckland, Auckland 1142, New Zealand

Lynnette R. Ferguson
Auckland Cancer Society Research Centre, FM & HS, University of Auckland, Auckland 1142, New Zealand
Discipline of Nutrition, FM & HS, University of Auckland, Auckland 1142, New Zealand
Nutrigenomics New Zealand, University of Auckland, Auckland 1142, New Zealand

Index